Pituitary Function and Immunity

Associate Professor
Department of Immunology
Faculty of Medicine
University of Manitoba
Winnipeg, Manitoba, Canada

CRC Press, Inc.
Boca Raton, Florida

Library of Congress Cataloging in Publication Data
Main entry under title:

Pituitary function and immunity.

   Bibliography: p.
   Includes index.
   1. Immunity—Endocrine aspects.   2. Pituitary
hormones—Physiological effect.   3. Immune response—
Regulation.   I. Berczi, Istvan.
QR182.P57   1986   616.07'9   85-9694
ISBN-0-8493-6107-9

   Direct all inquiries to CRC Press, Inc., 2000 Corporate Blvd., N.W., Boca Raton, Florida, 33431,

International Standard Book Number 0-8493-6107-9

Library of Congress Card Number 85-9694
Printed in the United States

PREFACE

Pathologists suspected at the beginning of this century that the thymus might be subject to hormonal regulation. Subsequent observations in animals revealed that the extirpation of some endocrine organs, such as the gonads, induced changes in the size of the thymus and of other lymphoid organs. These findings triggered a series of experiments in the 1930s and 1940s, which were aimed at the elucidation of hormonal influences on lymphoid tissue. At that time, the function of lymphoid organs was unknown and knowledge of the endocrine system was limited, which hampered seriously the development of rational approaches to this problem. This difficulty, coupled with primitive and inefficient methodology, led to confusion and eventual disbelief in hormonal immunoregulation.

Until recently the accumulation of biomedical knowledge was confined within the limits of various disciplines, whereas interdisciplinary research lagged behind. However, it is becoming eminently clear that the creation of disciplines was merely the reflection of our intellectual limitations in understanding biomedicine and that further advancement is possible only through building interdisciplinary bridges, which enable us to view natural phenomena in their true complexity. Thus, it became obvious that neurology and endocrinology examine different facets of the same regulatory mechanism, now frequently referred to as the neuroendocrine system.

The immune system is still regarded by many as autonomous, with an elaborate self-regulatory mechanism, which is influenced only superficially, if at all, by neuroendocrine factors. Presumably, this view stems from the ability of lymphocytes to mount immune reactions in vitro and also to migrate into diseased tissues, or even to mucosal surfaces, and to function in such environments where neurohormonal regulation might be grossly disturbed or nonexistent. Nevertheless, some basic and clinical scientists suspected all along that interaction and coordination must exist between these two systems. Thus, ever since transplantation immunity has been discovered, it was clear that the conceptus in mammals is an allograft equivalent, yet it survives, despite the recognition of paternal antigens of the fetus by the maternal immune system. Also, it has been well known for some time that mammals and birds protect their offspring against environmental pathogens by the transfer of specific antibodies through the egg, placenta and/or milk. This elaborate mechanism, which is vital for the survival of the species, could hardly have evolved without a delicate coordination of reproduction, a neurohormonally regulated function, with the immune system. Clinical observations revealed that certain autoimmune diseases are prevalent in females. Furthermore, some diseases in which psychosomatic factors have been identified, such as rheumatoid arthritis, also have underlying immune abnormalities. These facts point to the inevitable conclusion that interaction between the neuroendocrine and immune systems is a necessity, and that it has to be elucidated, it we are to understand immune function in the context of homeostasis of the organism.

This volume examines the role of the pituitary gland in the regulation of the immune system using an interdisciplinary approach. Introductory chapters are provided for the reader, which are intended to bridge the gaps between disciplines. It is my sincere hope that this book will catalyze the reformation of prevailing views about immunoregulation and about the integration of the immune system into the overall function of the body.

I. Berczi

THE AUTHOR/EDITOR

Dr. Istvan Berczi is Associate Professor of Immunology of the University of Manitoba Health Sciences Center in Winnipeg, Canada. He received his D.V.M. degree from the Veterinary School of Budapest, Hungary in 1962, and his Ph.D. in 1972, from the Department of Immunology, Faculty of Medicine, University of Manitoba.

Dr. Berczi is a member of several professional societies and scientific organizations that include the Canadian Society for Immunology, the American Association of Immunologists, the American Association for Cancer Research, the Transplantation Society, the New York Academy of Sciences and the American Association for the Advancement of Science. He authored or co-authored over 60 articles in referred journals, most of which are related to Immunology or Cancer Immunology. He serves on the Advisory Board of the Journal of Experimental and Clinical Cancer Research and has served as advisor to various granting agencies that include the National Cancer Institute at NIH, the Medical Research Council of Canada, the National Sciences and Engineering Council of Canada. He also serves as a reviewer for papers published in the Canadian Medical Association Journal.

Dr. Berczi's major research interest lies with hormal regulation of the immune system. Other activities in his laboratory are related to the production of monoclonal antibodies and the immunobiology of cancer. His research program has been supported over the years by the Medical Research Council of Canada, the National Cancer Institute of Canada, the Manitoba Heart Foundation, Winnipeg Clinic Research Institute, the National Institutes of Health, the St. Boniface Research Foundation, the National Sciences and Engineering Council of Canada, and the Arthritis Society of Canada. He has been the recipient of the Visiting Scientist Award by the Medical Research Council of Canada in 1980, in support of his sabbatical research at the Dept. of Tumor Biology, Karolinska Institute, Stockholm, Sweden.

CONTRIBUTORS

Robert Ader, Ph.D.
Dean's Professor, Director
Division of Behavioral and
  Psychosocial Medicine
Department of Psychiatry
University of Rochester School of
  Medicine and Dentistry
Rochester, New York

Istvan Berczi, D.V.M., Ph.D.
Associate Professor
Department of Immunology
Faculty of Medicine
University of Manitoba
Winnipeg, Manitoba, Canada

Hugo O. Besedovsky, M.D.
Senior Investigator
Medizinische Abteilung
Schweizerisches Forschungsinstitut
Davos-Platz, Switzerland

Dana Bovbjerg, Ph.D.
Instructor in Immunology
Department of Medicine
Cornell University Medical College
New York, New York

David A. Clark, M.D., Ph.D.,
  F.R.C.P. (C)
Associate Professor and MCR Scientist
Departments of Medicine, Obstetrics
  and Gynecology, and Host Resistance
  and Reproductive Biology Programs
McMaster University
Hamilton, Ontario, Canada

Adriana del Rey, Ph.D.
Senior Investigator
Medzinische Abeilung
Schweizerisches Forschungsinstitut
Davos-Platz, Switzerland

Thomas J. Gerstenberger, Ph.D.
Teaching Fellow
Department of Psychology
Kent State University
Kent, Ohio

Eva Nagy, M.D.
Lecturer
Department of Immunology
Univesity of Manitoba
Winnipeg, Manitoba, Canada

Benjamin H. Newberry, Ph.D.
Professor
Department of Psychology
Kent Ohio University
Kent, Ohio

Elizabeth S. Raveche, Ph.D.
Senior Investigator
National Institute of Arthritis,
  Diabetes, Digestive, and Kidney
  Diseases
National Institutes of Health
Bethesda, Maryland

Ernst Sorkin, Ph.D.
Professor
Medizinische Abteilung
Schweizerisches Forschungsinatitut
Davos-Platz, Switzerland

Alfred D. Steinberg, M.D.
Chief, Cellular Immunology
National Institute of Arthritis,
  Diabetes, Digestive and Kidney
  Diseases
Bethesda, Maryland

ABBREVIATIONS

A	—	Adrenalin
ACTH	—	Adrenocorticotropic hormone
ADCC	—	Antibody-dependent cellular cytotoxicity
ADH	—	Antidiuretic hormone
ADP	—	Adenosine diphosphate
Adrx	—	Adrenalectomy
AIPF	—	Anaphylactoid inflammation promoting factor
ATP	—	Adenosine triphosphate
ATS	—	Anti-thymocyte serum
AVP	—	Arginine vasopressin
BCG	—	Bacille Calmette-Guerin
BGG	—	Bovine gammaglobulin
BGH	—	Bovine growth hormone
BPRL	—	Bovine prolactin
BRC	—	Bromocriptine
C_3	—	Component C_3 of complement
cAMP	—	Cyclic 3′, 5′ - adenosine monophosphate
CBG	—	Corticosteroid binding globulin
cGMP	—	Cyclic 3′, 5′ - guanosine monophosphate
CG	—	Chorionic gonadotropin
CH	—	Constant portion of heavy chain
CL	—	Constant portion of light chain
CNS	—	Central nervous system
Con-A	—	Concanavalin A
C. parvum	—	Corynebacterium parvum
CRH	—	Corticotropin-releasing hormone
CSF	—	Colony stimulating factor
CTL	—	Cytotoxic T lymphocytes
DES	—	Diethylstilbestrol
2-DG	—	2-Deoxyglucose
DHT	—	Dihydrotestosterone
DLN	—	Draining lymph nodes
DNA	—	Deoxyribonucleic acid
DNCB	—	Dinitrochlorobenzene
DNP	—	Dionitrophenol
DTH	—	Delayed type hypersensitivity
E. coli	—	Escherichia Coli
EBV	—	Epstein Barr virus
ECF	—	Eosinophil chemotactic factor
ECF-A	—	Eosinophil chemotactic factor of anaphylaxis
EPF	—	Early pregnancy factor
ESF	—	Erythropoietin stimulating factor
ESP	—	Eosinophil stimulation factor
EV	—	Estradiol valerate
Fc	—	Cristalizing fraction of immunoglobulin
FSH	—	Follicle stimulating hormone
GAF	—	Glucocorticoid antagonizing factor
GF	—	Germ-free
GH	—	Growth hormone
GH-RF	—	Growth hormone releasing factor

GH-RIH	—	Growth hormone release-inhibiting hormone
PGE_1	—	Prostaglandin E_1
PHA	—	Phytochaemagglutinin
PIH	—	Prolactin inhibiting hormone
PL	—	Placental lactogen
PNA	—	Peanut agglutinin
poly A:U	—	Polyadenylic-polyuridylic acid
poly I- poly C	—	Polyinosinic-polycytidylic acid
poly I:C	—	Polyinosinic-polycytidylic acid
PPD	—	Purified protein derivative
PRL	—	Prolactin
PTH	—	Parathyroid hormone
PWM	—	Pokeweed mitogen
RES	—	Reticuloendothelial system
RNA	—	Ribonucleic acid
RPRL	—	Rat prolactin
S. aureus	—	*Staphylococcus aureus*
s.c.	—	Subcutaneous
SC	—	Secretory component
20 αSDH	—	20 α Hydroxysterioid dehydrogenase
SLE	—	Systemic lupus erythematosus
Slp	—	Sex-linked protein
S. mansoni	—	*Schistosoma mansoni*
SP	—	Substance P
SPF	—	Specific pathogen-free
SPG	—	Syngeneic pituitary graft
SRBC	—	Sheep red blood cells
SRS-A	—	Slow reactive substance of anaphylaxis
ssDNA	—	Single stranded deoxyribonucleic acid
GIF	—	Glucocorticoid increasing factor
GMP	—	Guanosine monophosphate
GRMF	—	Glucosteroid response modifying factor
GTP	—	Guanosine triphosphate
GVH	—	Graft-vs.-host
GVHR	—	Graft-vs.-host-reaction
H	—	Heavy (chain of immunoglobulin)
^{3}H-DHA	—	^{3}H-dihydroalperenolol
^{3}H-SP	—	^{3}H-spiroperidol
HCG	—	Human chorionic gonadotropin
HGH	—	Human growth hormone
HLA	—	Human histocompatibility antigen
HPL	—	Human placental lactogen
HRBC	—	Horse red blood cells
Hypox	—	Hypophysectomy/ized
^{125}I-HYP	—	^{125}I-hydroxybenzyl pindolol
Ia	—	Immune response associated (antigens)
IGF	—	Insulin-like growth factor
Ig-SC	—	Immunoglobulin secreting cells
IL-1	—	Interleukin 1
IL-2	—	Interleukin 2
i.m.	—	Intramuscular
i.p.	—	Intraperitoneal

Ir	—	Immune response (genes)
ITP	—	Idiopathic thrombocytopenic purpura
K	—	Killer
KLH	—	Keyhole limpet hemocyanin
L	—	Light (chain of immunoglobulin)
LH	—	Luteinizing hormone
LH-RH	—	Lutenizing hormone-releasing hormone
LPH	—	Lipotrophin
LPS	—	Lipopolysaccharide
MBSA	—	Methylated bovine serum albumin
MC	—	Methyl cholanthrene
MCF	—	Macrophage chemotactic factor
MHC	—	Major histocompatibility complex
MIF	—	Macrophage migration inhibitory factor
MLC	—	Mixed lymphocyte culture
MLR	—	Mixed lymphocyte reaction
MMF	—	Macrophage mitogenic factor
MP	—	Methylprednisoline
MSH	—	Melanocyste-stimulating hormone
NA	—	Noradrenaline
NK	—	Natural killer
NTA	—	Natural T cell antibody
NZB	—	New Zealand black
NZW	—	New Zealand white
OV	—	Ovariectomy/ized
PDGF	—	Platelet-drived growth factor
PFC	—	Plaque-forming cells
TA	—	Trimacinolone acetonide
T_3	—	3, 5, 3′ - Triiodo-L-thyronine, triiodothyronine
T_4	—	3, 5, 3′, 5′ - Tetraiodo-L-thyronine, thyroxin
TCGF	—	T cell growth factor
TFM	—	Testicular feminized male mice
TK	—	Thymidine kinase
TL	—	Thymus leukemia antigen
TRH	—	Thyrotropin-releasing hormone
TSH	—	Thyroid-stimulating hormone
VIP	—	Vasoactive intestinal polypeptide

ACKNOWLEDGMENTS

The pareparation of this volume was greatly facilitated by the help, advice, and criticism of my colleagues, associates, and friends, particularly by Dr. K. Kovacs, Department of Pathology, University of Toronto, Dr. Eva Nagy, G. E. Wren, and C. McKenzie, Department of Immunmology, University of Manitoba, and G. Jaczina. The devoted secretarial and excellent editorial assistance of Mrs. Yvonne Yowney is greatly acknowledged. The sustained encouragement by Dr. A. H. Sehon, Head, Department of Immunology and Dr. H. G. Friesen, Head, Department of Physiology, Faculty of Medicine, University of Manitoba was extremely helpful. A special thanks to my wife, Anna, and my family, for their support and understanding during these trying months, which gave strength in critical moments of this effort. Financial support for the production of this monograph was provided, in part, by Sandoz Pharmaceuticals and from grants awarded by the Medical Research Council and the Arthritis Council and the Arthritis Society of Canada to I. Berzci.

TABLE OF CONTENTS

Chapter 1

THE IMMUNE SYSTEM AND ITS FUNCTION

I. Berczi

TABLE OF CONTENTS

I. INTRODUCTION

The science of immunology was founded by Jenner's observations in 1798 on the protection against smallpox by inoculation with cowpox. His experiments were prompted by the widely held impressions that those individuals who had had cowpox, which is a benign disease, were not affected in subsequent smallpox epidemics. To test this belief, he inoculated a boy with pus from a cowpox lesion of a dairy maid. Some weeks later, when the boy was reinoculated with infectious pus from a patient suffering from smallpox, the disease failed to occur. Repetition of the experiment many times led to Jenner's classic report that vaccination (vacca = cow) leads to immunity against smallpox. Jenner's finding was not extended for about 100 years until Pasteur rediscovered the general principles underlying vaccination. During his studies on chicken cholera, Pasteur happened to inoculate some chickens with an old culture of the causative bacterium *(Pasturella aviseptica)*, and these animals failed to develop disease. When the same chickens were reinoculated with a fresh culture, which was known to be pathogenic, they again failed to become ill. These observations were soon applied to many other infectious diseases; various procedures have been used to destroy the viability or to attenuate the virulence of pathogenic organisms for the purpose of vaccination.

Another giant of medical science, Robert Koch, discovered that guinea pigs infected with the tubercle bacillus will display a local reaction if injected intradermally with culture fluids of *Mycobacterium tuberculosis* ("Koch phenomenon"). Chase and Landsteiner showed in 1945 that this type of allergic reaction, classified later as delayed-type hypersensitivity, can only be transferred from one animal to another by living cells (cell-mediated immunity), whereas other immune reactions can be transmitted by serum (humoral immunity).

The ability of responding rapidly to infectious agents, or to other foreign materials (antigens), with the synthesis of specific proteins (antibodies) and/or production of specific effector cells has been encountered only in vertebrates.[1] This adaptive immune response is of vast importance for survival as it constitutes the principal means of defense against pathogenic microorganisms, parasites, and possibly against neoplastic disease.[2] Our knowledge of immunity in invertebrates is rudimentary, but it appears that these animals can also recognize foreign materials. Transplant failures in coelentarates were attributed to the existence of a defense mechanism similar to that of graft rejection in higher animals.[3] Earthworms are able to destroy grafts from donors of the same or different species. This graft rejection is characterized by specificity and anamnesis and can be transferred with immune cells (coelomocytes).[4-6] Insects can also develop immunity rapidly with the appearance of nonprotein antibacterial factors produced by antigenic stimulation, while in general, arthropods fail to recognize tissue grafts as foreign.[7]

Studies on the immune systems of mammals and birds revealed that lymphocytes have the ability to recognize and respond to antigens. There are two major categories of lymphocytes: those that mature in the thymus (T lymphocytes), and those that become immunocompetent in the bursa of Fabricius (birds) or in the bone marrow (mammals, B lymphocytes). All lymphocytes arise from the multipotential stem cells, which reside in the bone marrow.[8] Both T and B lymphocytes can be divided to subsets according to their functions. T lymphocytes can develop into immune effector cells, (e.g., killer T cells and delayed hypersensitive T cells) and also play a fundamental role in the regulation of immune responses (helper and suppressor T cells). The chief function of B lymphocytes is antibody formation. Antibodies are fixed to the surface of all leukocytes (T cells, B cells, monocytes, macrophages, polymorphonuclear leukocytes) via F_c receptors and serve as specific recognition units of the antigen. This amplification mechanism permits the recruitment of leukocytes for the defense of the host against intruders as well as being involved in the regulation of immune responses (feedback mechanism). Other soluble mediators derived from lymphoid cells, called lymphokines, also play essential roles in immune defense and immunoregulation. A family of serum proteins belonging to the complement and properdin system is also integrated into immune defense as well as into the regulation of immune reactions. Furthermore, evidence is rapidly increasing that the immune system interacts with a variety of other cells and organs in the body. Of special interest to us is the interactions with the neuroendocrine system.

II. CELLS OF THE IMMUNE SYSTEM

A. Development of Immunocytes

In both birds and mammals, hemopoietic stem cells first appear in the yolk sac. Later in embryonic development, the hemopoietic cells migrate through the blood stream to colonize the liver in mammals and the spleen in both birds and mammals, before they home to their permanent residence in the bone marrow. It was demonstrated[9-11] that the morphologically and functionally very different cells of the erythrocyte, lymphocyte, monocyte-macrophage, and granulocyte series all originate from the same multipotential stem cells. Since all the cells of the blood have finite life spans, some of the small resting stem cells are committed on a regular basis to become progenitors of the various cell types by an unknown mechanism, in order to maintain normal values of blood cells. Progenitor cells are larger than stem cells; they actively synthesize DNA, and they differentiate into mature cells of the lineage they are committed to under the influence of specific hormones and microenvironmental factors. For instance, erythropoietin is known as the major hormone responsible for the generation of red blood cells, colony stimulating factor (CSF), and governs the production of granulocytes and macrophages.

Progenitor cells of the T cell lineage home to the thymus in order to proceed with further differentiation and maturation. The mechanism of homing is not understood in detail, but is presumed to be mediated by cell surface receptors. The stromal framework of the thymus is formed from epithelial cells of the third and fourth pharyngeal pouches during embryonic life. The thymic microenvironment enables the committed stem cells to differentiate into mature T lymphocytes. Hormones secreted by thymic epithelial cells (thymopoietin, thymosine, etc.) as well as cell-to-cell contact appear to play important roles in T cell differentiation.[12,13] A number of thymic hormones and biologically active factors have been described to date awaiting further characterization and determination of biological activity.

In birds, progenitors of B lymphocytes home to the bursa of Fabricius, a pouch that is attached to the intestine near the cloaca. Although much less studied, the maturation of B cells in the bursa appears to follow a similar pattern to that of T cell maturation. Bursopoietin[14] is the presumed hormone having a major regulatory effect. In mammals B lymphocytes differentiate from their progenitors within the bone marrow.

The thymus, bursa, and the bone marrow, which are preoccupied with antigen-independent lymphopoiesis, are known as the primary lymphoid organs. Mature T and B lymphocytes from these organs home to the secondary lymphoid organs, namely the spleen, lymph nodes, and mucosal lymphoid tissues, where some of them will undergo further antigen-driven differentiation, as required.

B. Lymphocytes

B and T lymphocytes cannot be distinguished morphologically in the resting state. Morphological differences will occur, however, after activation. In addition, a number

Table 1

SOME PROPERTIES OF LEUKOCYTES, MAST CELLS AND PLATELETS

Properties	Cell Types							
	T	B	Mf	Ba	Eo	Ne	Ma	Pl
Antigen receptor	+	+	−	−	−	−	−	−
Ig content	−	+	−	−	−	−	−	−
E rosette	+	−	−	−	−	−	−	−
Differentiation Ag	+	+	+	+	+	+	+	+
Fc receptor	+	+	+	+	+	+	+	+
C′ receptor	±	+	+	+	+	+	+	+[a]
Phagocytosis	−	−	+	+	+	+	−	−
Response to mitogens	+	+	+	−	−	−	−	−
Adherence[b]	−	−	+	+	+	+	+	−

Note: T = T lymphocytes, B = B lymphocytes, Mf = macrophages, Ba = basophilic leukocutes, Eo = eosinophilic leukocytes, Ne = neutrophilic leukocytes, Ma = mast cells, Pl = platelets, Fc = fragment of immunoglobulins, C′ = complement, E = erythrocyte.

[a]   Only nonprimate platelets have C′ receptors.
[b]   Adherence to glass or plastic under tissue culture conditions.

of other criteria can be used for the detection and separation of lymphocyte subsets as summarized in Table 1.

1. T Lymphocytes

Mature immunocompetent T lymphocytes leave the thymus and settle in the spleen (where approximately 30% of the mononuclear cells are T cells), in the lymph nodes (approximately 60% of mononuclear cells), and also recirculate constantly (about 70% of mononuclear blood cells are T cells). The bone marrow also contains some T cells that are different from T cells of other sources with regard to their response to mitogens and to allogenic cells. When triggered, T cells will initiate DNA synthesis, which results in the accumulation of cytoplasmic RNA that can be stained by pyronin. The ultrastructure of T lymphoblasts is characterized by numerous polyribosomes, smooth endoplasmic reticulum, microfilaments, and microtubules. Activated cells frequently exhibit characteristic protrusions called uropods. T cells in comparison with B lymphocytes contain more lactate dehydrogenase isoenzyme-1, have a higher net negative surface charge, and are more susceptible to freezing and thawing and osmotic damage. They are also less adherent than B lymphocytes to various surfaces in tissue culture. T lymphocytes home specifically to the periarteriolar zone of white pulp in the spleen and to the paracortical area of lymph nodes. Long-lived and short-lived T lymphocytes can be distinguished. T cells lose their recirculating capacity when activated by antigen.

At least four functional classes of T lymphocytes may be distinguished: helper, suppressor, delayed-type hypersensitive, and cytotoxic T cells. Helper T cells are needed for the antigen-driven differentiation of all effector lymphocytes (delayed-type hypersensitive-, killer-, suppressor-T cells, and antibody-secreting B lymphocytes). Suppressor T cells effectively antagonize the initiation of new effector cells during the normal course of immune responses. Delayed-type hypersensitive T cells have the ability to migrate specifically to the sites of minor antigen deposits within the tissues. They secrete lymphokines that attract other mononuclear cells (macrophages) to the site and also activate the recruited cells for the elimination of antigenic microorganisms, or other antigenic material. Killer (cytotoxic) T cells are able to destroy target cells in an immunologically specific fashion in vitro and are involved in graft and tumor rejection, in defense against viruses, fungi, and certain bacteria, and are also responsible for some autoimmune reactions. In the mouse, these functional subsets of T lymphocytes can be readily distinguished according to their antigenic markers (Lyt and Ia antigens). Recently a series of monoclonal antibodies became available commercially that allow for similar functional distinction of human T lymphocytes on the basis of their specific antigenic surface markers. Monoclonal antibodies capable of distinguishing T cell subsets have also been produced against rat T lymphocytes.

T lymphocytes are able to recognize antigen specifically through their surface receptors. Numerous clones exist within the immune system that are able to recognize a variety of antigen determinants (epitopes). The recognition site of T cell antigen receptors appears to be very similar, if not identical, to the antigen-combining site of corresponding antibodies. However, the rest of the T cell receptors do not seem to be closely related to immunoglobulins. In addition to foreign antigens, some of the helper and suppressor T lymphocytes recognize class II histocompatibility (Ia) antigens, or immunoglobulin isotypes, allotypes, and idiotypes. Most killer T cells recognize class I histocompatibility determinants on their targets.

Regulatory T cells (helper and suppressor) appear to have receptors for the Fc portion of various classes and subclasses of immunoglobulin. Although the function of these receptors has not been fully elucidated, it seems certain that they are involved in immunoregulation. Apparently, some T cells have receptors for complement components as well, especially for C3. The function of complement receptors is largely unknown. A peculiar receptor that is present on most human T cells is the one recognizing sheep erythrocytes (Sheep Red Blood Cells (SRBC), E receptor). Human T cells bind SRBC under proper conditions, which leads to "rosette" formation. This reaction is widely used for the routine discrimination and even for the separation of human T cells from other mononuclear cell types. T cells from other species also bind foreign erythrocytes: marmoset and pig T cells bind to SRBC, guinea pig T cells to rabbit erythrocytes, cat T cells to rodent, dog T cells to human and guinea pig, and rat T cells to guinea pig erythrocytes.

Certain mitogens, such as concanavalin A, or phytohemagglutinin (PHA), stimulate T lymphocytes, whereas some other mitogens, such as pokeweed mitogen, are capable of stimulating both T and B cells. Stimulated cells will transform into blasts, synthesize DNA, divide, and secrete lymphokines. The reactivity of lymphocytes to various mitogens in vitro is used frequently for the evaluation of lymphocyte function, as well as for the generation of a variety of soluble products.

2. B Lymphocytes

In birds, B cells mature in the bursa of Fabricius that contains stem cells, mature B cells, and a small number of T cells. In comparison with mammals, the bursa is regarded as a bone marrow equivalent in birds. Bursal cells are able to respond immunologically when stimulated.

B lymphocytes may be small, medium sized (blasts, proplasmacyte), or large with abundant cytoplasm and characteristically eccentric nucleus (plasma cell). When stimulated, immunoglobulin production may start in association with free ribosomes in the cytoplasm. With continuing stimulation plasmacytes will evolve, which are characterized by a nucleus with coarse chromatin, a well-developed Golgi apparatus, and rough endoplasmic reticulum. Plasma cells secrete large amounts of immunoglobulin and are unable to return to the small lymphocyte stage, but rather, eventually die.

Although B lymphocytes are considered generally as nonadherent, they adhere loosely to nylon wool, which is used routinely for separating from T cells. Adherence to glass bead column and to acrylic acid polymer also has been reported. Human peripheral B cells form spontaneous rosettes with mouse red blood cells, which may be used as a B lymphocyte marker.

The most important marker of B cells is surface and cytoplasmic immunoglobulin. B cells switch the expression of Ig class during their differentiation: IgD is expressed first, then IgM, which is followed by either IgG or IgA, and perhaps IgE. B lymphocytes may also be classified as long-lived and short-lived.

In the chicken the periellipsoidal lymphoid tissue in the spleen is bursa-dependent. In mammals B cells are localized mainly in the germinal centers of the spleen (in the red pulp) and lymph nodes. Most B lymphocytes producing IgA are located in intimate anatomical relationship to mucous membranes, or glandular tissue. The bone marrow contains 30 to 40% B lymphocytes; in the spleen approximately 60% of the mononuclear cells are B cells, in the lymph nodes around 30%, and in the thymus there are very few B cells, if any (less than 2%).

The most important function of B lymphocytes is antibody formation. Besides antibody formation, B lymphocytes probably perform a number of other functions, which are not studied very well to date. It seems certain, however, that some B cells are able to secrete lymphokines and to trigger immunoregulatory events.

B cell clones recognize specific epitopes on the antigen by their surface immunoglobulin receptors (IgD and/or IgM). After the binding of polyvalent antigen to surface Ig, the complexes are redistributed on the cell surface, a contractile event occurs, and then the complexes are endocytosed and shed from the membrane. Eventually new receptors appear on the cell surface. This in vitro cycle, in the absence of cooperative cell interactions, does not lead to B cell differentiation into secreting plasma cells, whereas it does so when induced in the proper conditions involving helper cells. Virgin precursor cells have antigen receptors of the IgM class, regardless of the class of antibody eventually secreted. Exposure to antigen induces a shift in receptor class from IgM to IgG.

B lymphocytes also have Fc receptors for various immunoglobulin classes and for the C3 complement component. Various polysaccharides, such as lipopolysaccharide (LPS) from Gram-negative bacteria, pneumococcal polysaccharide SIII, levan from *Corynebacterium levaniformis* and dextran, can all function as B lymphocyte mitogens and are able to induce polyclonal antibody synthesis in vitro. These B cell mitogens function also as T-independent antigens, since they are able to initiate specific antibody formation without helper T cells. Pokeweed mitogen is capable of stimulating both B and T lymphocytes, whereas PHA is not mitogenic for B cells.

C. Macrophages and Monocytes

Arising from the bone marrow, monocytes circulate briefly and then, under steady-state conditions, randomly leave the blood stream or attach to the wall of sinusoids. Here they undergo a series of structural and functional alterations, leading to the formation of the tissue macrophage or histiocyte. Their tissue life span is relatively long, and they continue to actively synthesize a variety of macromolecules in response to environmental stimuli.

The nucleus is characteristically round-, or bean-shaped, and for this reason, macrophages and monocytes are often categorized as mononuclear phagocytes. The most characteristic morphological feature of these cells is the abundance of lysosomes in the cytoplasm. In activated macrophages the number of lysosomes, as well as the enzyme content of the lysosomes (acid phosphatase, beta-glucuronidase), is increased. In response to certain stimuli, such as foreign bodies, microbial infections, certain mycoses, parasites (e.g., leishmaniasis), macrophages can transform into multinucleated giant cells that arise through fusion of single cells. The spleen and lymph nodes contain a macrophage-related cell, characterized by cytoplasmic processes and named dendritic cells. Such cells do not contain large numbers of lysosomes and are not phagocytic. Dendritic cells are able to retain antigen on their surface through specifically bound antibody. Other macrophage-related cells are the Kupffer cells in the liver and Langerhans cells in the skin. Additional subclasses of macrophages have been proposed repeatedly, but are not firmly established as yet. The extensive network of macrophage-like cells throughout the body is often referred to as the reticuloendothelial system (RES).

Although mononuclear phagocytes do not have antigen receptors of their own, they seem to be able to recognize foreign materials by stereospecific receptors or by antibodies, and perhaps T cell factors (e.g., arming factor), fixed onto their surface through specific receptors. After the recognition of a soluble antigen, or other chemoattractant, macrophages and monocytes can migrate towards the source of the stimulus (chemotaxis). Macrophages are essential for the induction of both humoral- and cell-mediated immune reactions and also participate in immunoregulation. In addition, they play an important role in effector immune mechanisms through their phagocytic and cytotoxic activity. Mononuclear phagocytes express receptors for the complement factor C3b. Lymphokine receptors are also present on macrophages and monocytes.

Macrophages can be activated nonspecifically for cytotoxicity by a variety of agents, such as endotoxins, double-stranded RNA, poly I-poly C, bovine gamma globulin (BGG), purified protein derivative (PPD), Freund's complete adjuvant, pyran copolymer, and various microorganisms. Such nonspecifically activated macrophages have the capacity to recognize and destroy tumor cells and some other fast growing cell lines, while nonneoplastic (slow growing) cells are affected very little, or not at all. It is noticeable that many of the macrophage-activating substances listed above are also potent immunological adjuvants.

D. Killer Cells

Nonimmune effector cells are able to kill antibody coated target cells, which is called antibody-dependent cellular cytotoxicity (ADCC). The effector cells for ADCC possess receptors for the Fc portion of IgG antibodies and include macrophages, monocytes, and some lymphocytes.

Another category of killer cells that are capable of destroying tumor and cultured cell targets without antibody coating are designated as natural killer (NK) cells. NK cells are heterogeneous. Some of them appear to be T cell-related, although they develop in the bone marrow, rather than in the thymus.

E. Polymorphonuclear Leukocytes

Blood smears of man and animals stained with a Romanowsky-type technique, such as Giemsa's, May-Grunwald-Giemsa, or Wright's stain, exhibit white blood cells with segmented nuclei (polymorphonuclear cells) and with granules in their cytoplasm (granulocytes). In man, and in most domestic and laboratory animals, cells with three different granules may be distinguished: i.e., cells containing relatively small pink or pinkish blue granules are called neutrophils; those having larger bright red granules are designated as eosinophils; and the ones having large dark blue granules are named basophils. These basic cell types may be distinguished in mammals, birds, and even in the frog. The neutrophils of rabbits, golden hamsters, and chickens stain very similarly to that of eosinophils; therefore, they are often called pseudoeosinophils, rather than neutrophils. Rats, mice, and golden hamsters have practically no circulating basophilic granulocytes. All three classes of granulocytes are primarily blood cells and thought to penetrate tissues only after specific stimuli, such as inflammation, which may or may not be immunologically initiated.

Tissue mast cells will also be discussed here because of their functional similarities to basophilic leukocytes; however, their origin seems to be different in that at least a subset of mast cells is thymus dependent for differentiation. Tissue mast cells may be small and roundish, spindle- or star-shaped, and occasionally have extremely long processes. The nucleus has an ovoid shape and the cytoplasm contains numerous, large granules that stain metachromatically with basic aniline dyes. Mast cells occur almost exclusively in connective tissue, around small blood vessels, nerves, glandular ducts, and epithelial linings. They also migrate into the peritoneal fluid. The thymus may contain a significant number of mast cells located within the stroma. Lymph nodes contain mast cells in their capsule and septum. The spleen is poor in mast cells, though some may be found in the capsule and also in the stroma.

1. Basophilic Leukocytes

Although there is no doubt that basophilic leukocytes are integrated in various immune reactions, their exact functions have not been elucidated. Basophils fix IgE and possibly also IgG antibodies on their surface and can be triggered by antigen to release from their granules a variety of biologically reactive mediators, such as histamine, heparin, and enzymes. Certain split products of complement (anaphylatoxins), are also potent releasing agents. Little is known about the biological significance of the released substances, other than they cause serious symptoms in allergic individuals where excess amounts are released. Tissue mast cells appear to have an identical function. It has been proposed that basophils contribute to host resistance against parasites and tumors. Basophils have receptors for, and respond chemotactically to, a complement-derived (C5a) factor. Similar responses can be elicited by lymphocyte-derived chemotactic factors. Human basophils respond with chemotaxis to the enzyme, plasma kallikrein, and to culture fluids of bacteria.

The function of tissue mast cells is very similar, if not identical, to that of basophils. There is a well-known inverse relationship between basophil and mast cell frequency in various species; thus, mice and rats, in which basophils are vanishingly rare, have correspondingly greater number of tissue mast cells. This may be an indication that mast cells and basophils supplement each other. In addition to histamine and serotonin, mast cells of the rat, mouse, hamster, and ruminants also contain dopamine. Heparin is abundant in mast cells of all species. Other substances such as proteolytic enzymes and a chemotactic peptide for eosinophils, are also contained in mast cell granules. Mast cells may generate "slow reactive substance of anaphylaxis" (SRS-A) after exposure to antigen, or to anti-IgE antibodies. The content of mast cell granules may be released by specific cell-bound IgE antibodies after reaction with the antigen, by some complement components, or by basically-charged drugs and peptides. In addition to Fc receptors for IgE, mast cells also possess receptors for cleavage products of the third and fifth component of complement (C3a and C5a), which are formed during complement activation.

2. Eosinophilic Leukocytes

After 3 to 4 days of maturation from precursor cells and release from the bone marrow, the eosinophil spends only 3 to 4 hr in the blood stream en route to the tissue site, where it remains to complete a life cycle of 8 to 12 days. Eosinophils migrate to loose submucosal connective tissue, especially of the respiratory and gastrointestinal tracts. It has been long recognized that parasitic invasions and allergic reactions evoke eosinophilia. The accumulation of eosinophils at sites of immediate hypersensitivity reactions is due to an eosinophil chemotactic factor of anaphylaxis (ECF-A), which is released along with other chemical mediators from sensitized mast cells that have been challenged with specific antigens. Eosinophils have Fc receptors for IgM, IgG, IgA, and IgE. Eosinophils also respond to lymphokines, such as the eosinophil stimulation promoter (ESP), ECF-A, and eosinophil chemotactic factor (ECF).

3. Neutrophil Leukocytes

Neutrophils represent the vast majority of granulocytes, and hence they are often referred to as polymorphonuclears. Neutrophils contain two types of granules: azurophils and specific. The enzymes contained in specific granules function best at neutral pH, while the enzymes of azurophil granules have their pH optimum in the acid range. At present approximately 30 different enzymes and biologically active substances, contained by neutrophils, have been identified. The chemotactic factors of neutrophils affect eosinophils (ECF), macrophages, and platelets. At least some of the chemotactic activity generated by neutrophils could come from complement, after the release of a C5 cleaving enzyme.

One of the most important function of neutrophils is phagocytosis and subsequent digestion of foreign materials, including pathogenic microbes. Antibodies play an important role in the triggering of phagocytosis, since neutrophils specifically recognize immune complexes through their surface receptors for Fc and complement. After the ingestion of immune complexes, lysosomes merge with phagocytic vacuoles containing the foreign material and the resulting cytoplasmic organelle is called phagolysosome. During phagocytosis, lysosomal enzymes and other factors are released by neutrophils into the extracellular environment, which provoke acute inflammation. During the inflammatory process some neutrophils die, which leads to further release of phlogistic substances, and thus, the inflammation further escalates. Complement activation is not a prerequisite for enzyme release by neutrophils, but may enhance the process.

The importance of neutrophils in body defense is illustrated by the fact that malfunction, or neutropenia, results in unusual susceptibility to infection, especially those caused by Gram-positive bacteria. Various diseases caused by immune complexes such as glomerulonephritis, arthritis, lesions in the lungs, mycocardium, joints, and skin, are also due to a large extent to the damaging effect of neutrophils. Complement-derived chemotactic factors are the main attractants for neutrophils to the site of immune complex deposition.

F. Platelets

Platelets are nonnucleated cells of the blood present only in mammals. In lower vertebrates, and even in some mammalia of lower orders, the functional equivalent of the platelet is the nucleated thrombocyte. Platelets are cytoplasmic fragments of megakaryocytes, which originate from the multipotential hemopoietic stem cell. At least two hormones are involved in the regulation of megakaryocyte function, namely, megakaryocyte-colony stimulating factor and thrombopoietin. The former is believed to act on progenitor cells, whereas the latter influences megakaryocyte development.[15,16]

Platelets store and are capable of releasing a variety of substances that include proteins, identical or similar to plasma proteins, lysosomal enzymes, cationic proteins, platelet specific proteins, metabolically inactive nucleotides (ADP and ATP), biogenic amines, factors which alter blood vessel permeability, and the coagulation-stimulating lipid (platelet factor 3).[17,18] The recently discovered platelet-derived growth factor (PDGF) is a heat stable cationic polypeptide, consisting of two peptide chains linked by disulfate bridges and having a molecular weight of 28 to 33,000 daltons. It affects fibroblasts and other connective tissue-derived cells, glial cells, and osteoclasts. In vivo binding studies revealed uptake of ^{125}I-PDGF by the inner zone of the adrenal cortex and by the corpora lutea of the ovaries of pregnant mice, indicating a selective affinity of PDGF for steroid producing tissues. A polypeptide hormone derived from brain and pituitary, the fibroblast growth factor, has many properties that are strikingly similar to those of PDGF.[17,19,20]

Platelets express surface Fc receptors for the various subclasses of IgG,[21] and possibly also for IgE,[22] as well as for the Clq,[23] and the C3a[24] fragments of complement. Basophils and mast cells produce a platelet-activating factor, which is released specifically by IgE-mediated reactions to antigen.[25] Human lymphocytes stimulated by concanavalin A release factors that produce platelet aggregation and acceleration of clot retraction.[26] Apparently platelets are also capable of recognizing exposed subendothelial tissue via surface receptors.[27] C-reactive protein inhibits platelet aggregation and release reactions, activation of platelet factor 3 and platelet-dependent clot retraction.[28]

The principal role of the platelet is related to blood coagulation. Platelets adhere specifically to several substances such as collagen; they may aggregate and/or undergo a secretory response called the release reaction.[29] It is clear, however, that platelet aggregation and release can be triggered immunologically by immune complexes, activated complement components, and also by lymphokines. Thus, it is not surprising that platelets were shown to have a role in systemic anaphylaxis[30,31] and in graft rejection.[32] Moreover, mouse platelets were shown to lyse antibody-coated erythrocytes, but nucleated cells were unaffected. Most classes of mouse immunoglobulins can initiate the platelet-mediated lytic reaction.[33] The IgE mediated killing of schistosomes by human and rat platelets has also been observed recently.[23] Taking into consideration that platelets represent 34% of the leukocyte volume they may indeed exert a massive defense mechanism against parasites. Similarly, thrombocytes, which are three times more abundant than other circulating phagocytes, were identified as the primary circulating phagocytic cells in chickens.[34]

G. Other Cells
1. Red Blood Cells
Red blood cells in primates have receptors for complement components (C3b and C4b). Recent studies showed that human red blood cells are important participants in the handling of immune complexes,[35] and in all likelihood, play a fundamental role in the prevention of immune complex related complications in disease such as glomerulonephritis, arteritis, and arthritis.

2. Mucosal and Glandular Epithelial Cells
Certain cells of the gastrointestinal, respiratory, and genitourinary mucosa, and of exocrine glands (salivary, lacrimal), are intimately associated with immunoglobulin A-secreting plasma cells. These epithelial cells synthesize a peptide, called secretory component, which is also expressed on their surface. The dimeric IgA, released by the plasma cells, binds to the secretory component on the surface of the epithelial cells, which is followed by the uptake of IgA, and transit through the epithelial cells to the mucosal surface as intact secretory IgA. The secretory component protects the molecule from breakdown by proteolytic enzymes and increases its resistance to pH changes.[36]

3. Astrocytes, Epidermal, and Endothelial Cells
Astrocytes in the brain are apparently capable of presenting antigen to T lymphocytes.[37] A previously unrecognized antigen-presenting cell was found in the murine epidermis that is responsible for the UV radiation-related activation of suppressor immune mechanisms.[38] The endothelial cells form the interface between the blood and tissues, and thus, are in a unique position to regulate lymphocyte traffic and activation. The so-called high endothelial venules are capable of binding selectively, certain lymphocytes in peripheral lymph nodes and Peyer's patches in the gastrointestinal tract.[39] In addition, there is evidence to suggest that endothelial cells also play a role in lymphocyte activation.[40]

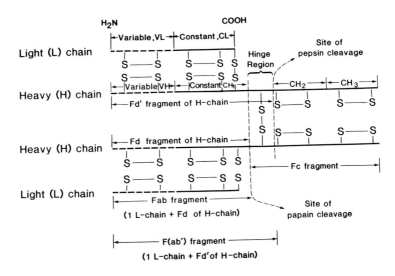

FIGURE 1. The scheme of IgG structure.

III. HUMORAL FACTORS OF IMMUNITY

A. Immunoglobulins

Tiselius and Kabat[41] analyzed serum proteins by electrophoresis and concluded that of the three separable globulin fractions of vertebrate sera (alpha-, beta-, and gammaglobulin), gammaglobulins showed an elevation in intensively immunized animals. Purified antibodies, isolated from specific precipitates with various antigen, were also identified as gammaglobulins. Antibody molecules are globular proteins containing carbohydrate and are commonly referred to as immunoglobulins. The term immunoglobulin is distinct and somewhat broader than gammaglobulin, since it includes proteins that extend into the β- and α-2 range of electrophoretic mobility. Immunoglobulins comprise a vastly heterogenous population of proteins, composed of antibodies of various molecular sizes and of widely different specificities.

All the classes and subclasses of immunoglobulins, from a variety of vertebrate species examined so far, contain two heavy (H) and two light (L) peptide chains in a special arrangement, which is shown in Figure 1, using IgG as an example. The molecule is sensitive to limited digestions with papain, which cleaves the molecule into two fragments, containing and L chain and the Fd fragment of the H chain. This is called the Fab fragment. The third fragment consists of two identical portions of the H chain and is called the Fc fragment, because it is crystallizable. Pepsin cleaves the molecule behind the inter H chain disulfide bonds, which yields F(ab')₂ fragments. The Fab portion contains the antigen binding site of the molecule, which is formed by V regions of both the H and L chains showing hyper variability of amino acid sequences. The remaining parts of H and L chains show much less variability and are called constant (C) regions. The four chains of the basic molecule are linked to each other covalently by disulfide bonds, the positions and numbers of which vary somewhat according to the various immunoglobulin classes and subclasses. The hinge regions of the Y shaped molecule allows for extreme flexibility of the antigen combining sites. Recent extensive analysis of immunoglobulin sequences revealed regions that have a certain amount of repetitiveness and are called domains. Light chains contain one variable (VL) and one constant (CL) domain, whereas heavy chains contain one variable (VH) and three constant domains (CH1, CH2, and CH3). Each domain forms a loop-like structure, which is due to the intrachain disulfide bonds, and is conceived as a separate functional entity. The IgM molecule contains an additional CH domain. The L chains of all immu-noglobulins fall into two chemically and antigenically different groups, known as *κ* and *λ*. In humans, and a variety of higher animals examined, there are five major classes of immunoglobulins known as IgA, IgD, IgE, IgG, and IgM, the H chains of which are class specific and designated by the corresponding Greek letters as *α, δ, ε, γ,* and *μ.* Furthermore, some of the immunoglobulin classes can be divided into sub-classes according to specific differences located in the carboxyterminal portions of the H chains. The major characteristics of human immunoglobulins are summarized in Table 2.

The Fc portions of all immunolgobulin classes and subclasses perform important biological functions, such as complement fixations, transplacental transfer, secretion, and binding to cells with Fc receptors: thus, trigger phagocytosis, target cell killing, and exert immunoregulatory function. Many of these functions are mediated by car-bohydrate moieties, rather than protein sequences.

Certain sequence variability of immunoglobulin molecules that can be detected by specific antibodies are classified as isotypes, allotypes, and idiotypes. The term isotype refers to variant molecules within an immunoglobulin class, (e.g., IgG1, IgG2, IgG3, and IgG4). Allotypic determinants are controlled by allelic genes and may be located in the C regions of H and L chains. In contrast, most of the idiotypic determinants are located in the V regions (antigen combining site). Apparently, the amino acid sequence that specifies the complementariness of different families of antibodies with the anti-genic determinant vary, depending on the clonal origin of antibodies. In other words, the sequence of hypervariable regions shows unique idiotypic determinants of the an-tibody molecule produced by a given clonal cell, which is seldom to be duplicated by another clone.

The heavy and light chains of immunoglobulins are produced in the rough endo-plasmic reticulum of B lymphocytes, and assembly begins in the cysternae. Carbohy-drate is added in the Golgi complex, after which the molecules are packed in secretory vesicles that fuse with the plasma membrane and become externalized and shed, or remain membrane-bound in order to function as an antigen receptor.

1. IgA

IgA is the major secretory immunoglobulin present in all mucose membrane secre-tions (bronchial, small intestine, vaginal), in parotid saliva, amniotic and lacrimal fluid, and also in the colostrum. In contrast to serum IgA, which is a monomer, the secretory IgA has a dimeric form joined by J chain and excreted against a concentra-tion gradient by specialized epithelial cells that add a secretory component to the mol-ecule. Secretory IgA is resistant to proteolysis and to pH changes and represents the host's first line of defense against infections and other harmful agents, which come into contact with mucous membranes. It was also proposed that IgA protects other immune systems from extensive stimulation via the gastrointestinal tract.

2. IgD

IgD is a minor serum component, is susceptible to proteolytic degradation, heat denaturation, and has a short half-life. Antibody activity could only be demonstrated by indirect methods and IgD is only able to activate complement by the alternate path-way. The major function of IgD is to serve as an antigen receptor on the membrane of B lymphocytes.

3. IgE

IgE is present in serum in trace amounts only, and was known as the reagin respon-sible for allergic reactions, until biochemically identified.[42] Tonsils, adenoids, bron-

Table 2
SUMMARY OF SOME PROPERTIES OF HUMAN IMMUNOGLOBULINS

	IgG	IgA	IgM	IgD	IgE
Synonyms	γG, 7S, γ_2, γ_{ss}	γA, β_2A, γ_1A	γM, 19S, β_2M, γ_1M	γD	γE, IgND
Physicochemical properties					
Sedimentation constant	6.5—7.0	7, 10, 13, 15, 17	18—20, 30	6.2—6.8	8
Molecular weight	150,000	180,000; 385,000*ᵃ	900,000	183,000	196,000
Total carbohydrate (%)	2.9	7.5	11		10
Immunochemical properties					
Heavy-chain classes	γ	α	μ	δ	ε
Light-chain types	κ, λ	κ, λ	κ, λ	κ, λ	κ, λ
Molecular formula	$\gamma_2\kappa_2$, $\gamma_2\lambda_2$	$\alpha_2\kappa_2$, $\alpha_2\lambda_2$ $(\alpha_2\kappa_2)2SC^a$; $(\alpha_2\lambda_2)2SC^{*a}$	$(\mu_2\kappa_2)5$; $(\mu_2\lambda)5$	$\delta_2\kappa_2$, $\delta_2\lambda_2$	$\varepsilon_2\kappa_2$, $\varepsilon_2\lambda_2$
Number of subclasses known	4	2	2	1	1
Biological values					
Serum conc. (mg%)	800—1680	140—420	50—190	0.3—10	0.0017—0.006
Synthesis rate (mg/kg/day)	20—40	2.7—5.5	3.2—16.9	0.03—14.9	
Catabolic rate (% I.V. pool/day)	4—7	14—34	14—25	18—60	
Distribution (% in I.V. pool)	48—62	40	65—100	63—86	
Antibody activity	Yes	Yes	Yes	Yes	Yes
Placental passage	Yes	No	No	No	No
Presence in cerebrospinal fluid	Yes	Yes	No		
Complement fixation	Yes	No	Yes	No	No?

ᵃ In exocrine secretions, IgA has a dimeric structure and an attached secretory component (SC).

chial and peritoneal lymph nodes, and the respiratory and gastrointestinal mucosa contain numerous IgE plasma cells, but very few can be found in the spleen or in the subcutaneous lymph nodes, and none in peripheral blood and bone marrow. Tissue mast cells, basophils, lymphocytes, macrophages, and possibly even platelets, have specific Fc receptors for IgE. Heating of IgE antibodies to 56°C for 30 min destroys their binding capacity to cellular receptors. The major function of IgE is to equip various cells of the leukocyte series with antigen specific receptors (homocytotropic antibody), and such cells in turn will participate actively in various immune and inflammatory reactions. The role of IgE in host defense against various parasites is well documented.

4. IgG

IgG is the major class of immunoglobulins comprising about 85% of the total immunoglobulins in man. About 50% of IgG is located extravascularly; therefore, it is also the major component of humoral immunity in tissues. In man four subclasses of IgG can be identified, which share common antigenic determinants specifying the IgG class, but each subclass possesses unique antigenic determinants not shared by any of the other subclasses. The number of disulfide bonds between the H chains varies among these subclasses, and the L chain is linked at different positions to the γ-2, γ-3, and γ-4 chains. Evidence is increasing to suggest that these four subclasses of IgG have different biological functions, although the relationship between function and structure is still under investigation. IgG is less efficient in complement fixation and agglutination than IgM; thus, the neutralization of soluble antigens, both in the extravascular and intravascular space, may be considered as its main function.

5. IgM

IgM is a pentamer of five basic immunoglobulin units held together by disulfide bonds and a J chain. A single molecule contains ten combining sites if a small molecule is used as antigen, but only five combining sites are demonstrable for macromolecular antigens, possibly because of steric interference. Because of the large molecular size (M stands for macroglobulin), IgM is localized almost entirely in the vascular space and the concentration in the tissue is only 1/16 of that in the blood. IgM is 100 times more efficient in lysing red cells than IgG by the activation of complement, and also a very efficient agglutinator, suggesting that it is especially well adapted for handling bacteria and other particulate antigens. In addition, monomeric IgM molecules also serve as membrane bound receptors for B lymphocytes.

6. Antibody Diversity

Ever since the enormous heterogeneity of antibodies were recognized in terms of specificity, avidity, classes, and subclasses, it remained a mystery how such diversity was achieved at the genetic level. Numerous theories have been generated and these can be divided into two major groups. The first group of theories, or germ line theories, states that genes coding for antibody specificity are passed from generation to generation. A serious conceptual problem of these theories was that according to some very conservative calculations a prohibitively large proportion of mammalian genome would be committed to the maintenance of antibody response. The second group of theories allows only a limited number of immunoglobulin genes to be passed from generation to generation and suggests that diversity is generated through somatic mutation. However, there was no precedent for a mechanism that could generate such an extensive mutation. Recently, the riddle of antibody diversity has been solved, using modern technology in genetics.[43-47] It became clear that the immunoglobulin molecule is the product of multiple genes, some of which code for variable regions and others for the constant regions of the molecule. A number of mechanisms such as gene translocation, recombination, excision, and splicing are involved at the genetic level in the generation of antibody specificity and diversity. These mechanisms also permit the switching of antibody classes by the same B lymphocyte, while maintaining antibody specificity. In this case, the same V region genes first are associated with the constant region genes of IgM, which later on may be switched to the C genes of IgG, or to the C genes of some other immunoglobulin class. Translocation and rearrangement is mediated by specific joining genes at the DNA level and splicing occurs at the RNA level, in order to bring together the specific gene segments for translation. It is easy to see that these alterations could generate a vast repertoire of different chain sequences. The possible combinations alone could account for the extensive diversity of antibody molecules.

B. Complement

The complement system[48,49] comprises at least 13 different plasma proteins, which play an important role in immunological and nonimmunological host defense. The immunological defense system involves nine proteins (C1, C2, C3, C4, C5, C6, C7, C8, C9) that execute the complement reaction according to the so-called classical pathway. IgM and IgG (with the exception of IgG4 antibodies) expose a receptor site on their Fc portion for complement, after combination with the specific antigen. This receptor is recognized by the first complement component, which is followed by the activation of C4, C2, C3, and C5, by enzymatic cleavage, each component is being a pro-enzyme that can act on a number of molecules of the next component in the system after activation. Once C5 is cleaved to C5a and C5b, C5b initiates the membrane attack complex that is a self-assembling process, involving the remaining complement components. Apparently, certain peptides of the C5b, 6, 7, 8, and 9 complex are inserted during this process into the phospholipid bilayer of the membrane, so as to form a channel of about 55 to 100 Å in diameter, which allows the escape of cytoplasmic components leading to cell death.

The nonspecific pathway of complement activation does not involve antibodies, but rather, it can be triggered by a variety of polysaccharides including the LPS (endotoxin) membrane component of Gram-negative bacteria and also by aggregated proteins. This alternate pathway of activation involves properdin factors B and D, an enzyme that cleaves C3b, and a cofactor that accelerates this cleavage. The system is capable of activating C3 and from there on the sequence of the reaction is identical to that of the classical pathway.

In addition to the selfsustained killing of certain target cells, such as cells of animals or gram-negative bacteria, certain cleavage products (C3a, C5a) exert important biological activities that include mediator release from basophilic leukocytes and mast cells (anaphylatoxins), release of hydrolytic enzymes from neutrophils, chemotactic, and phagocytosis-stimulating effects on neutrophils, eosinophils, and monocytes. These factors are capable of producing muscle contraction by acting directly on smooth muscle cells. All these effects are mediated by specific membrane receptors of the reacting cells. Recent investigations revealed that many of the complement components are produced by monocyte-macrophages, and that lymphocytes and mononuclear phagocytes are also capable of activating complement while expressing membrane receptors for the bioactive fragments. This provides for yet another amplification system of local immune reactivity, utilizing complement components that play a role in lymphocyte stimulation and the activation of mononuclear phagocytes.[50] Indeed, evidence is increasing that complement fragments are involved in the regulation of immune responses.[51,52] Moreover, the complement system bridges immune mediated reactions with the coagulation cascade, as well as with inflammatory reactions.[53]

C. Lymphokines, Interleukins, and Cytokines

The term *lymphokines* [54,55] was created to designate soluble mediators of nonimmunoglobulin nature produced primarily by T lymphocytes. After some time it has been realized that other cells also secrete soluble mediators and the term *monokine* is used by some for factors elaborated by the monocyte-macrophage lineage. The term *cytokine* solves this problem by referring to all soluble mediators. Most lymphokines regulate a variety of functions of leukocytes, or of some other target cells such as osteoclasts, liver, and brain cells (e.g., endogenous pyrogen). Recently the mediators of cell interaction and regulation during immune responses have been named *interleukins.* [56] Most of these mediators are highly potent, short-range factors that are present in lymphoid tissues only in trace amounts. For this reason, their isolation and characterization is slow and difficult. A few of them, such as interleukin 2 for instance, have already been purified and characterized. [57] Many of these substances satisfy the criteria of classical hormones, i.e., they are secreted by highly specialized cells in order to alter the activity of target cells at the DNA level, which is mediated by specific receptors. Interestingly enough, some lymphokines and peptide hormones appear to be related structurally and may exert similar functions on specific targets. [58]

Over 90 biological activities, attributed to lymphokines, have been described to date. Some of the more frequently detected lymphokines may be grouped as follows.

1. Growth factors that include mitogenic, proliferation, blastogenic, and colony stimulating factors
2. Differentiation factors
3. Activating factors that include helper, enhancing, potentiating, stimulator, and inducing factors
4. Inhibitory factors including suppressor, clone inhibitory, proliferation inhibitory, and counter-inhibitory factors
5. Chemotactic factors
6. Immobilizing and migration inhibitory factors
7. Macrophage aggregating and fusion factors
8. Interferon
9. Lymphotoxin, macrophage cytotoxicity factor and macrophage arming factor
10. Endogenous pyrogen

IV. ANTIGENS

In general, lymphokines are specific for their target cells, e.g., there are separate growth factors for B and T lymphocytes, separate chemotactic factors for monocytes, eosinophilic, neutrophilic, or basophilic leukocytes, etc. Some of the helper and suppressor cell factors are antigen specific while others are also able to recognize histocompatibility antigens, idiotypes, and allotypes on the surface of their target cells. Much remains to be done in the field of lymphokine analysis, which may well include mediators for the interaction of the neuroendocrine and immune systems.

All substances capable of eliciting an immune response are defined as *antigens.* [59] The response induced may manifest as immunity (elicited by an immunogen) or tolerance (induced by a tolerogen). Depending on the conditions of antigen-lymphocyte interactions, the same compound may function as an immunogen, tolerogen, or both (e.g., by the induction of partial or split tolerance). Antibodies, or immune effector cells, generated during an immune response will have the potency of interacting specifically with the antigen, and also frequently with chemically related (cross-reactive) compounds. A memory exists for most antigens that were encountered by the immune system in the past, and a faster, more efficient immune response is induced upon secondary exposure (secondary or anamnestic reaction). The duration of this memory is variable. A great variety of small molecules that are not capable of inducing an immune response on their own are designated as haptens. Haptens may be rendered immunogenic, if covalently linked to an antigenic carrier molecule, or tolerogenic if coupled with a tolerogenic carrier.

According to traditional views, only substances foreign to the body are immunogenic, whereas self components are not. There is ample experimental evidence to show that this is not the case; rather, self reactive clones exist, but normally are suppressed by immunoregulatory mechanisms. Such clones can be activated by a variety of mitogens and become reactive in autoimmune disease.

A. Soluble Antigens

A great number of substances that include proteins, polysaccharides, lipo- and glycoproteins, and nucleic acids can function as potent immunogens. According to our current understanding, some minor regions (5 to 6 amino acids or sugars) on the immunogenic macromolecule, called antigenic determinants or epitopes, interact specifically with the antigen receptors of lymphocyte clones that have the ability to recognize them.[80] This interaction is mediated by noncovalent forces (charge, hydrophobic, hydrophilic, etc.),. and is required, but by no means is sufficient, for triggering an immune response. Experiments with synthetic antigens revealed that a minimum of two sufficiently spaced epitopes will allow for the cell interactions necessary to trigger an immune response. In general, the more epitopes present in a macromolecule, the stronger is its immunogenicity. Polysaccharides, which are simply polymers of sugar molecules, are immunogenic only at a high molecular weight, while polypeptides consisting of a variety of amino acids may be immunogenic as small molecules. Simple chemicals, including a number of drugs, may induce immune reactions after repeated skin contact (skin sensitizers) or internal application (drug allergy). These substances are nonimmunogenic by themselves; however, they react with host proteins, which leads to the formation of immunogenic conjugates. A variety of antigens, frequently of polysaccharide nature (e.g., lipopolysaccharide of Gram-negative bacteria, pneumococcal polysaccharide, dextran) function as B lymphocyte mitogens. These substances induce polyclonal antibody synthesis and are capable of eliciting specific antibody formation without T lymphocyte help, which is needed for most other antigens. These substances are called thymus-independent antigens and are capable of functioning as thymus-independent carriers as well. The immune system of some animal strains, and of some humans is unable to respond to certain antigens due to genetically determined factors.

B. Histocompatibility Antigens

The idea of transplanting tissues or organs for the correction of injuries, or other defects, is as old as medicine itself. The early trials of allotransplantation failed without exception, whereas autografts were permanently accepted. Gorer in 1937 was the first to observe that mice belonging to a particular inbred strain will produce antibodies against the tissues of animals which belong to a different inbred strain. In the 1940s, Medawar and co-workers, showed that the rejection of skin allografts is also an immunological phenomenon. The antigens responsible for graft rejection were named transplantation antigens and were studied extensively in inbred strains of mice with the aid of alloantisera. Due to the contribution of numerous workers, it became gradually clear that an entire region of chromosome 17 in the mouse and of chromosome 6 in man, contains a series of genes that code for the major histocompatibility (MHC) antigens, responsible for rapid graft rejection, as well as for a number of other products that are involved in immune function. A schematic map of the MHC region of mouse and man is shown in Figure 2. On the basis of their products, three classes of

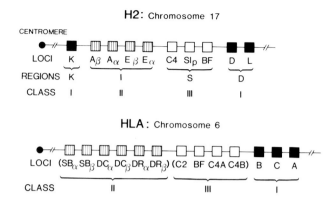

FIGURE 2.   The major histocompatibility region of mouse and man.

genes are recognized. Class I genes (K,D,L in the mouse and A,B,C in man) code for a single polypeptide chain of 44,000 daltons mol wt, which is membrane bound and is present on all nucleated cells, as well as on red blood cells of mice, but not of man. This molecule contains three external domains, a transmembrane region, and a cytoplasmic domain. A serum protein of 12,000 daltons mol wt, called β_2-microglobulin, is associated through noncovalent forces permanently with Class I histocompatibility antigens. Two types of Class II molecules, (A and E), are recognized in the mouse. Each contain an α chain (34,000 daltons) and a β chain (29,000 daltons). Both are membrane bound and associated with each other with two extracellular domains each, a transmembrane region and an intracellular domain. In man three Class II molecules, (DC, DR, and SB) comprised of α and β chains in a similar fashion, are known to date. The third group of genes (Class III) code for soluble serum proteins that include the complement component C4 and sex-linked protein. Class I and Class II histocompatibility antigens, β_2-microglobulin and immunoglobulin molecules, show homology, indicating that these gene families were derived from a common ancestor. Recent evidence suggests that the antigen receptor of T lymphocytes is also a member of this super gene family.[60,61]

Killer T cells mediating antiviral immunity, graft, and possibly also tumor rejection, recognize Class I histocompatibility antigens and will kill aberrant cells having altered histocompatibility antigens (allografts, tumor cells) or virus related antigens on their surface. The products of Class II genes mediate regulatory cell interactions (inducer, helper, suppressor) during immune reactions, and for this reason, are also called immune response (Ir) genes and their products immune-associated (Ia) antigens. The regions of the chromosome containing Ir genes is called the I region. The genetically controlled inability of a variety of mouse strains to respond to certain antigens has frequently been mapped into the I region.[60,62] In addition to lymphocytes and the monocyte-macrophage lineage, Ia antigens are also expressed on nonlymphoid tissues, which include epidermal Langerhans' cells, erythrocyte and granulocyte precursors in the bone marrow, epithelial cells lining the intestinal tract, the bile duct, the respiratory and urinary tract, cells of the parotid and submandibular glands, and the lactating mammary gland. Spermatozoa, but not the trophoblast, and oligodendrocytes of the brain express Ia antigens in the mouse. Human endothelial cells from the umbilical vein could be induced to express Ia-like antigens by treatment of primary cultures with the lectin, phytohemagglutinin.

Recent findings indicate that in addition to their role in immune reactions, MHC genes may have a general role in cell communication, mediated by cell-to-cell interaction and by a variety of ligands, including peptide hormones (glucagon, insulin, endorphin).[63,64] Interestingly enough, testis size and testosterone levels in inbred strains of mice were also found to be MHC-dependent.[65] Furthermore, certain inborn errors of metabolism, such as the deficiency of 21-hydroxylase (which causes abnormal steroid metabolism in the adrenal) and hemochromatosis, are also MHC-linked.[66,67]

Minor histocompatibility antigens, blood group substances, embryonic and fetal antigens, organ specific and differentiation antigens, tumor antigens, and species specific antigens cannot be discussed here because of space limitations.

V. THE IMMUNE RESPONSE

A. Cell Interactions During Immune Reactions

Although there are still many gaps in our understanding of the immune response and its regulation, certain basic principles are reasonably well established. It is clear that three major categories of cells participate in the generation of effector immune function to thymus-dependent antigens, which represent the overwhelming majority of immunological stimuli. The three cell types are: antigen-presenting cells, helper/inducer cells, and effector cell precursors.[68,70]

The cells presenting the antigen are generally considered to be members of the monocyte-macrophage lineage, although some of them seem to be highly specialized. Apparently, these cells have the capacity to recognize foreign material (antigen) in a nonspecific fashion, although they also bind antibodies through their Fc receptors and antigen specific (arming) T cell factors. It was proposed[60] that Ia molecules interact specifically with a limited number of amino acid sequences of protein antigens and thus, fix the antigen molecule to the cell surface. The antigen may or may not be processed (partially digested) prior to its association with the cell surface. Usually the majority of antigenic molecules are degraded and eliminated completely, and only a minor fraction is presented to immunocytes. The presented antigen will be recognized by certain clones of T lymphocytes that have receptors compatible with the presented epitopes. Numerous studies indicate that this recognition takes place in the context of the presenting Ia molecule.[70] This recognition leads to cell-to-cell contact (antigen bridging) and to the release of interleukins, which is followed by the proliferation and differentiation of antigen responsive immature helper/inducer T lymphocytes. These T cells will act in turn on effector cell precursors (T and B lymphocytes) and induce growth and differentiation again in conjunction with the antigen. A schematic outline of the antigen driven differentiation of effector T lymphocytes is presented in Figure 3. The major steps involved in the humoral immune response appear to be identical, although it is clear that the growth and differentiation factors for B lymphocytes are not identical with those of effector T cell precursors. During antigen presentation, as well as during helper-precursor cell interactions, Ia molecules and immunoglobulin determinants (idiotype, allotype, isotype) are also recognized specifically by T cells. Although the antigen-mediated bridging of cells has been demonstrated morphologically, numerous experiments indicate that cell-to-cell contact is not an absolute requirement during the immune response, since antigen specific and nonspecific factors are capable of mediating the entire sequence of events.

The generation of suppressor T lymphocytes, which regulate all immune responses, is also the result of the interaction of antigen-presenting inducer and precursor cells, as outlined in Figure 3. Suppressor T cells may be antigen specific, but may also be directed to idiotypic, allotypic, or isotypic determinants of B lymphocytes, and possibly also to similar determinants of T lymphocytes. They inhibit immune responses during the early stages of initiation. Recently T cells interfering with suppressor cell development were also identified and were named contra-suppressor cells.[71]

As predicted originally by Jerne,[72] immune phenomena are governed by a network

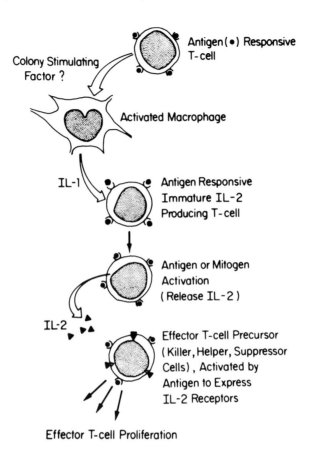

FIGURE 3.   Schematic diagram of interleukin function in cellular immune response.[57]

interaction of various immunocytes.[69,73] Normally an antigenic stimulus leads to the development of immune effector mechanisms, which is followed by suppressor mechanisms. Predominantly or exclusively effector or suppressor responses are also known, however, which are frequently genetically determined. These reflect abnormalities of cell interactions during the immune response. Unresponsiveness to a given antigen (immunological tolerance) may reflect the lack of clones capable of recognizing the antigen specifically, or could be the result of an overwhelming suppressor cell response. Self tolerance, which is maintained by suppressor cells, also can be broken experimentally, indicating the permanent presence of autoreactive lymphocyte clones. Early studies on immunoregulation indicated that IgG antibodies exert a feedback inhibitory effect on the immune response. This can be explained in part by the activation of phagocytic cells through immune complexes, which leads to the rapid elimination of the antigen. However, it also became clear that immune complexes are potent stimulators of suppressor cells. Recent evidence suggests that certain kinds of antigen-presenting cells, such as the dendritic cells in spleen and lymph nodes and the Langerhans cells in the skin, preferentially induce immunity, whereas other macrophage-like cells induce suppression and/or tolerance rather than immunity. Differences in the immune response, due to the route of antigen application, may in fact be related to the anatomic distribution of antigen-presenting cells. For instance, it was shown that feeding an antigen to animals, or injection into the portal vein, leads to the induction of tolerance rather than immunity. This could reflect the predominance of antigen-presenting cells within the gastrointestinal tract, and/or in the liver, that favor the generation of suppressor cells. On the other hand, the well-known effectiveness of intradermal immunization, both for cell-mediated and humoral immune reactions, could be explained with the extreme potency of Langerhans cells to induce immune reactions.

The so-called T-independent antigens, many of which are derived from pathogenic microorganisms, do not require the participation of helper T lymphocytes in order to elicit an antibody response. Most, if not all, of these substances are capable of polyclonal lymphocyte activation. Although the mechanism of action of T-independent antigens has not been elucidated in full detail, it appears that in addition to the antigen signal, these substances are capable of delivering mitogenic signals to the cell, which normally would come from regulatory cell interaction. The response to T-independent antigens is regulated by suppressor T cells and polyclonal B cell activation leads to massive rebound suppression, which could serve to the advantage of pathogens that possess this potential.[74] A variety of serum factors that include lipoproteins, alpha globulin, alpha fetoprotein, vitamins, microelements, essential amino acids, and other nutritional factors also have an effect on immunocompetence. The hormones secreted or regulated by the pituitary gland are of special interest as factors of immunoregulation not originating within the immune system.

B. Immune Effector Mechanisms

Traditionally humoral and cell-mediated immune reactions were distinguished on the basis that humoral immunity can be transferred to normal animals by serum, whereas cell-mediated immunity can only be transmitted by lymphocytes. This classification is highly artificial because both types of responses occur to most immunogens. The ultimate mission of immune effector mechanisms is to defend the host against pathogenic microbes and toxic agents through specific recognition, followed by neutralization, destruction, and/or elimination. The recognition step may be achieved by specific antibodies or by lymphocytes, and thus, we may divide the effector mechanisms accordingly.

1. Antibody-Mediated Mechanisms

The first line of defense on mucosal surfaces is mediated by secretory IgA antibodies. Presumably these antibodies can prevent the penetration of microbes into tissues by the interference of their interaction with tissue receptors, through surface alteration and/or aggregation, or agglutination. The IgE-mast cell-basophil system, which is also preferentially associated with mucosal surfaces and exocrine glands, is considered to be the second line of defense (gate-keeper) against intruders. This system is extremely sensitive to minute amounts of antigen. IgE-mediated mechanisms are assumed to provide defense against parasitic infestations. Apparently, IgE antibodies are capable of triggering macrophages, or eosinophilic granulocytes for the killing of parasites. The activation of the complement, cascade, which in turn interacts with a variety of biological systems, appears to be the major function of IgM and to a lesser extent of IgG. This is a marvelous humoral mechanism for the specific destruction of foreign cells. In addition, complement components are known to activate phagocytic cells (opsonization). IgM and IgG antibodies are also efficient in virus neutralization, possibly through the alteration of receptor molecules. IgG is the major immunoglobulin class in serum and tissue fluids and, in addition to complement fixation and neutralization reactions, it is known to activate all phagocytic cells as well as to trigger antibody-dependent cytotoxic reaction. Humoral immunity is considered to be effective against most microorganisms, with the exception of intracellular parasites, which require cell-mediated immunity for complete defense.

2. Cell-Mediated Mechanisms

Killer T lymphocytes are known to mediate graft and tumor rejection and to be instrumental in host defense against viruses and certain bacteria, such as *Mycobacterium, Bucella,* and *Listeria.* Apparently, the elimination of intracellular parasites from the body requires the killing of harboring cells. Another important cell-mediated effector mechanism is delayed-type hypersensitivity. This reaction is mediated by a special subset of effector T lymphocytes that are not capable of cytotoxic reactions, but rather, have the ability of homing to sites of antigen deposits within tissues and to attract mononuclear phagocytes to the site through the secretion of chemotactic factors. The macrophages, and to some extent other phagocytic cells that migrate to the site, will then be activated by T cell-derived lymphokines for the destruction and/or elimination of the antigen. In contrast with the rapid appearance of IgE-mediated allergic reactions after the deposition of the antigen in the skin (immediate hypersensitivity), this cell-mediated immune reaction requires 24 to 48 hr to develop (delayed-type hypersensitivity). The third type of immune effector cells that are capable of recognizing specific targets are called natural killer (NK) cells. As indicated by their name, these cells are present in nonimmunized animals and man, and can recognize and kill a variety of cellular targets that have altered surface moieties. At least some of the NK cells are T cell-related, although they appear to be heterogenous. The mechanism of their differentiation and target recognition is unknown at the present time. NK cells are readily activated by interferon, which suggests a role for these cells in viral immunity. They are also considered to be important in host defense against tumors.

C. The Effect of Immune Mechanism on Other Systems

Osteoclasts appear to be macrophage-related cells that are regulated, in part, by interleukin-like substances.[75] Furthermore, certain lymphokines are known to promote hematopoietic cell proliferation and differentiation.[76] Monocyte-macrophages produce procoagulant molecules under the influence of T cell-derived factors.[77] Immune mechanisms were also indicated in the production of acute phase proteins by the liver.[78] Finally, the possible role of immune mechanisms in mammalian reproduction has also been suggested.[79]

REFERENCES

1. Smith, R. T., Miescher, P. A., and Good, R. A., Eds., *Phylogeny of Immunity,* University of Florida Press, Gainesville, 1966.
2. Burnet, F. M., *Immunological Surveillance,* Pergamon Press, Oxford, 1970.
3. Campbell, R. C. and Bibb, C., Transplantation in coelenterates, *Transplant. Proc.,* 2, 202, 1970.
4. Chateaureynaud-Duprat, P., Specificity of allograft reaction in *Eisemia foetida, Transplant. Proc.,* 2, 222, 1970.
5. Cooper, E. L., Specific tissue graft rejection in earthworms, *Science,* 166, 1414, 1969.
6. Cooper, E. L., Transplantation immunity in helminths and annelides, *Transplant. Proc.,* 2, 216, 1970.
7. Hink, F., Immunity in insects, *Transplant. Proc.,* 2, 233, 1970.
8. Greaves, M. F., Owen, J. J. T., and Raff, M. C., *T and B lymphocytes, Origins, Properties and Roles in Immune Responses,* American Elsevier, New York, 1973.
9. Till, J. E. and McCullock, E. A., A direct measurement of the radiation sensitivity of normal mouse bone marrow cells, *Radiat. Res.,* 14, 213, 1961.
10. Wu, A. M., Till, J. E., Siminovitch, L., and McCulloch, E. A., A cytological study of the capacity for differentiation of normal hemopoietic colony-forming cells, *J. Cell. Physiol.,* 69, 177, 1967.

11. Wu. A. M., Till, J. E., Siminovitch, L., and McCulloch, E. A., Cytological evidence for a relationship between normal hemopoietic colony-forming cells and cells of the lymphoid system, *J. Exp. Med.*, 127, 455, 1968.
12. Brodniewicz-Proba, T., Perreault, C., and Potworowski, E. F., Thymic microenvironmental factor: solubilization and preliminary characterization, *Mol. Immunol.*, 20, 137, 1983.
13. Goldstein, A. L., Low, T. L. K., Zatz, M. M., Hall, N. R., and Naylor, P. H., Thymosins, *Clin. Immunol. Allergy,* 3, 119, 1983.
14. Brand, A., Gilmour, D. G., and Goldstein, G., Lymphocyte-differentiating hormone of bursa of Fabricius, *Science,* 193, 319, 1976.
15. Tavassoli, M., Megakaryocyte — platelet axis and the process of platelet formation and release — a review, *Blood,* 55, 537, 1980.
16. Williams, N. and Levine, R. F., The origin, development and regulation of megakaryocytes, *Br. J. Haematol.*, 52, 173, 1982.
17. Niewiarowski, S., Proteins secreted by the platelet, *Thromb. Haemos.,* 38, 924, 1977.
18. Pfueller, S. F. and Luscher, E. F., The effect of immune complexes on blood platelets and their relationship to complement activation, *Immunochemistry,* 9, 1151, 1972.
19. Ross, R. and Vogel, A., The platelet-derived growth factor — a review, *Cell,* 14, 203, 1978.
20. Heldin, C. H., Westermark, B., Mellstrom, K., Johnsson, A., Ek, B., Nister, M., Betsholtz, C., Ronnstrand, L., and Wasteson, A., Platelet-derived growth factor. Structural and functional aspects, *Surv. Synth. Pathol. Res.,* 1, 153, 1983.
21. Henson, P. M. and Spiegelberg, M. L., Release of serotonin from human platelets induced by aggregated immunoglobulins of different classes and sublcasses, *J. Clin. Invest.,* 52, 1282, 1973.
22. Joseph, M., Auriault, C., Capron, A., Vorng, H., and Vines, P., A new function for platelets: IgE-dependent killing of schistosomes, *Nature (London),* 303, 810, 1983.
23. Suba, E. A. and Csako, G., C1q (C1) receptor on human platelets: inhibition of collagen-induced platelet aggregation by C1q (C1) molecules, *J. Immunol.,* 117, 304, 1976.
24. Becker, S., Hadding, U., Schorlemmer, H. U., and Bitter-Suermann, D., Demonstration of high-affinity binding sites for C3a anaphylatoxin on guinea-pig platelets, *Scand. J. Immunol.,* 8, 551, 1978.
25. Benveniste, J., Camussi, J., Mencia-Huerta, J. M., and Polonsky, J., Isolation and partial characterization of PAF, *Ann. Immunol. Inst. Pasteur,* C128, 259, 1977.
26. Coeugniet, D. and Bendixen, G., Lymphokines and thrombosis. I. Thrombocyte aggregating activity released by human lymphocytes stimulated with concanavalin-A, *Acta Allergol.,* 31, 94, 1976.
27. Nurden, A. T. and Caen, J. P., Annotation — membrane glycoproteins and human platelet function, *Br. J. Hameatol.,* 38, 155, 1978.
28. Fiedel, B. A., Simpson, R. M., and Gewurz, H., Effects of C-reactive protein on platelet function. III. The role of cAMP, contractile elements, and prostaglandin metabolism in CRP-induced inhibition of platelet aggregation and secretion, *J. Immunol.,* 119, 877, 1977.
29. Droller, M. J., Ultrastructure of platelet release reaction in response to various aggregating agents and their inhibitors, *Lab. Invest.,* 29, 595, 1973.
30. Fesus, L., Csaba, B., and Muszbek, L., Platelet activation factor, the trigger of haemostatic alterations in rat anaphylaxis, *Clin. Exp. Immunol.,* 27, 512, 1977.
31. Pinckard, R. N., Halonen, M., Palmer, J. D., Butler, C., Shaw, J. O., and Henson, P. M., Intravascular aggregation and pulmonary sequestration of platelets during IgE-induced systemic anaphylaxis in the rabbit: abrogation of lethal anaphylactic shock by platelet depletion, *J. Immunol.,* 119, 2185, 1977.
32. Burrows, L., Haimov, M., Aledort, L., Leiter, E., Nirmul, G., Shanzer, H., Taub, R., and Glabman, S., The platelet in the obliterate vascular rejection phenomenon, *Transplant. Proc.* 5, 157, 1973.
33. Soper, W. D., Bartlett, S. P., and Winn, H. J., Lysis of antibody-coated cells by platelets, *J. Exp. Med.,* 156, 1210, 1982.
34. Chang, C.-F. and Hamilton, P. B., The thrombocyte as the primary circulating phagocyte in chickens, *J. Reticuloendothel. Soc.,* 25, 585, 1979.
35. Medof, M. E., Lam, T., Prince, G. M., and Mold, C., Requirement for human red blood cells in inactivation of C3b in immune complexes and enhancement of binding to spleen cells, *J. Immunol.,* 130, 1336, 1983.
36. Tomasi, T. B. and Grey, H. M., Structure and function of immunoglobulin A, *Prog. Allergy,* 16, 181, 1972.
37. Fontana, A., Fierz, W., and Wekerle, H., Astrocytes present myelin basic protein to encephalitogenic T-cell lines, *Nature (London),* 307, 273, 1984.
38. Granstein, R. D., Lowy, A., and Greene, M. I., Epidermal antigen-presenting cells in activation of suppression: identification of a new functional type of ultraviolet radiation-resistant epidermal cell, *J. Immunol.,* 132, 563, 1984.

39. Andrews, P., Ford, W. L., and Stoddart, R. W., Metabolic studies of high-walled endothelium of postcapillary venules in rat lymph nodes, *Ciba Found. Symp.,* 71, 211, 1980.
40. Roska, A. K., Johnson, A. R., and Lipsky, P. E., Immunologic function of endothelial cells: guinea pig aortic endothelial cells support mitogen-induced T lymphocyte activation, but do not function as antigen-presenting cells, *J. Immunol.,* 132, 136, 1984.
41. Tiselius, A. and Kabat, E. A., An electrophoretic study of immune sera and purified antibody preparations, *J. Exp. Med.,* 69, 119, 1939.
42. Ishizaka, K., Human reaginic antibodies, *Ann. Rev. Med.,* 21, 187, 1970.
43. Sakano, H., Rogers, J. H., Hüppi, K., Brack, C., Traunecker, A., Maki, R., Wall, R., and Tonegawa, S., Domains and the hinge region of an immunoglobulin heavy chains are encoded in separate DNA segments, *Nature (London),* 277, 627, 1979.
44. Sakano, H., Maki, R., Kurosawa, Y., Roeder, W., and Tonegawa, S., Two types of somatic recombination are necessary for the generation of complete immunoglobulin heavy-chain genes, *Nature (London),* 286, 676, 1980.
45. Sakano, H., Kurosawa, Y., Weigert, M., and Tonegawa, S., Identification and nucleotide sequence of a diversity DNA segment (D) or immunoglobulin heavy-chain genes, *Nature (London),* 290, 562, 1981.
46. Davis, M. M., Kim, S. K., and Hood, L. E., DNA sequences mediating class switching in immunoglobulins, *Science,* 209, 1360, 1980.
47. Weigert, M., Perry, R., Kelley, D., Hunkapiller, T., Schilling, J., and Hood, L., The joining of V and J gene segments creates antibody diversity, *Nature (London),* 283, 497, 1980.
48. Fearon, D. T. and Austen, K. F., The human complement system. Biochemistry, biology and pathobiology, *Essays Med. Biochem.,* 2, 1976.
49. Müller-Eberhard, H.-J. and Schreiber, R. D., Molecular biology and chemistry of the alternative pathway of complement, *Adv. Immunol.,* 29, 1, 1980.
50. Sundsmo, J. S., The leukocyte complement system, *Fed. Proc.,* 41, 3094, 1982.
51. Weiler, J. M., Ballas, Z. K., Needleman, B. W., Hobbs, M. V., and Feldbush, T. L., Complement fragments suppress lymphocyte immune responses, *Immunol. Today,* 3, 238, 1982.
52. Egwang, T. G. and Befus, A. D., The role of complement in the induction and regulation of immune responses, *Immunology,* 51, 207, 1984.
53. Thaler, M. S. and Klausner, R. D., *Medical Immunology,* Lippincott, New York, 1977.
54. de Weck, A. L., Kristensen, F., and Landy, M., Eds., *Biochemical Characterization of Lymphokines,* Academic Press, New York, 1980.
55. Rocklin, R. E., Bendtzen, K., and Greineder, D., Mediators of immunity: lymphokines and monokines, *Adv. Immunol.,* 29, 55, 1980.
56. Moller, G., Ed., Interleukins and lymphocyte activation, *Immunol. Rev.,* Vol. 63, 1982.
57. Gillis, S., Interleukin 2: biology and biochemistry, *J. Clin. Immunol.,* 3, 1, 1983.
58. Blalock, J. E.,. The immune system as a sensory organ, *J. Immunol.,* 132, 1067, 1984.
59. Sela, M., Ed., *The Antigens,* Vols. 1—4, Academic Press, New York, 1979.
60. Benacerraf, B., Role of MHC gene products in immune regulation, *Science,* 212, 1229, 1981.
61. Steinmetz, M. and Hood, L., Genes of the major histocompatibility complex in mouse and man, *Science,* 222, 727, 1983.
62. Katz, D. and Benacerraf, B., Eds., *The Role of the Products of the Histocompatibility Gene Complex in Immune Responses,* Academic Press, New York, 1976.
63. Edidin, M., MHC antigens and non-immune functions, *Immunol. Today,* 4, 269, 1983.
64. Farid, N. R., Ed., *HLA in Endocrine and Metabolic Disorders,* Academic Press, New York, 1981.
65. Ivanyi, P., Hampl, R., Starka, L., and Mickova, M., Genetic association between H-2 gene and testosterone metabolism in mice, *Nature (London) New Biol.,* 238, 280, 1972.
66. New, M. I., Dupont, B., and Levine, L. S., HLA and adrenal disease, in *HLA in Endocrine and Metabolic Disorders,* Farid, N. R., Ed., Academic Press, New York, 1981, 177.
67. Simon, M., Fauchet, R., Hespel, J.-P., Brissot, P., Genetet, B., and Bourel, M., Idiopathic hemochromatosis and HLA, in *HLA in Endocrine and Metabolic Disorders,* Farid, N. R., Ed., Academic Press, New York, 1981, 291.
68. Möller G., Ed., Accessory cells in the immune response, *Immunol. Rev.,* Vol. 53, 1980.
69. Gershon, R. K., Immunoregulation circa 1980: some comments on the state of the art, *J. Allergy Clin. Immunol.,* 66, 18, 1980.
70. Rosenthal, A. S., Current concepts: regulation of the immune response — role of the macrophage, *N. Engl. J. Med.,* 303, 1153, 1980.
71. Gershon, R. K., Eardley, D. D., Durum, S., Green, D. R., Shen, F.-W., Yamauchi, K., Cantor, H., and Murphy, D. B., Contrasuppression. A novel immunoregulatory activity, *J. Exp. Med.,* 153, 1533, 1981.
72. Jerne, N. K., Towards a network theory of the immune system, *Ann. Immunol.,* C125, 373, 1974.

73. Gershon, R. K., Symposium: immune regulation, *Fed. Proc. Fed. Am. Soc. Exp. Biol.,* 38, 2051, 1978.
74. Tsukuda, K., Berczi, I., and Klein, G., Human B lymphocytes activated by Epstein-Barr Virus (EBV) or by mitogens suppress nitrogen induced immunoglobulin production, *J. Immunol.,* 126, 1810, 1981. 1810, 1981.
75. Mundy, G. R., Monocyte-macrophage system and bone resorption, *Lab. Invest.,* 49, 119, 1983.
76. Watson, J. D., Mochizuki, D. Y., and Gillis, S., Molecular characterization of interleukin 2, at symposium: molecular characterization of lymphokines that promote hematopoietic cell proliferation and differentiation, *Fed. Proc. Fed. Am. Soc. Exp. Biol.,* 42, 2747, 1983.
77. Helin, H. J., Fox, R. I., and Edgington, T. S., The instructor cell for the human procoagulant monocyte response to bacterial lipopolysaccharide is a Leu-3a + T cell by fluorescence-activated sorting, *J. Immunol.,* 131, 749, 1983.
78. Jamieson, J. C., Kaplan, H. A., Woloski, B. M. R. N. J., Hellman, M., and Ham, K., Glycoprotein biosynthesis during the acute-phase response to inflammation, *Can. J. Biochem. Cell Biol.,* 61, 1041, 1983.
79. Prehn, R. T. and Lappé, M. A., An immunostimulation theory of tumor development, *Transplant. Rev.,* 7, 26, 1971.
80. Burnet, 1959.

GENERAL REFERENCES

1. *Cold Spring Harbor Symposia on Quantitative Biology,* Vol. 41 (Parts 1 and 2), Cold Spring Harbor Laboratories, Cold Spring Harbor, New York, 1976.
2. Greenwalt, T. J. and Janieson, G. A., Eds., *Granulocyte. Function and Clinical Utilization.* Vol. 13, Alan R. Liss, New York, 1977.
3. Myrvik, Q. and Weiser, R., Eds., *The Fundamentals of Immunology,* 2nd ed., Lea & Febiger, Philadelphia, 1984.
4. Paul, W. D., Ed., *Fundamental Immunology,* Raven Press, New York, 1984.
5. Selye, H., *The Mast Cells,* Butterworths, Reading, Mass., 1965.
6. Schermer, S., *The Blood Morphology of Laboratory Animals,* Davis, Philadelphia, 1967.

Chapter 2

THE PITUITARY GLAND

Eva Nagy

TABLE OF CONTENTS

I. INTRODUCTION

In 1877 Claude Bernard[1] was the first to point out that all living creatures tend to preserve constant conditions of life in their internal environment, which he termed "milieu interieur". Walter Cannon reached the same conclusion during his studies of blood glucose levels[2] and used the term "homeostasis" to denote steady states in living organisms that are maintained by complex physiologic mechanisms. The powerful regulatory forces that are involved in the maintenance of homeostasis in the internal milieu, despite often adverse environmental conditions, were studied by Hans Selye. He emphasized that animals have a remarkable ability to cope with various environmental stress situations and termed this phenomenon the general adaptation syndrome.[3] Recently, Austin called attention to the existence of homeostatic regulatory mechanisms within the immune system, namely in complement mediated reactions and in the mast cell-eosinophil-axis.[4]

It is well-known that the nervous system, together with the endocrine system, regulate directly or indirectly the internal environment of higher organisms and also mediate their adaptation to various factors in their surroundings.

II. BRIEF DESCRIPTION OF THE PITUITARY GLAND

The pituitary gland is located in the base of the skull in the sella turcica, a cavity within the sphenoid bone, and is attached to the hypothalamus with a stalk. The pituitary is a small organ; it weighs about 0.5 g in man and it may approach 1 g in weight during pregnancy. We distinguish the anterior lobe of pituitary that is also called adenohypophysis, and the posterior lobe, or neurohypophysis, and an intermediate portion or pars intermedia. The anterior lobe amounts to approximately 75% of the total weight of the gland. The pars intermedia is missing or is present in traces (2%) in man. The pituitary gland is embryologically derived from cells of both stomodeal ectoderm (Rathke's pouch) and neural ectoderm of the floor of the forebrain.[5] By the 12th week of intrauterine life, the pituitary is identifiable macroscopically, secretory granules appear in the cytoplasm of adenohypophyseal cells, and pituitary hormones can be detected by radioimmunoassay.

The blood supply of the pituitary gland originates from branches of the superior hypophyseal artery, which is a branch of the internal carotid artery. Venous blood enters the pituitary by an important *portal system,* the so-called gomitoli, which are comprised of short terminal arterioles with strong muscluar walls surrounded by a dense capillary network. The capillaries drain into long portal veins that flow down the pituitary stalk to enter into the sinusoidal capillaries of the anterior lobe. The inferior hypophyseal arteries anastomose with each other. These vessels represent the major blood supply to the posterior pituitary and also contribute an arterial input to capillaries that drain into the short portal veins. The venous drainage of the pituitary gland enters into the internal jugular vein. The direction of blood flow in the portal veins is from the median eminence to the pituitary. Neuronal secretions of hypothalamus reach the adenohypophysis through these vessels (Figure 1).

The posterior lobe of the pituitary consists of secretory nerve fibers descending from the supraoptic and paraventricular nuclei, while the anterior lobe consists of cells that can be stained with traditional hematoxylin and eosin stains as acidophils, basophils, and chromophobes.

The cytologic classification of adenohypophyseal cell types was made more accurate by the combination of immunocytochemical and immunoelectron microscopic techniques. By the combination of these methods, it became possible to identify the type of hormone secreted by each pituitary cell; therefore, they can now be classified ac-

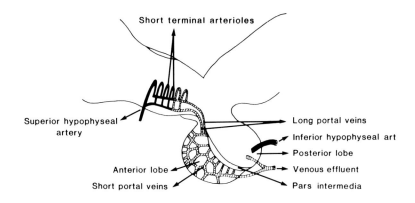

FIGURE 1. Relationship of pituitary and its blood supply to neighboring structures.

cording to their function.[6] (See Table 1.) It has also been proposed that in addition to the functional cells, a so-called pituitary stem cell may also exist.[7]

III. AN OVERVIEW OF PITUITARY FUNCTION AS PART OF THE NEUROHORMONAL REGULATORY SYSTEM

A. Hypophyseal Hormones and Their Function

To a great extent it was due to the pioneering studies of Cushing and associates that the concept of the pituitary gland as "conductor of the endocrine orchestra" gained prominence.[8] These workers demonstrated first that the pituitary gland, while not essential for life, normally exerts an important influence on the metabolic processes of the body. Subsequent studies revealed the importance of pituitary function in the development of sexual organs and behavior.[8]

Three hormones, namely vasopressin, oxytocin and neurophysin, are known to be released by the posterior lobe of pituitary, while as many as nine different hormones (listed in Table 2) are produced by the adenohypophysis.

Chemically, these hormones can be classified into three major groups according to their sequence homology. ACTH, α-MSH, and β-LPH belong to one such group that is formed from a large common precursor protein, proopiomelanocortin. It has recently been discovered that β-LPH is the prohormone for morphine-like peptides named endorphins. The second related group consists of TSH, LH, and FSH, all of which contain two chains. The α-chains of these hormones are virtually identical, whereas the β-chains of each hormone differ both in configuration and in molecular weights. The β-chains are inactive by themselves, but they confer biological specificity when combined with an α-chain. Growth hormone (GH) and prolactin (PRL) represent the third related group of pituitary hormones.

1. Growth Hormone (GH)

Young rats treated with pituitary extract will grow large (gigantism). This experimental result can be repeated with different kinds of animals. The daytime GH level in adult man is less than 3 ng/mℓ. The serum level of GH rises during sleep. The symptoms of GH excess depends on age in both animals and humans. If it occurs before epiphyseal union, the linear growth may be enormous (over 200 cm). If the GH excess occurs after epiphyseal union, acromegaly will result. It is caused most often by a tumor of acidophil cells of the anterior pituitary. The symptoms and signs of acromegaly develop insidiously over many years. The tumor is often large with suprasellar

Table 1
ADENOHYPOPHYSEAL CELLS AND THEIR FUNCTION

Cell type	Size (μ in diameter)	Hormone secreted
Somatotroph	350—500	Growth hormone (GH)
Lactotroph	275—350	Prolactin (PRL)
Thyrotroph	50—100	Thyroid stimulating hormone (TSH)
Gonadotroph	275—375	Follicle stimulating hormone (FSH)
		Luteinizing hormone (LH)
Corticotroph — Lipotroph	375—550	Adrenocorticotropic hormone (ACTH)
		β-Melanocyte stimulating hormone (βMSH)
		Endorphins
		β-Lipotrophin (βLPH)
Nonsecretory	Small, variable	Degranulated secretory cells

Table 2
THE NINE HORMONES OF THE ADENOHYPOPHYSIS

Group and hormone	No. of amino acids	Mol wt
1. Thyrotropin (TSH) (thyroid stimulating hormone)	211	32,000
Follitropin (FSH) (follicle stimulating hormone)	210	32,000
Lutotropin (LH, ICSH) (luteinizing hormone, interstitial cell stimulating hormone)	204	32,000
2. Lactotropin (PRL) (prolactin)	199	23,500
Somatotropin (GH) (growth hormone)	191	22,650
3. β-Lipotropin (βLPH)	91	9,500
Adrenocorticotropin (ACTH) (adrenocorticotropic hormone)	39	4,500
β-Melanotropin (βMSH) (melanocyte stimulating hormone)	22	2,000
Endorphins	15—30	

extension. X-ray examination usually reveals an enlarged sella, a lantern jaw, and overbite of the lower incisors. Bitemporal hemianopsia, diabetes mellitus, thickening of the soft tissues, and acral enlargement of the head are the characteristic symptoms.

Dwarfism occurring at the beginning of life is caused either by the lack of GH or decreased secretion of GH. If it is caused later on by infection, supracellar cyst or chraniopharyngeoma: hypophyseal destruction, infantilism, and dwarfism (Lorain-Levi's syndrome) will develop.

GH increases blood sugar by antagonizing the action of insulin and maintains a positive nitrogen balance. GH increases lipolysis, free fatty acids, ketone body production, glomerulus filtration, and serum level of Na, K,Cl,P. GH does not act on its target organ directly. It affects tissues by the stimulation of somatomedins in the liver. The known somatomedins are similar in structure and in function to insulin.

2. Adrenocorticotropic Hormone (ACTH)

ACTH increases the synthesis and release of adrenocortical steroids, primarily cortisol. Hypophysectomy causes atrophy of the adrenal cortices and the decrease of corticosteroid synthesis and release. Extra-adrenal effects of ACTH are lipolysis, ketosis, early hypoglycemia, and late insulin resistance. These symptoms can be demonstrated in adrenalectomized animals. The first 13 amino acids in ACTH are identical to that of the amino acid sequence of α-MSH. As a result ACTH has MSH activity, namely, it enhances the pigmentation of the skin. In addition, ACTH is believed to play an important role in adaptation to various stress conditions. Normal serum level of ACTH in man at 8:00 a.m. is <80 pg/mℓ. Patients with relatively high plasma ACTH concentration (200 to 300 pg/mℓ) develop Cushing's disease that is due to hypercorticalism, secondary to the inappropriate secretion of ACTH by the pituitary.

In Cushing's disease the most constant symptom is obesity and a moon-shaped plethoric face. The skin is often dry and readily bruised and lacerated with minor trauma. Purple striae appear in the skin of the lower abdomen. Most patients have mild hypertension and ankle edema due to the mineralocorticoid effect of excess glucocorticoid. Osteoporosis is common; diabetes mellitus occurs in about 20% of cases. Increased androgen secretion presents in the female with acne and hirsutism. Oligomenorrhea and amenorrhea result from suppression of pituitary gonadotropins.

In the absence of ACTH secretion, the adrenal zona fasciculata atrophies and Addisons's syndrome will develop. Weakness, fatigue, anorexia, and weight loss are almost universal. Postural hypotension, sometimes syncope, occur due to mineralocorticoid insufficiency and salt depletion.

3. Melanocyte-Stimulating Hormone (MSH)

MSH is secreted by cells located in the pars intermedia of the hypophysis and they are also dispersed in the neurohypophysis in humans. There are three other known substances with MSH activity besides ACTH: α-MSH, β-MSH, and β-LPH (β-lipotropin). The endorphins (α, β, γ) appear to be parts of a larger molecule identical to β-lipotropin. This large peptide molecule also contains a segment identical to β-melanocyte-stimulating hormone, which includes a segment identical to ACTH. The rapid degradation of β-endorphin in the brain raises the possibility that this peptide is acting as a neurotransmitter. α-MSH has not been detected in normal plasma. β-MSH is present in the normal plasma in a concentration of 0.1 ng/mℓ.

4. Thyroid-Stimulating Hormone (TSH)

TSH stimulates the synthesis, storage, and release of hormones of the thyroid gland. Calcium ion is necessary for TSH's effect on the thyroid cells. The normal serum level of TSH in man is <5 μU/mℓ. In the thyroid gland TSH affects all phases of iodine metabolism, increasing the capacity of the I⁻ pump. First it stimulates the I⁻ efflux, then the I⁻ uptake is increased. TSH accelerates the synthesis of thyroglobulin. It also effects both carbohydrate and phospholipid metabolism. First it stimulates glucose utilization and oxygen consumption. Glucose is required for synthesis of thyroglobulin and of proteins. It has stimulatory effects on protein synthesis as well.

The excess production of TSH by pituitary tumors is very rare, but when it occurs, it causes hyperthyroidism that is more common in females than in males. The common symptoms of hyperthyroidism are weight loss despite normal or increased appetite, irritability, heat intolerance, excessive perspiration, tremor, palpitation, fatigue, muscle weakness, oligomenorrhea, amenorrhea, and eye complaints.

Hypopituitarism or hypothalamic disease may be caused by a large variety of lesions. Reduced secretion of TSH causes thyroid atrophy (central hypothyroidism). The symptoms are poor cold tolerance, fatigue, weight gain, dry skin, slow speech and movement, hoarse voice, thin lateral eyebrows, and slow heart rate. Amenorrhea, galactorrhea, and anemia may also occur.

5. Gonadotropins

Follicle-stimulating hormone (FSH) and luteinizing hormone (LH) are glycoprotein hormones. FSH is responsible for control of gametogenesis stimulating the granulosa cells of the ovary and the Sertoli cells of the testis. LH is responsible for control of sex hormone synthesis. It luteinzes mature graafian follicles in the ovary that have discharged their egg, and also acts on the Leydig cells of the testis. Normal levels of gonadotropins in plasma include

1. Women, mature, and premenopausal (except at ovulation) — FSH: 5 to 30 μU/ mℓ, LH: 5 to 25 μU/mℓ
2. Ovulatory surge — FSH: 5 to 20 μU/mℓ, LH: 15 to 40 μU/mℓ
3. Postmenopausal — FSH: 40 μU/mℓ, LH: 40 μU/mℓ
4. Men mature — FSH: 5 — 20 μU/mℓ, LH 5 to 20 μU/mℓ
5. Children of both sexes — FSH: 5 μU/mℓ, LH: 5 μU/mℓ

The loss of pituitary gonadotropins leads to gonadal atrophy. In men, libido and potency decrease, sperm cells disappear from the semen, and pubic, axillary hair, and beard growth is decreased. In women, menstruation ceases.

On rare occasions pituitary adenomas that secrete FSH, LH have been reported to cause precocious puberty. The disorders that cause true isosexual precocity result from disturbance of the hypothamlamic pituitary axis. In girls, breast development begins before the age of 7 years and menstruation before the age of 9.

6. Chorionic Gonadotropin (CG)

CG is also composed of two peptide chains (α and β), and it is produced by tropho-blastic cells that maintain the corpus luteum of pregnancy. Increased levels of CG are found in women with hydatidiform mole and choriocarcinoma as well. At approximately 10 weeks of gestation the CG reaches the maxmium level: 100 IU/mℓ. After 120 days of gestation the CG persists at a level of 20 IU/mℓ. If the level of CG rises above 500 to 600 IU/mℓ of plasma, the diagnosis is neoplastic trophoblastic disease. The gonadotropic hormones can restore spermatogenesis and testosterone in men with hypopituitarism.

7. Prolactin (PRL)

The amino acid sequence of human and other animal prolactins has recently been established.[9] The PRL level in the serum increases during pregnancy, reaching maximum level at the third trimester. PRL is needed for the initiation and maintenance of lactation in a properly prepared mammary gland. Normal level of serum PRL in men is 6 to 8 ng/mℓ, in women 9 to 15 ng/mℓ, if the serum PRL level is greater than 200 ng/mℓ prolactinoma is almost always indicated.

Prolactinomas are the most common secretory tumors of the pituitary. Women with microadenomas usually have amenorrhea with or without galactorrhea. Amenorrhea and galactorrhea may follow pregnancy (Chiari-Fommel syndrome) or be without pregnancy (del Castillo's syndrome). Men with pituitary tumors have loss of libido and potency. Visual impairment and headache may occur in both sexes.

Clinical evidence of PRL deficiency is only recognized in post-partum necrosis of the pituitary (Sheehan's syndrome). Obstetric bleeding or shock can cause pituitary necrosis. Post-partum enlargement of the breasts and lactation are lacking. Pubic and axillary hair fail to grow; menstruation, if it returns at all, is infrequent. If the pituitary necrosis is extended, severe panhypopituitarism may develop.

8. Placental Lactogen (PL)

PL is secreted by the syncytiotrophoblast of placenta. It has both lactogenic and somatotrophic properties. The principal role of PL is the insulin antagonism. It may be responsible for the development of diabetic ketoacidosis in pregnant women.

9. Vasopressin and Oxytocin

The neuroendocrine function of the posterior pituitary was suggested less than 100 years ago. Vasopressin (antidiuretic hormone-ADH) and oxytocin have been characterized and synthesized by du Vigneaud.[10,11]

Both oxytocin and vasopressin are octapeptides, synthesized by nerve cells located in the supraoptic and in the paraventricular nuclei of the hypothalamus and transported to the posterior pituitary where they are stored and released. Vasopressin plays an important regulatory role in water conservation and maintenance of body fluid osmolality, blood volume, and blood pressure. In healthy adults, plasma vasopressin concentration correlates with plasma osmolality. The average serum osmolality is 288 mOsm/kg. In this case the plasma vasopressin is around 1 pg/ml. Oxytocin is a regulator of lactation (milk ejection) and of uterine smooth muscle contraction. Oxytocin level of plasma in men and preovulatory women: 0.5 to 2 μU/ml, ovulating women: 2 to 4 μU/Ml, lactating women: 5 to 10 μU/ml. Increased plasma osmolality is a powerful stimulus for release of vasopressin. The hypertonic environment of the collecting ducts results in water reabsorption, tending to reduce plasma osmolality. Pathological deficiency of vasopressin results in an increased plasma osmolality and excretion of large volumes of pale, dilute urine with secondary polydipsia. This condition is called diabetes insipidus.

Vasopressin excess is characterized by a plasma osmolality lower than that of urine. This may be caused by ectopic secretion of vasopressin and is called the syndrome of inappropriate antidiuretic hormone secretion. The patient is usually asymptomatic until the plasma sodium falls to less than 120 mmol/ℓ when the clinical features of water intoxication appear.

B. Hypothalamic-Releasing Hormones and Their Role in the Regulation of Hypophysis

Several decades ago, transplantation studies indicated that hypophyseal function is dependent on hypothalamic influences.[12,13] The pituitary removed from direct contact with median eminence loses the capacity to synthesize and release most of its hormones. Based on this evidence, Green and Harris[14] postulated that neurohormonal substances might originate in the median eminence of the tuber cinereum and thus, regulate secretion of anterior pituitary hormones. Subsequent work by Schally and co-workers[15,16] and by Guillemin and Peterson[17,18] and by others led to the detection of a number of hypothalamic factors controlling the release of pituitary hormones (Table 3). Thyrotropin-releasing hormone (TRH) was identified and biochemically analyzed in 1969,[19,20] gonadotropin-releasing hormone (LH-RH) in 1971,[21] growth hormone release-inhibiting hormone (GH-RIH) in 1973,[22] corticotropin-releasing hormone (CRH) in 1981-82,[23-25] and growth hormone-releasing factor (GH-RF) identified in 1965[26] and characterized in 1980-83.[27-30]

Some of these factors have already been identified chemically, e.g., TRH consists of (pyro)glu-His-Pro-amide or 2-pyrolidone-5-carboxylyl-His-Pro-amide. The luteinizing hormone-releasing and follicle stimulating hormone-releasing hormone consist of ten amino acids, and the GH-RIH (somatostatin) is a tetradecapeptide. The corticotropin-releasing factor is a hypothalamic 41-residue polypeptide. The endocrine function of the hypothalamus has been the subject of several recent reviews.[31-36]

The regulation of the six generally accepted pituitary hormones by neuroendocrine factors is summarized in Table 4.

It is interesting that dopamine, which is a well-known neurotransmitter, has been found to inhibit PRL synthesis.[34] Furthermore, TRH, LH-RH, CRH, and somatostatin, each of which originally were isolated from extracts of the hypothalamus, actually occur throughout the CNS, including the spinal cord. However, this does not imply that these peptides are randomly distributed. Several groups of researchers have shown that each of these compounds has a unique distribution pattern, and they have been

Table 3

HYPOTHALAMIC HORMONES CONTROLLING THE RELEASE OF PITUITARY HORMONES

Name	No. of amino acids	Abbreviation used	Function
Corticotropic releasing hormone	41	CRH	Release of ACTH
Growth hormone releasing hormone	40,44	GH-RH	Release of GH
Somatostatin			
Growth hormone release inhibiting hormone	14	GH-RIH	Inhibition of GH and TSH release
Thyrotropin releasing hormone	3	TRH	Release of TSH and PRL
Dopamine			
Prolactin release inhibiting hormone		PIH	Inhibition of PRL release
Luteinizing hormone releasing hormone and follicle stimulating hormone releasing hormone	10	LH-RH or Gn-RH	Release of FSH and LH

separately identified by immunocytochemistry in axonal tracts and neuronal bodies in well-characterized anatomical formation of the CNS. In addition, the endocrine pancreas in all vertebrates secretes somatostatin that in turn can inhibit the secretion of gastrin, secretin, cholecystokinin, pepsin, and HCl by acting directly at the level of gastric mucosa. TRH has been found recently in extracts of the stomach and of the duodenum.[18] It has been postulated that all peptide hormone-producing cells are derived from the neuralectoderm, as are all neurons, which could explain the occurrence of various peptides in the brain as well as in endocrine cells in other tissues. Morphological studies indicated a very punctual localization for these peptides that implied a very short range role for these substances (peptidergic synapses). Guillemin[18] proposed that these peptides, called hormones earlier, do not fit the definition of a hormone any more. Rather, they seem to be candidates of neurotransmitters. Hokfelt et al.[37] has concluded that some neurons may contain both peptides and one of the catecholamines, a classical neurotransmitter. These recent discoveries serve the conceptual basis for the mechanism of neuroendocrine regulation of various bodily functions including immune reactions.

C. Hormones and Their Mechanism of Action

In 1905 Starling[38] defined hormones as chemical messengers that are made in one tissue (ductless gland) and carried through the blood to stimulate another tissue. However, this classical definition does not fit a number of substances that are recognized today as hormones. At present, there is no generally accepted definition of hormones, although Raacke[39] has attempted recently to create such a definition. He proposed that a substance be classified as a hormone if it satisfies the following criteria:

1. That it be normally produced endogenously by specific cells, but that it also be active if supplied exogenously
2. That it acts as a chemical messenger or signal among different kinds of cells, that is, that it be produced by one kind of cell, and exert its biological activity on another type.
3. That it exert its effect through or as part, of a regulatory complex that acts directly on the genome

Hormones stimulate their target cells through hormone receptors that are able to

Table 4

THE REGULATION OF
PITUITARY SECRETION BY
HYPOTHALAMIC
RELEASING AND
INHIBITORY HORMONES

Pituitary hormone	Releasing hormone	Inhibiting hormone
ACTH	CRH	—
GH	GH-RH	GH-RIH
TSH	TRH	—
PRL	TRH	DOPAMINE
FSH, LH	LH-RH	—

combine with their respective hormones specifically and with high affinity (with dissociation constants in the range of 10^{-9} to $10^{-11} M$). The receptors for polypeptide hormones and catecholamines are located in the plasma membrane, whereas those for steroid and thyroid hormones are located in the cytoplasm and/or the nucleus.[39-43] In addition, the presence of hormone receptors at other locations has been postulated: intracellular gonadotropin receptors, thyroid hormone receptors in mitochondria, and insulin receptors in the nucleus and other intracellular structures.[41-43]

The concentration and affinity of hormone receptors are critical factors in determining the response of a given target tissue to the respective hormone. A high concentration and /or affinity of receptors, should be in general, though not necessarily, accompanied by high sensitivity to the respective hormone, whereas hormone insensitivity would occur when the concentration and/or affinity of hormone receptors is low. In the mouse, an X-linked mutation (tfm) interferes with normal androgen-dependent differentiation of XY males, causing a female phenotype in spite of the presence of testosterone producing testes. The tfm mutation renders all the target organs of testosterone completely or almost completely unresponsive to androgens attributable to a defect in the androgen receptor.[44] A similar syndrome of testicular feminization occurs in man.[45] Moreover, an absence of human GH receptors has been postulated as the basic defect in Laron dwarfism, a human disease in which there are clinical features of GH deficiency, but the blood levels of this hormone are actually elevated.[46] In general, cells that lack functionally active hormone receptors are resistant to hormone action. However, the mere presence of hormone receptors is not sufficient to guarantee cell response to the hormone since subsequent cellular events are required for the manifestation of hormone action. These cellular events are incompletely understood at the present time. It is clear that steroid and thyroid hormones, which are able to pass through the plasma membrane readily, combine with their receptor proteins intracellularly, and then this hormone-receptor complex exerts its biological effect. Direct interaction with DNA, structural alteration of chromatin, binding to nuclear riboprotein particles, modification of histones, modification of nonhistone nuclear proteins, and modification of RNA polymerase activities all have been proposed for the mechanism of action of these hormones. In addition, various investigators suggested that steroid and thyroid hormones regulate RNA translation as well, which may take place through modification of tRNAs, change in the attachment of amino acids to tRNA, through affection of polysomes, change in translation initiation factors, modification of ribosome proteins, modification of ribosomal RNA maturation, and changes in messenger RNA stability.[42,43]

The prevailing view of the mode of action of peptide hormones is that they combine with specific external receptors in the membrane of their target cells, which causes allosteric activation of a membrane-localized adenyl cyclase, and that the resulting cyclic 3′,5′-adenosine monophosphate (cAMP) acts as a second messenger as originally proposed by Sutherland and co-workers[47] In addition, cyclic 3′,5′-guanozine monophosphate (cGMP), prostaglandins, polyamines (putrescine, spermidine, spermine), monoamines, calcium, and other ions have been proposed as second messenger. The experimental evidence is especially strong for the interaction of hormone receptors with the cAMP and cGMP system.[34,48,49]

The idea of the second messenger has been criticized recently by Raacke[39] who pointed out that it is difficult, if not impossible, to explain the specific action of hormone on their target cells with a nonspecific intracellular messenger such as cAMP. For example, in fat cells the cAMP is stimulated by epinephrine, by ACTH, TSH, LH, GH, secretin, vasoactive intestinal peptide, and dexamethasone and inhibited by insulin, oxytocin and prostaglandins. In order to achieve hormone specificity, Raacke proposed that cAMP would have to combine with a specific protein.

Raacke's theory was constructed on the assumption that protein hormones do not enter their target cells. However, recent studies with insulin,[36,45] β-MSH,[51] epidermal growth factor,[50,52] parathyroid hormone,[53] gonadotropins,[54] prolactin,[55] and nerve growth factor[56,57] showed that protein or peptide hormones do in fact enter the cell after combination with their specific surface receptors.

The penetration of target cells by peptide hormones would justify the existence of intracellular insulin receptors, which were found to be distinct from those on the plasma membrane, and which were detected in the nucleus smooth and rough endoplasmic reticulum, and in the Golgi apparatus.[41] It has been proposed that insulin receptors located on the plasma membrane of target cells mediate short term effects such as the stimulation of membrane transport and the change of membrane potential. On the other hand, the long term effects of insulin (such as activation and inhibition of enzymes, the increase of protein synthesis, the inhibition of protein degradation, and the modulation of DNA and RNA synthesis in the nucleus) is better explained by the internalization of insulin that may then act through its intracelluar receptors.[41] However, the exact mechanism of entry is not known, and thus, it is quite possible that hormones bring their surface receptors in with them when they enter cells. This raises the question of whether the receptors may have a biological function in the cells, in addition to the hormones that are assumed to be biologically active. Recent evidence shows that the insulin receptor may be responsible for many of insulin's effects. It was found that when cells were exposed to antibodies to the insulin receptor, they behaved in many respects as though they were exposed to insulin. The receptor antibody could cause not only the short-term effects of insulin, but at least one of the long-term effects, namely the induction of an enzyme known as lipoprotein lipase. The antibody to the insulin receptor binds to the receptor, but bears no chemical resemblance to insulin. One must assume that when the antibody receptor reaction occurs, it causes the receptor to change its shape, which in turn could exert its effect on the cell.[58] It is also possible that antibodies can trigger the internalization of insulin receptors similar to that of the specific hormone.

The number and perhaps the affinity of hormone receptors on target cells is regulated by the specific hormone itself. For example, elevation of circulating insulin levels causes a decrease in the number of insulin receptors in target tissues,[59,60] In the obese-hyperglycemic mice, there is a marked resistance to insulin action, hyperinsulinemia, and the plasma membranes have a marked decrease in the capacity for insulin binding. However, when such obese mice are fasted and insulin levels decrease, insulin receptors increase toward normal.[61,62] The mechanism of this autoregulation can now be explained easily by assuming that cells exposed to excess hormone internalize and degrade rapidly hormone-receptor complexes, in order to avoid over-responding to the hormone. On the other hand, they gain receptors when there is little hormone around, in order to make it more likely that they will pick up the hormones required. In addition to autoregulation, coordinated regulation (interaction of a steroid and peptide hormone to effect the number of receptors for the same or a different peptide hormone) and heteroregulation (regulation by one hormone of receptors for an entirely different hormone) of hormone receptors has been postulated with some supporting experimental evidence.[42,43]

REFERENCES

1. Bernard, C., Lecons sur les phénomènes de la vie communs aux animaux et aux vegétaux, J. B. Balliere et Fils, Paris, 1877.
2. Cannon, W. B., Some general features of endocrine influence on metabolism, *Am. J. Med. Sci.,* 171, 1, 1926.
3. Selye, H., General adaptation syndrome and disease of adaptation, *J. Clin. Endocrinol.,* 6, 117, 1946.
4. Austin, K. F., Homeostasis of effector systems which can also be recruited for immunologic reactions, *J. Immunol.,* 121, 793, 1978.
5. Atwell, W. J., The development of the hypophysis cerebri in man, with special reference to the pars tuberalis, *Am. J. Anat.,* 37, 159, 1926.
6. Pelletier, G., Robert, F., and Hardy, J., Identification of human anterior pituitary cells by immunoelectron microscopy, *J. Clin. Endocrinol. Metab.,* 46, 534, 1978.
7. Ezrin, C., Kovacs, K., and Horvath, E., A functional anatomy of the endocrine hypothalamus and hypophysis, *Med. Clin. N. Am.,* 62, 229, 1978.
8. Crow, S. J., Cushing, H. W., and Homans, J., Experimental hypophysectomy, *Bull. Johns Hopkins Hosp.,* 21, 127, 1910.
9. Shome, B. and Parlow, A. F., Human pituitary prolactin: the entire linear amino acid sequence, *J. Clin. Endocrinol. Metab.,* 45, 1112, 1977.
10. du Vigneaud, V., Ressler, C., Swan, J. M., Roberts, C. W., Katsoyannis, P. G., and Gordon, S., The synthesis of an octapeptide amide with the hormonal activity of oxytocin, *J. Am. Chem. Soc.,* 75, 4879, 1953.
11. du Vigneaud, V., Gish, D. T., Katsoyannis, P. G., and Hess, G. P., Synthesis of the pressor-antidiuretic hormone, arginin-vasopressin, *J. Am. Chem. Soc.,* 80, 3355, 1958.
12. Greep, R. O., Functional pituitary grafts in rats, *Proc. Soc. Exp. Biol. Med.,* 34, 754, 1936.
13. Harris, G. W. and Jacobsohn, D., Functional grafts of anterior pituitary gland, *Proc. R. Soc. London Ser. B,* 139, 263, 1952.
14. Green, J. D. and Harris, G. W., The neurovascular link between the neurohypophysis and adenohypophysis, *J. Endocrinol.,* 5, 136, 1947.
15. Schally, A. V., Arimura, A., and Kastin, A. J., Hypothalamic regulatory hormones, *Science,* 179, 341, 1973.
16. Schally, A. V., Aspects of hypothalamic regulation of the pituitary gland, *Science,* 202, 18, 1978.
17. Peterson, R. E. and Guillemin, R., The hormones of the hypothalamus, *Am. J. Med.,* 57, 591, 1974.
18. Guillemin, R., Peptides in the brain: the new endocrinology of the neuron, *Science,* 202, 390, 1978.
19. Bler, J., Enzmann, F., Folkers, K., Bowers, C. Y., and Schally, A. V., The identity of chemical and hormonal properties of the thyrotropin-releasing hormones and pyroglutamyl histidyl-proline amide, *Biochem. Biophys. Res. Commun.,* 37, 705, 1969.
20. Burgess, R., Dunn, T. F., Desiderio, D., and Guillemin, R., Structure moléculaire du facteur hyposhalamigne hypophysiotrope TRF d'origine ovine: mise en évidence par spectromètre de masse de la séquence PCA-His-Pro-NH₂, *C. R. Acad. Sci. (Paris),* 269, 1870, 1969.
21. Matsuo, H., Baba, Y., Nair, R. M. G., Arimura, A., and Schally, A. V., Structure of the porcine LH- and FSH-releasing hormone. I. The proposed amino acid sequence, *Biochem. Biophys. Res. Comm.,* 43, 1334, 1971.
22. Brazean, P., Vale, W., Burgus, R., Ling, N., Butcher, M., Rivier, J., and Guillemin, R., Hypothalamic polypeptide that inhibits the secretion of immunoreactive pituitary growth hormone, *Science,* 179, 77, 1973.
23. Rivier, J., Characterization of a 41-residue ovine hypothalamic peptide that stimulates secretion of corticotropin and β-endorphin, *Science,* 213, 1394, 1981.

24. Vale, W., Primary structure of corticotropin-releasing factor from ovine hypothalamus, *Proc. Natl. Acad. Sci. U.S.A.,* 78, 6517, 1981.
25. Huang, W. Y. Chang, R. C. C. Redding, T. W., Vigh, S., and Schally, A. V., Purification and characterization of the corticotropin-releasing factor (CRF) from porcine hypothalami, *Fed. Proc. Fed. Am. Soc. Exp. Biol.,* 41, 1458, 1982.
26. Dharinval, A. P. S., Krulich, L., Katz, S. H., and McCann, S. M., Purification of growth hormone-releasing factor, *Endocrinology,* 77, 932, 1965.
27. Frohman, L. A., Szabó, M., Berelowitz, M., and Stachura, M. E., Partial purification and characterization of a peptide with growth hormone releasing activity from extra pituitary tumors in patients with acromegaly, *J. Clin. Invest.,* 65, 43, 1980.
28. Spics, J., River, J., Torner, M., and Vale, W., Sequence analysis of a growth hormone-releasing factor from a pancreatic islet tumor, *Biochemistry,* 21, 6037, 1982.
29. Sykes, J. E. and Lowry, P. J., Purification of a high-molecular-weight somatoliberin (growth hormone-releasing factor) from pig hypothalami, *Biochem. J.,* 209, 643, 1983.
30. Bohlen, P., Brazeau, P., Block, B., Ling, N., Gaillard, R., and Guillemin, R., Human growth hormone-releasing factor (GRF): evidence for two forms identical to tumor derived GRF-44-NH$_2$ and GRF-40, *Biochem. Biophys. Res. Commun.,* 114, 930, 1983.
31. Besser, G. M., Hypothalamus as an endocrine organ, *Br. Med. J.,* 3, 560, Part I, 1974; 613, Part II, 1974.
32. Malarkey, W. B., Recently discovered hypothalamic-pituitary hormones, *Clin. Chem.,* 22, 5, 1976.
33. Reichlin, S., Regulation of the endocrine hypothalamus, *Med. Clin. N. Am.,* 62, 235, 1978.
34. Labrie, F., Lagoie, L., Ferland, L., Beanlien, M., Massicotte, J., and Raymond, V., New aspects of the control of pituitary hormone secretion, *Ann. Clin. Res.,* 10, 109, 1978.
35. Locke, W., Control of anterior pituitary function, *Arch. Intern. Med.,* 138, 1541, 1978.
36. de la Fuente, J. R. and Rosenbanm, A. H., Psychoendocrinology, *Mayo Clin. Proc.,* 54, 109, 1979.
37. Hokfelt, T., Elfvin, G., Elde, R., Schultzberg, M., Goldstein, M., and Luft, R., Occurrence of somatostatin-like immunoreactivity in some peripheral sympathetic nonandrenergic neurons, *Proc. Natl. Acad. Sci. U.S.A.,* 74, 3587, 1977.
38. Starling, E. H., The chemical correlation of the functions of the body, I-IV, *Lancet,* 2, 339, 423, 501, 579, 1905.
39. Raacke, I. D., Protein hormones and the eucaryotic genome: a general theory of hormone action, *Perspect. Biol. Med.,* 21, 139, 1977.
40. Williams, D. L., The estrogen receptor: a minireview, *Life Sci.,* 15, 583, 1974.
41. Goldfine, I. D., Isulin receptors and the site of action of insulin, *Life Sci.,* 23, 2639, 1978.
42. Pimentel, E., Cellular mechanisms of hormone action. I. Transductional events, *Acta Cient. Venez.,* 29, 73, 1978.
43. Pimentel, E., Cellular mechanisms of hormone action. II. Posttransductional events, *Acta Cient. Venez.,* 29, 147, 1978.
44. Attardi, B. and Ohno, S., Cytosol androgen receptor from kidney of normal and testicular feminized (Tfm) mice, *Cell,* 2, 205, 1974.
45. Weisberg, M. G., Malkasian, G. D., and Pratt, J. H., Testicular feminization syndrome, *Am. J. Obstet. Gynecol.,* 107, 1181, 1970.
46. Jacobs, L. S., Sneid, D. S., Garland, J. T., Laron, Z., and Daughaday, W. H., Receptor-active growth hormone in Laron dwarfism, *J. Clin. Endocrinol. Metab.,* 42, 403, 1976.
47. Haynes, R. C., Sutherland, E. W., and Rall, T. W., The role of cyclic adenylic acid in hormone action, *Recent Prog. Horm. Res.,* 16, 121, 1960.
48. Cho-Chung, Y. S., On the interaction of cyclic AMP-binding protein and estrogen receptor in growth control, *Life Sci.,* 24, 1231, 1979.
49. Levitzki, A. and Helmreich, E. J. M., Hormone-receptor-adenylate cyclase interactions, *FEBS Lett.,* 101, 213, 1979.
50. Schlessinger, J., Shechter, Y., Willingham, M. C., and Pastan, I., Direct visualization of binding, aggregation and internalization of insulin and epidermal growth factor on living fibroblastic cells, *Proc. Natl. Acad. Sci. U.S.A.,* 75, 2659, 1978.
51. Varga, J. M., Moellmann, G., Fritsch, P., Godawska, E., and Lerner, A. B., Association of cell surface receptors for melanotropin with the Golgi region in mouse melanoma cells, *Proc. Natl. Acad. Sci. U.S.A.,* 73, 559, 1976.
52. Carpenter, G. and Cohen, S., ^{125}I-labeled human epidermal growth factor: binding, internalization and degradation in human fibroblasts, *J. Cell. Biol.,* 71, 159, 1976.
53. Nordquist, R. E. and Palmieri, G. M. A., Intracellular localization of parathyroid hormone in the kidney, *Endocrinology,* 95, 229, 1974.
54. Conn, P. M., Conti, M., Harwood, J. P., Dufan, M. L., and Catt, K. J., Internalization of gonadotropin-receptor complex in ovarian luteal cells, *Nature (London).,* 274, 598, 1978.

55. Nolin, J. M. and Witorsh, R. J., Detection of endogenous immunoreactive prolactin in rat mammary epithelial cells during lactation, *Endocrinology,* 99, 949, 1976.

56. Stockel, K., Paravicini, U., and Thoenen, H., Specificity of the retrograde axonal transport of nerve growth factor, *Brain Res.,* 76, 413, 1974.

57. Anders, R. Y., Ingming, J., and Bradshaw, R. A., Nerve growth factor receptors: identification of distinct classes in plasma membranes and nuclei of embryonic dorsal root neurons, *Proc. Natl. Acad. Sci. U.S.A.,* 74, 2785, 1977.

58. Kalata, G. B., Polypeptide hormones: what are they doing in cells, *Science,* 201, 895, 1978.

59. Huang, D. and Cuatrecasas, P., Insulin-induced reduction of membrane receptor concentrations in isolated fat cells and lymphocytes, *J. Biol. Chem.,* 250, 8251, 1975.

60. Soll, A. H., Goldfine, L. D., Roth, J., Kahn, C. R., and Neville, D. M., Thymic lymphocytes in obese (ob-ob) mice: a mirror of the insulin receptor defect in liver and fat, *J. Biol. Chem.,* 249, 4127, 1974.

61. Kahn, C. R., Neville, D. M., and Roth, J., Insulin receptor interaction in the obese-hyperglycemic mouse: a model of insulin resistance, *J. Biol. Chem.,* 284, 244, 1973.

62. Kahn, C. R. and Roth, J., Cell membrane receptors for polypeptide hormones: application to the study of disease states in mice and man, *Am. J. Clin. Pathol.,* 63, 656, 1975.

Chapter 3

PITUITARY MALFUNCTION AND IMMUNE ABNORMALITIES

I. Berczi

TABLE OF CONTENTS

I. INTRODUCTION

In his original description of the stress syndrome, Hans Selye[1] noted that various nocuous agents cause similar organic changes in rats, namely, enlargement of the adrenals, the involution of the thymus and lymphoid organs, and gastric erosions. This observation can be considered as the first evidence for the influence of neurohormonal mechanisms on the immune system. However, at the time neither the function of thymus, nor of lymphoid organs was known, and thus, the impact of this finding on immunology has been greatly delayed. Subsequently numerous experiments have shown that, indeed, stress alters a variety of immune reactions.[2,3]

II. HYPOTHALAMIC LESIONS

Szentivanyi and Filipp[4] observed that focal lesions of the tuberal region of hypothalamus protected guinea pigs against anaphylactic shock. Further experiments in guinea pigs and rabbits revealed that such hypothalamic lesions inhibited the production of circulating and tissue fixed antibodies, as well as provided protection against anaphylactic shock due to passively transferred antibody.[5] Other workers observed that hypothalamic lesions in commonly used laboratory animals (rabbits, guinea pigs, rats) inhibit the production of complement fixing antibodies,[6] delayed-type cutaneous hypersensitivity reactions,[7] the response of peripheral blood and spleen lymphoid cells to mitogens,[8,9] and caused decreased splenic natural killer cell activity.[10] Moreover, electrical stimulation of the hypothalamus led to increased thymus and spleen weight as well as increased humoral and cell-mediated immune reactivity.[11] Dann and co-workers[12] found that tuberal hypothalamic lesions stimulated allograft reactivity in rats. Hypophysectomy did not modify further the effect of tuberal lesions. The involvement of direct neural pathway(s) was suggested. On the other hand, Cross et al.[13,10] observed that the immunomodulatory effect of hypothalamic lesions is mediated predominantly, but not exclusively, by the pituitary gland. Besedovsky and co-workers[14] observed that during immune reactions the electrical activity of individual neurons in the ventrum medial hypothalamus of rats increased over 100% of base line activity. The authors predicted the existence of feedback signals emitted by the activated immune system towards the hypothalamus. The influence of the CNS on various immune phenomena has been reviewed repeatedly.[2,15,16]

III. PITUITARY DWARFISM

The first indication for the role of pituitary hormones in immune phenomena came from studies on the Snell-Bagg strain of recessive pituitary dwarf mouse. Baroni and co-workers[17,18] observed that dwarf animals exhibited an early involution of the thymus, cellular depletion in the bone marrow, and the peripheral lymphoid tissues. The primary (IgM) antibody response to sheep red cells was depressed, whereas the secondary (IgG) response reached normal levels. Treatment of dwarf animals with a combination of growth hormone (GH) and thyroxin prevented thymus involution and cellullar depletion of lymph nodes and bone marrow. The humoral antibody response was also normalized. Fabris and co-workers[19,20] made similar observations with regards to changes of lymphoid organs in hypopituitary Snell-Bagg mice. They emphasized that the immunodeficiency present in these mice was primarily the consequence of an arrested ontogenic development of the thymus, due to GH deficiency. In addition to deficient antibody formation, they also observed a prolonged survival of skin grafts in dwarf animals. The maximum life span of such immunodeficient mice could be extended from 110 to 300 to 400 days by the transfer of lymphocytes from normal adult donors. The beneficial effect of treatment with normal donor thymocytes and bone marrow cells either alone or in combination was further enhanced by hormonal treatment. GH, thyroxin, and luteotropic hormone were found to be beneficial for the restoration of leukocyte counts, the antibody response, and skin graft rejection. Hormone treatment was ineffective if dwarf mice were thymectomized in adult age.

Duquesnoy and co-workers[21] confirmed the observations of previous investigators with regard to immune deficiencies of the Snell-Bagg dwarf mouse. Severe lymphopenia, decreased antibody response, and graft-vs.-host (GVH) reactivity of dwarf spleen cells were observed. The lymphoid organs of dwarf animals were small and generally depleted of small lymphocytes, but serum immunoglobulins appeared to be within normal ranges. Schneider[22] found that the thymuses in Snell-Bagg pituitary dwarf mice were normal. Dwarf mice developed delayed-hypersensitivity reactions to oxazolone. The author suggested that these results, which are in contrast to other studies, may be due to differences in the husbandry of mouse colonies and that the immunological deficiencies described previously may not necessarily be a condition accompanying dwarfism. Dumont and co-workers[23] examined T and B lymphocytes in Snell-Bagg dwarf mice. There was no clear-cut qualitative or quantitative alteration in the intrathymic lymphocyte population of dwarf mice using the parameters of receptors for peanut agglutinin, physical analysis, and reactivity to phytohemagglutinin and concanavalin A. In the spleen of dwarf mice the number of T cells was slightly higher and B cells lower, but with similar response to T and B cell mitogens. However, when expressed as a function of body weight, the numbers of splenic T and B lymphocytes in untreated mice were about half the corresponding values in GH and thyroxin treated animals, or in normal littermates. It was suggested that in adult life developmental hormones exert little direct effect on the thymus, but influence the size of the pool of both peripheral T and B lymphocytes.

Duquesnoy[24] studied the Ames strain of recessive pituitary dwarf mice and found lymphocyte depletion and involution of the thymus, peripheral lymphoid tissue lymphopenia, and wasting syndrome with death at a young age. The appearance of IgM and IgG hemolytic plaque-forming cells after immunization with sheep erythrocytes was delayed and significantly less in dwarf mice than in normal littermates. The GVH reactivity of spleen cells in young Ames x AKR/F$_1$ hybrid mice was significantly lower in dwarf animals. However, there was no marked deficiencies in serum immunoglobulins and the colony-forming capacity of bone marrow cells was normal. The author suggested that in the Ames dwarf mouse the stem cell population in the bone marrow is normal, whereas the thymus-dependent lymphoid system is deficient.

A high frequency of wasting disease was observed among the offspring of inbred Weimaraner dogs. The affected pups had small thymuses, their antibody production and phytohemagglutinin (PHA) response were impaired. Such immunodeficient pups lacked a normal increase of plasma growth hormone after stimulation with clonidine, indicating concurrent abnormalities of the thymus dependent immune function and GH regulation.[25]

IV. HYPOPHYSECTOMY

In 1930, Smith[26] observed that the thymus of rats ceased to grow immediately after hypophysectomy (Hypox) and regressed in long survivors to less than half of the controls. In contrast, the thymuses of partially hypophysectomized rats showed an absolute loss in weight no greater than those of controls. Subsequent studies on the influence of Hypox on various immune reactions have yielded controversial results. Thus, hypophysectomized mice and rats were shown to exhibit a decreased antibody response,[26-30] while others found no change in antibody production[31-34] to various antigens. Similarly, it was reported that hypophysectomy had no effect on allogeneic skin graft survival,[12,28] whereas in another study, graft survival was prolonged in hypophysectomized rats.[35] Hypophysectomized rats required a greater dose of dinitrochlorobenzene in order to achieve a response equivalent to that of normal rats, as measured by the lymph node weight and lymphocyte proliferation assays.[36] The natural killer cell activity in spleens of mice and rats was also reduced after hypophysectomy.[10,37] Hypox rats did not develop adjuvant arthritis.[38]

Duquesnoy et al.[39] studied in rats the effect of hypophysectomy on immunological recovery after sublethal irradiation. Recovery of leukocyte count, antibody formation, and skin allograft rejection was defective after sublethal irradiation in adult hypophysectomized animals.

Bilder and Denckla[40] reported that 4-week-old rats rejected xenografts in 6 days, whereas the rejection time of 64-week-old animals averaged 13.4 days. After hypophysectomy and thyroxin treatment, 64-week-old rats rejected xenografts in 6.5 days. The same group of investigators[41] reported that long-term hypophysectomized rats responded better to immunization with sheep red blood cells (SRBC) than did their age-matched unoperated litter mates. Corticosterone, deoxycorticosterone, thyroxin, and bovine GH were given to hypophysectomized rats chronically in these experiments. Similar experiments were performed by Harrison et al.[42] in hypophysectomized C57BL/6J mice. The operated animals were maintained on hormone substitutes and on mineral supplemented drinking water. Corticosterone, deoxycorticosterone, and thyroxin were given chronically. For 3 to 7 weeks before responses to PHA and SRBC were tested, only minerals were given in the water, and the above named hormones plus bovine GH were injected. Hypophysectomy and endocrine supplementation in 8 to 9-month-old retired male breeder mice improved some, but not all, T-dependent functions tested at 15 months of age. Spleen cell responses to PHA and delayed-type hypersensitivity response to SRBC improved to levels shown by young controls. The tested animals had larger thymuses and much higher ratios of cortex/medulla areas than did age-matched controls. The life span of treated animals was reduced.

Pauly and Scheving[43] studied daily leukocyte rhythms in normal and hypophysectomized rats that were exposed to different light-dark schedules. Hypophysectomized animals exhibited lymphocytosis, but maintained the rhythm characteristic of lymphocytes. Hypophysectomy greatly modified, but did not abolish, rhythmic changes of eosinophil and neutrophil granulocytes.

During our initial investigations, a general immunodeficiency was detected in hypophysectomized rats.[44] Antibody production against ARBC, skin response to dinitrochlorobenzene, and the development of adjuvant arthritis were all markedly suppressed, and the survival of skin allografts was prolonged in hypophysectomized animals. Subsequent experiments, to be discussed later in detail, indicated that ectopically transplanted pituitary grafts, or treatment with GH, prolactin (PRL), or placental lactogen are equally capable of restoring the immunocompetence of hypophysectomized rats.

Tonic inhibition by dopamine, which is produced in the hypothalamus, is the dominating regulatory factor of PRL secretion. For this reason, ectopically transplanted pituitary glands secrete significant amounts of PRL, whereas other pituitary hormones are not secreted, due to the lack of hypothalamic releasing factors.[45] Residual pituitary tissue remaining after incomplete hypophysectomy may secrete PRL in amounts sufficient to maintain the immune reactivity of operated animals. This may be the major reason for the controversial finding of investigators studying the effect of hypophysectomy on immune reactions. Similarly, the PRL status of the various sublines of dwarf mice may be different, which could account, at least in part, for the discrepancy of the findings.

V. RELEVANT OBSERVATIONS IN MAN

There is some evidence in the literature for the influence of the pituitary gland on various immune phenomena in man. The immunosuppressive effects of ACTH and adrenal corticosteroids was discovered by Hench and co-workers[46] during the treatment of patients with rheumatoid arthritis. Their findings have since been substantiated extensively both in experimental animals and in patients, and ACTH and adrenal corticosteroids are commonly used today for the treatment of patients with various inflammatory and immune conditions. Furthermore, the hyperactivity of the pituitary — adrenal axis (Cushing's disease) is associated with immunological deficiency.[47,48]

Pathologists observed long ago that acromegaly is associated with thymic and lymphatic hyperplasia.[49] Recently an association was found between X-linked hypogammaglobulinemia and isolated GH deficiency.[50] The immunodeficiency was characterized by the absence of specific antibody production in vivo and impaired immunoglobulin secretion in vitro. Of the four patients examined three lacked circulating B lymphocytes. All the patients had deficient GH responses to insulin and arginine or methyldopa.

Patients with isolated GH deficiency had increased proportions of suppressor/cytotoxic T lymphyocytes and surface Ig bearing B lymphyocytes. Proliferative response to PHA and Con-A activated suppressor cells were normal. However, in mixed lymphocyte reactions, T cells from three or four patients responded poorly.[51]

Direct evidence of the association of PRL abnormalities with immune function in man is lacking with the possible exception of the findings of Ferrari et al.[52] These investigators observed that autoimmune thyroid disorders were far more frequent in hyperprolactinemic women than in the general population.

The cellular and humoral immune response in ten patients with various types of hypopituitarism has been evaluated. The immune function of patients was comparable to controls, except for a slight defect in phagocytic function.[53] Cases of inflammatory bowel disease (Crohn's disease) and eosinophilic gastroenteritis associated with hypopituitarism have been described. The case of eosinophilic gastroenteritis could be reversed completely by replacement therapy with cortisone.[54,55] The association of hypothalamic hypopituitarism with rheumatologic symptoms has also been described.[56] It is likely, that with our increasing understanding of the role of pituitary hormones in immune phenomena, the number of relevant clincial observations will increase substantially.

REFERENCES

1. Selye, H., A syndrome produced by diverse nocuous agents, *Nature (London)*, 138, 32, 1936.
2. Solomon, G. F., Amkraut, A. A., and Kasper, P., Immunity, emotions and stress, *Ann. Clin. Res.*, 6, 313, 1974.
3. Solomon, G. E., Immunologic abnormalities in mental illness, in *Psychoneuroimmunology*, Ader, R., Ed., Academic Press, New York, 1981, 259.
4. Szentivanyi, A. and Filipp, G.,. Anaphylaxis and the nervous system. II, *Ann. Allergy*, 16, 143, 1958.
5. Filipp, G. and Szentivanyi, A., Anaphylaxis and the nervous system. III, *Ann. Allergy*, 16, 306, 1958.
6. Korneva, E. A. and Khai, L. M., Effect of destruction of hypothalamic areas on immunogenesis, *Fed. Proc., Fed. Am. Soc. Exp. Biol.*, 23, T88, 1964.

7. Macris, N. T., Schiavi, R. C., Camerino, M. S., and Stein, M., Effect of hypothalamic lesions on immune processes in the guinea pig, *Am. J. Physiol.,* 219, 1205, 1970.

8. Keller, S. E., Stein, M., Camerino, M. S., Schleifer, S. J., and Sherman, J., Suppression of lymphocyte stimulation by anterior hypothalamic lesions in the guinea pig, *Cell. Immunol.,* 52, 334, 1980.

9. Roszman, T. L., Cross, R. J., Brooks, W. H., and Markesbery, W. R., Hypothalamic immune interactions. II. The effect of hypothalamic lesions on the ability of adherent spleen cells to limit lymphocyte blastogenesis, *Immunology,* 45, 737, 1982.

10. Cross, R. J., Markesbery, W. R., Brooks, W. H., and Roszman, T. L., Hypothalamic-immune interactions. Neuromodulation of natural killer activity by lesioning of the anterior hypothalamus, *Immunology,* 51, 399, 1984.

11. Janković, B. D., Jovanova, K., and Markovic, B. M., Effect of hypothalamic stimulation on the immune reactions in the rat, *Period. Biol.,* 81, 211, 1979.

12. Dann, J. A., Wachtel, S. S., and Rubin, A. L., Possible involvement of the central nervous system in graft rejection, *Transplantation,* 27, 223, 1979.

13. Cross, R. J., Brooks, W. H., Roszman, T. L., and Markesbery, W. R., Hypothalamic-immune interactions: effect of hypophysectomy on neuroimmunomodulation, *J. Neurol. Sci.,* 53, 557, 1982.

14. Besedovsky, H., Sorkin, E., Felix, D., and Haas, H., Hypothalamic changes during immune response, *Eur. J. Immunol.,* 7, 323, 1977.

15. Stein, M., Schiavi, R. C., and Camerino, M., Influence of brain and behavior on the immune system, *Science,* 191, 435, 1976.

16. Fauman, M. A., The central nervous system and the immune system, *Biol. Psychiatr.,* 17, 1459, 1982.

17. Baroni, C. D., Fabris, N., and Bertoli, G., Effects of hormones on development and function of lymphoid tissues. Synergistic action of thyroxin and somatotropic hormone in pituitary dwarf mice, *Immunology,* 17, 303, 1969.

18. Baroni, C. D., Pesando, P. C., and Bertoli, G., Effects on hormones on development and function of lymphoid tissues. II. Delayed development of immunological capacity in pituitary dwarf mice, *Immunology,* 21, 455, 1971.

19. Fabris, N., Pierpaoli, W., and Sorkin, E., Hormones and the immunological capacity. III. The immunodeficiency disease of the hypopituitary Snell-Bagg dwarf mouse, *Clin. Exp. Immunol.,* 9, 209, 1971.

20. Fabris, N., Pierpaoli, W., and Sorkin, E., Hormones and the immunological capacity. IV. Restorative effects of developmental hormones or of lymphocytes on the immunodeficiency syndrome of the dwarf mouse, *Clin. Exp. Immunol.,* 9, 227, 1971.

21. Duquesnoy, R. J., Kalpaktsoglou, P. K., and Good, R. A., Immunological studies on the Snell-Bagg pituitary dwarf mouse, *Proc. Soc. Exp. Biol. Med.,* 133, 201, 1970.

22. Schneider, G. B., Immunological competence in Snell-Bagg pituitary dwarf mice: response to the contract-sentitizing agent oxazolone, *Am. J. Anat.,* 145, 371, 1976.

23. Dumont, F., Robert, F., and Bischoff, P., T and B lymphocytes in pituitary dwarf Snell-Bagg mice, *Immunology,* 38, 23, 1979.

24. Duquesnoy, R. J., Immunodeficiency of the thymus-dependent system of the Ames dwarf mouse, *J. Immunol.,* 108, 1578, 1972.

25. Roth, J. A., Lomax, L. G., Altszuler, N., Hampshire, J., Kaeberle, M. L., Shelton, M., Draper, D. D., and Ledet, A. E., Thymic abnormalities and growth hormone deficiency in dogs, *Am. J. Vet. Res.,* 41, 1256, 1980.

26. Smith, P. E., Effect of hypophysectomy upon the involution of the thymus in the rat, *Anat. Rec.,* 47, 119, 1930.

27. Lundin, P. M., Action of hypophysectomy on antibody formation in the rat, *Acta Pathol. Microbiol. Scand.,* 48, 351, 1960.

28. Enerback, L., Lundin, P. M., and Mellgren, J., Pituitary hormones elaborated during stress. Action on lymphoid tissues, serum proteins and antibody titres, *Acta Pathol. Microbiol. Scand.,* Suppl. 144, 141, 1961.

29. Gisler, R. H. and Schenkel-Hulliger, L., Hormonal regulation of the immune response. II. Influence of pituitary and adrenal activity on immune responsiveness *in vitro, Cell. Immunol.,* 2, 646, 1971.

30. Comsa, J., Schwarz, J. A., and Neu, H., Interaction between thymic hormone and hypophyseal growth hormone on production of precipitating antibodies in the rat, *Immunol. Commun.,* 3, 11, 1974.

31. Nagareda, C. S., Antibody formation and the effect of X-radiation on circulating antibody levels in the hypophysectomized rats, *J. Immunol.,* 73, 88, 1954.

32. Kalden, J. R., Evans, M. M., and Irvin, W. J., The effect of hypophysectomy on the immune response, *Immunology,* 18, 671, 1970.

33. Thrasher, S. G., Bernardis, L. L., and Cohen, S., The immune response in hypothalamic-lesioned and hypophysectomized rats, *Int. Arch. Allergy Appl. Immunol.,* 41, 813, 1971.

34. Tyrey, L. and Nalbandov, A. V., Influence of anterior hypothalamic lesions on circulating antibody titres in the rat, *Am. J. Physiol.*, 222, 179, 1972.
35. Comsa, J., Leonhardt, H., and Schwarz, J. A., Influence of the thymus-corticotropin-growth hormone interaction on the rejection of skin allografts in the rat, *Ann. N.Y. Acad. Sci.*, 249, 387, 1975.
36. Prentice, E. D., Lipscomb, H., Metcalf, W. K., and Sharp, J. G., Effects of hypophysectomy on DNCB-induced contact sensitivity in rats. *Scand. J. Immunol.*, 5, 955, 1976.
37. Saxena, Q. B., Saxena, R. K., and Adler, W. H., Regulation of natural killer activity in vivo. III. Effect of hypophysectomy and growth hormone treatment on the natural killer activity of the mouse spleen cell population, *Int. Arch. Allergy Appl. Immunol.*, 67, 169, 1982.
38. Toivanen, P., Siikala, H., Laiho, P., and Paavilainen, T., Suppression of adjuvant arthritis by estrone in adrenalectomized and ovariectomized rats, *Experientia*, 23, 560, 1967.
39. Duquesnoy, R. J., Mariani, T., and Good, R. A., Effect of hypophysectomy on immunological recovery after sublethal irradiation of adult rats, *Proc. Soc. Exp. Biol. Med.*, 131, 1076, 1969.
40. Bilder, G. E. and Denckla, W. D., Restoration of ability to reject xenografts and clear carbon after hypophysectomy of adult rats, *Mech. Ageing Dev.*, 6, 153, 1977.
41. Scott, M., Bolla, R., and Denckla, W. D., Age-related changes in immune function of rats and the effect of long-term hypophysectomy, *Mech. Ageing Dev.*, 11, 127, 1979.
42. Harrison, D. E., Archer, J. R., and Astle, C. M., The effect of hypophysectomy on thymic aging in mice, *J. Immunol.*, 129, 2673, 1982.
43. Pauly, J. E. and Scheving, L. E., Daily leukocyte rhythms in normal and hypophysectomized rats exposed to different environmental light-dark schedules, *Anat. Rec.*, 153, 349, 1965.
44. Nagy, E. and Berczi, I., Immunodeficiency in hypophysectomized rats, *Acta Endocrinol.*, 89, 530, 1978.
45. Chen, C. L., Amenomori, Y., Lu, K. H., Voogt, J. L., and Meites, J., Serum prolactin levels in rats with pituitary transplants or hypothalamic lesions, *Neuroendocrinology*, 6, 220, 1970.
46. Hench, P. S., Kendall, E. C., Slocumb, C. H., and Polley, H. F., Effect of hormone of adrenal cortex (17-hydroxyl-11-dehydrocorticosterone; compound E) and of pituitary adrenocorticotrophic hormones on rheumatoid arthritis; preliminary report, *Ann. Rheum. Dis.*, 8, 97, 1949.
47. Britton, S., Thoren, M., Sjoberg, H. E., The immunological hazard of Cushing's syndrome, *Br. Med. J.*, 4, 678, 1975.
48. Liddle, G. W., The adrenals, in *Textbook of Endocrinology*, 6th ed., Williams, R. H., Ed., W. B. Saunders, Philadelphia, 1981, 249.
49. Ahlqvist, J., *Endocrine Influences on Lymphatic Organs, Immune Responses, Inflammation and Autoimmunity*, Almqvist & Wiksell, Stockholm, 1976, 80.
50. Fleisher, T. A., White, R. M., Broder, S., Nissley, S. P., Blaese, R. M., Mulvihill, J. J., Olive, G., and Waldmann, T. A., X-linked hypogrammaglobulinemia and isolated growth hormone deficiency, *N. Engl. J. Med.*, 302, 1429, 1980.
51. Gupta, S., Fikrig, S. M., and Noval, M. S., Immunological studies in patients with isolated growth hormone deficiency, *Clin. Exp. Immunol.*, 54, 87, 1983.
52. Ferrari, C., Boghen, M., Paracchi, A., Rampini, P., Raiteri, F., Benco, R., Romussi, M., Codecasa, F., Mucci, M., and Bianco, M., Thyroid autoimmunity in hyperprolactinaemic disorders, *Acta Endocrinol.*, 104, 35, 1983.
53. Ramos-Zepeda, R., Kretschmer, R., Lopez-Osuna, M., Parra-Covarrubias, A., and Perez-Pasten, A., Evaluation of immunological function in human hypopituitarism, *Arch. Invest. Med.*, 4, 197, 1973.
54. Green, J. R. B., O'Donoghue, D. P., Edwards, C. R. W., and Dawson, A. M., A case of apparent hypopituitarism complicating chronic inflammatory bowel disease, *Acta Paediatr. Scand.*, 66, 643, 1977.
55. Haeney, M. R. and Wilson, R. J., Co-existent eosinophilic gastroenteritis and hypothalamic-pituitary dysfunction, *Postgrad. Med. J.*, 53, 411, 1977.
56. Yunus, M., Masi, A. T., and Allen, J. P., Hypothalamic hypopituitarism presenting with rheumatologic symptoms, *Arthritis Rheum.*, 24, 632, 1981.

Chapter 4

THE INFLUENCE OF PITUITARY-ADRENAL AXIS ON THE IMMUNE SYSTEM

I. Berczi

TABLE OF CONTENTS

I. INTRODUCTION

Early investigators noted that administration of highly purified ACTH preparations induced thymic involution, splenic atrophy, and lymphopenia in several species of animals. ACTH was not effective in adrenalectomized animals, and lymphatic tissue atrophy could be maintained for long periods by continuous treatment with large amounts of ACTH or cortisone.[1] In this chapter the influence of ACTH and related peptides, of adrenal hormones on immunocytes, and immune phenomena will be reviewed.

II. ACTH AND RELATED PEPTIDES

A. ACTH

1. Rabbit

Some of the earliest observations with regards to the effect of ACTH on inflammatory and immune responses were made in rabbits. Thus, Berthrong et al.[2] showed that cardiovascular lesions produced by anaphylactic hypersensitivity were inhibited by ACTH treatment. Bjornedoe et al.[3] described that treatment of rabbits with ACTH and cortisone reduced their antibody respose to pneumococcal antigens. Similar reductions occurred when the hormones were administered at the beginning of immunization or after immunization was well advanced. Hormone treatment was followed by atrophic changes in lymphoid tissue and a decrease in the number of mononuclear cells. Malkiel and Hargis[4] showed that ACTH and cortisone given in physiological doses to rabbits prior to and during, the period of immunization with bovine serum albumin inhibited antibody formation as measured by the quantitative precipitin reaction. ACTH caused a marked diminution of the antibody titer and cortisone induced an almost complete suppression. Germuth and co-workers[5] studied the effect of ACTH and cortisone on antibody formation and on the development of Arthus type hypersensitivity. Both hormones suppressed circulating antibody formation, cortisone being more effective than ACTH. The Arthus reaction itself was unaffected if treatment was started when serum antibody concentrations were high. The authors concluded that ACTH and cortisone reduced circulating antibody by inhibiting antibody formation rather than by promoting antibody destruction. Kass and co-workers[6] also observed that ACTH in sufficient dosage depressed the production of antibodies in rabbits in a similar fashion to that of hydrocortisone.

Fever is now regarded by some as a lymphokine induced reaction of the nervous system that amplifies immunological body defenses against intruding pathogens. It is interesting to note that the central administration of ACTH reduced fever in rabbits in doses that have no effect on afebrile effect of ACTH.[7]

2. Mouse

Similar observations were made in mice with regards to the effect of ACTH on immune reactions. Hayes and Dougherty[8] observed that ACTH or cortisone suppressed the formation of antibodies to horse serum in a dose-dependent fashion. The greater the amount of antigen administered, the more hormone was required to suppress antibody formation. The kinetics of antibody production was not altered by hormone treatment, and cessation of treatment at 9, 11, or 17 days after antigen administration was followed by a prompt resumption of antibody synthesis. Newsom and Darrach[9,10] showed that ACTH, when administered at sufficiently high doses, suppressed the formation of hemolytic antibodies in mice. This inhibition of antibody production could be overcome by increasing the dose of antigen. Corticosterone exerted a similar inhibitory effect on the formation of hemolysins. Medawar and Sparrow[11] studied the effects of ACTH and cortisone on skin graft survival in mice. The injection of 1 mg/day of ACTH in a slow absorption medium prolonged graft survival by 50%, which was equivalent to the effect of 0.4 mg/day of cortisone acetate. ACTH was ineffective in adrenalectomized mice. Female mice were slightly less responsive to cortisone and ACTH than were males.

Spry[12] observed that in rats infused with ACTH the output of lymphocytes from the thoracic duct was decreased, and when radioactively labeled thoracic duct lymphocytes were injected, they were inhibited from recirculating into the lymph. The author concluded that the recirculation of lymphocytes is related to adrenal steriod output.

3. Rat

Hayashida and Li[13] administered ACTH to rats during the period of immunization with fraction IA of *Pasteurella pestis* in a daily dose just sufficient to prevent body weight increase relative to the nontreated group. Antibody formation was significantly depressed in hormone treated animals. The administration of growth hormone simultaneously with ACTH maintained body weight at the level slightly above that of the controls and resulted in an effective counteraction of the antibody depression produced by ACTH.

We examined the effects of ACTH on various immune reactions in rats. ACTH in 10 μg daily doses (equivalant to 0.01 IU) lowered significantly the antibody response of normal rats to sheep red blood cells (SRBC) while the impaired response of hypophysectomized animals was unaffected. When 20 μg of ACTH was given daily, which is considered by many as a *physiological* dose, further reduction occurred in the antibody response of normal animals.[14] Hypophysectomized rats do not develop contact sensitivity reactions to dinitrochlorobenzene (DNCB) unless given prolactin (PRL) or growth hormone (GH). ACTH treatment does not influence the poor reactivity of Hypox animals, but antagonizes the restoration of reactivity, if applied jointly with either PRL or GH.[15] The development of adjuvant arthritis is inhibited by hypophysectomy in rats, but normal arthritic reaction occurs if the animals are treated with PRL or GH. Additional treatment with ACTH inhibits this restoration.[16] Treatment of rats with the dopaminergic ergot alkaloid bromocriptine (BRC) inhibited the induction of contract sensitivity to DNCB, of adjuvant arthritis and experimental allergic encephalitis, and suppressed the antibody response to SRBC and to bacterial lipopolysaccharides (LPS). The immunocompetence of BRC suppressed animals could be restored by additional treatment with either PRL or GH. Treatment with ACTH antagonized the restoring effect of PRL and GH.[17] These experiments indicate that ACTH has a suppressive effect on humoral cell mediated and autoimmune reactions, and that it acts antagonistically with GH and PRL on the immune system.

4. Man

Ever since the discovery of Hench and co-workers[18] of the therapeutic action of ACTH and cortisone in rheumatoid arthritis, these two hormones have been applied in medicine for the treatment of various inflammatory conditions and of diseases with underlying immune abnormalities. The vast amount of clinical observations have been reviewed periodically[19,20] and it is well recognized that the effect of these hormones on immune reactions is complex.

Several clinical observations suggest that in man therapeutic doses of ACTH seldom affect antibody levels. Thus, the production of protective antibody against pneumococcal polysaccharide was unaltered during treatment with ACTH and cortisone,[21] and precipitin formation to the same antigen in patients receiving cortisone treatment for rheumatoid arthritis was not inhibited.[22] Similarly ACTH and cortisone did not reduce the development of diphtheria antitoxin following toxoid injections.[23] However, it has been reported repeatedly that the course of acquired hemolytic anemia improved significantly with ACTH and cortisone treatment; this was associated with a reduction in antibody titers.[24,25] Several investigators have established in both clinical and in experimentally induced serum sickness that ACTH or cortisone inhibit the disease at doses that produce no alternation in the response of skin to test dose of antigens.[26-31] Cortisone and ACTH in dosages sufficient to inhibit the tuberculin reaction were without effect on the titer of hemagglutinating antibodies.[32,33]

5. Other Species

ACTH treatment of guinea pigs sensitized with heat-killed tubercle bacilli suppressed skin reactivity to tuberculin. Furthermore, guinea pigs treated with ACTH showed suppression of inflammation but not necrosis produced by intracutaneous application of turpentine oil. ACTH produced marked eosinopenia and lymphopenia in guinea pigs.[33] ACTH, when given daily s.c. to guinea pigs in a slow release medium, prolonged the survival of skin grafts similar to that obtained with cortisone.[34]

ACTH administration to cattle injected with a vaccinal strain of bovine viral diarrhea virus weakened their resistance to this pathogen. ACTH administered separately caused a depression of lymphocyte mitogenesis in response to selected mitogens.[35]

The response of peripheral blood leukocytes in 3-week-old chickens to ACTH injection was biphasic; a leucopenia, after 1 hr and a marked leucocytosis was observed between 4 to 12 hr after hormone administration. The leucopenic response was due to the reduction in the number of circulating lymphocytes whereas the leucocytosis response was caused by a large increase in the number of polymorphonuclear cells.[36]

B. Opioid Peptides

The existence of endogenous opiates was first predicted from the presence of specific morphine receptors in brain tissue. Subsequently two pentapeptides, called met-enkephalin and leu-enkephalin that were specific for morphine receptors, have been isolated. Soon it was recognized that met-enkephalin has sequence identity with a portion of the pituitary hormone, β-lipotropin, which turned out to be the prohormone of the pituitary opiates: α-, β-, and γ-endorphins are derived by enzymatic cleavage from a common precursor molecule called proopiomelanocortin, and their secretion is regulated jointly by the feedback action of glucocorticoids. The cerebral enkephalins function as neurotransmitters, and are synthesized and regulated independently of pituitary opiates. (Please see Chapter 2 for more details and references.)

The presence of opiate receptors on human lymphocytes and platelets has been demonstrated by the specific binding of ^{3}H-naloxone, which is a close chemical and conformational congener of morphine. Naloxone is specific for μ-type opioid receptors.[37]

Individuals addicted to opiate drugs were found to be immunodeficient, which was associated with a significant depression of the number of T lymphocytes in the peripheral blood as measured by E rosette formation. At the same time an increase in the absolute number of null lymphocytes (not expressing any T or B cell markers) was detected. A 1 to 3 hr incubation of addict-derived lymphocytes with naloxone (10^{-6} to $10^{-7}M$) reversed both T cell depression and null cell increase by allowing the null cells to express E receptors. This conversion of null to T lymphocytes was also reflected in the increase of DNA synthesis to phytohemagglutinin (PHA) stimulation.[38] Others observed that morphine and dextromoramide inhibited the percentage of active E rosettes. This effect was specifically inhibited by naloxone.[39] Methionine-enkephalin was found to increase significantly the active E rosettes from lymphoma patients as well. Leucine-enkephalin increased active E rosettes only at a single low concentration. Neither enkephalins altered significantly the total number of E rosettes.[40]

The mitotic response of human peripheral blood lymphocytes to PHA was suppressed significantly by morphine[41] and also by β-endorphin. Suppression by β-endorphin was not blocked by pretreatment with naloxone.[42] On the other hand, β endorphin enhanced the proliferation response of rat spleen cells to concanavalin A and PHA. This enhancing effect of β-endorphin was dose-dependent and occurred at concentrations similar to those found in rat plasma. The potentiating effect of β-endorphin was not influenced by naloxone. Alpha-endorphin and [D-Ala^2, Met^5] enkephalin did not affect the proliferative responses of rat spleen cells to mitogens. None of the peptides tested had any effect on resting spleen cells or on the response to a mixture of LPS and dextran sulfate, which are mitogenic for B lymphocytes.[43] Methionine-enkephalin and leucine-enkaphalin enhanced the mitogenic response of mouse lymphocytes to PHA at 10^{-8} and 10^{-10} mg/mℓ concentration, respectively.[44]

Human natural killer (NK) cell activity was significantly enhanced by both β-endorphin and methionine-enkephalin. Leucine-enkephalin, α-endorphin, and morphine did not augment NK activity. Naloxone inhibited the augmentation of cytotoxicity produced by β-endorphin and met-enkephalin.[45] On the other hand, splenic NK cells activity in rats was suppressed by the opioid, but not the nonopioid form of stress. This suppression was blocked by naltrexone. Similar suppression of NK activity could be induced by high doses of morphine.[46]

β-Endorphin and met-enkephalin were found to stimulate human mononuclear cell chemotaxis in a bimodal fashion with peak activities occurring at 10^{-12} and $10^{-8}M$ concentrations. Removal of glass adherent cells from the responding population resulted in a loss of chemotactic response to β-endorphin. Infusion of β-endorphin into the cerebral ventricle of rats caused the immigration of macrophage-like cells into the ventricle, which is consistent with the in vitro chemotactic effect of β-endorphin.[47]

Postaglandin E_1 inhibits the release of serotonin from rat mast cells after an antigen challenge. Morphine, β-endorphin, and met-enkephalin reversed this effect of PGE_1. Naloxone antagonized this action of opioid peptides.[48]

Finally, it has been observed that β-endorphin binds specifically to the terminal complexes (C5b-9) of human complement.[49]

III. ADRENAL HORMONES

A. The Effect of Adrenalectomy on Immunocytes and Immune Responses

In thymic-irradiated bone marrow shielded rats adrenalectomy (Adrx) accelerated the repopulation of the thymus with precursor cells.[50] In mice Adrx caused the depletion of T lymphocytes from lymph nodes, whereas the thymus was increased in size and blood leukocytes increased in number. This effect appeared reversible.[51] Adrx decreased the accumulation of adoptively transferred T cells to the bone marrow and reduced the graft-vs.-host (GVH) reactivity of bone marrow cells in mice.[52]

Spleen cells from Adrx male rats exhibited enhanced responsiveness to a variety of mitogens, whereas lymph node cells from the same animals manifested decreased mitogenic responsiveness in comparison with controls. Antibody-dependent cytotoxic and NK cell activities were significantly decreased in both the spleen and lymph nodes of Adrx animals. Alteration of normal leukocyte circulatory and homing patterns were suggested by which Adrx produces differential effects on lymphoid cells in various organs of the immune system.[53]

Handling and bleeding of adult male Sprague-Dawley rats every 10 min, for 60 min resulted in eosinopenia after the first sampling, which reached a nadir of 63% by 40 min. This eosinopenia could be prevented by Adrx or Hypox.[54]

Recently, Keller et al.[55] demonstrated that stress is capable of inducing suppression of lymphocyte response to PHA in Adrx rats. This finding suggests that adrenal independent mechanisms participate in the suppression of lymphocyte function by stressors. Stress induced lymphopenia, however, was found to be adrenal dependent.

Treatment of rats for 3 weeks with aminoglutethimide, which inhibits adrenal steroidogenesis, led to a marked increase in the number of circulating lymphocytes.[56] Adrx, or treatment with aminoglutethimide, enhanced the delayed-hypersensitivity response of mice to SRBC.[51] Similarly, Adrx and the glucocorticoid synthesis inhibitor, metyrapone, abolished the suppression caused by immobilization stress of delayed-type hypersensitivity reaction to SRBC in mice. In contrast, the immobilization induced increase in contact sensitivity to 2,4-dinitro-1-fluorobenzene was still observed after hormonal modification. Similar results were observed whether the mice were given metyrapone or adrenalectomized before or after sensitization.[57]

A pair of congeneic mouse strains (C57BL/10Sm and B10.129) were studied, in which females reject allografts more consistently and more rapidly than males. Adrx, gonadectomy, and combined gonadectomy-Adrx substantially increased the strength of rejection by males and to a lesser extent, the strength of rejection by females. Adrx and gonadectomized Adrx males and females showed essentially similar rejection patterns.[58] Splenic enlargement was observed in adult C57BL/6J mice at 7, 14, and 21 days after Adrx. Splenic enlargement was enhanced further by the injection of allogeneic spleen cells to Adrx recipients at 14 days. Both the splenic enlargement following Adrx and its modification by injection of allogeneic cells were abolished by injection of cortisone acetate.[59] Heim and co-workers[60] studied the influence of thymectomy and

Adrx on GVH reaction (GVHR) in mice. It was concluded that adrenal gland hypersecretion contributed to the T lymphocyte induced tissue damage in this condition. However, Adrx performed 24 hrs before the induction of GVHR in mice resulted in early and/or increased incidence of disease in various strain combinations, which could be prevented by the administration of corticosterone acetate.[61]

In a series of experiments, Levine and co-workers[62-64] demonstrated that Adrx aggravated experimental allergic encephalomyelitis in rats and also accelerated its passive transfer. Adrx, shortly after onset of clinical signs, was uniformly lethal to rats within 2 days. If Adrx was postponed until the 3rd to 5th day, most rats survived and showed a complete or incomplete remission, followed by relapse. However, Adrx did not induce relapses when the disease was produced with aqueous antigen or by passive transfer with lymphoid cells. It was suggested that relapses are due to persistent antigenic stimulus from water in oil inocula, which are influenced by adrenal homeostatic mechanisms.

Enhanced production of IgE antibodies has been observed in Adrx rats.[65] Furthermore, T cell deficient nude rats exhibited a very poor antibody response to horse red blood cells (HRBC) even after treatment with the thymic hormone, thymosin fraction 5. Normal response occured after additional Adrx.[66]

Besedovsky and co-workers[67] suggested that the adrenal gland is involved in the phenomenon of antigenic competition. Rats injected first with HRBC and 5 days later with SRBC showed a strong antigenic competition. Adrx rats injected in a similar manner had five times more PFC when compared with the sham-operated controls. Adrx or sham-operated animals receiving only SRBC showed no difference in plaque-forming cells (PFC) numbers. Six days after HRBC injection to normal rats, a fivefold increase in corticosterone blood level was measured, and a strong decrease was noted on day 11. The role of corticosteroids in antigenic competition was further supported by in vitro experiments.

B. Glucocorticoids

Selye[68] demonstrated first the thymus atrophy in rats following the administration of adrenocortical extracts. This observation was soon confirmed by Carriere et al.[69] and by Ingle.[70] Cortisone (or compound E) was first isolated in 1935 by Kendall and co-workers. Dougherty[1] analyzed the older literature with regard to the effect of adrenocorticosteriods on lymphoid tissue and concluded that corticosterone and its derivatives, dehydrocorticosterone and compound E of Kendall, were effective in the production of acute lymphatic tissue involution. Of these compounds, cortisone seemed to be most active. Advances in the biochemistry of adrenal corticosteroids and the well established suppressive effect of cortisone on lymphoid tissue on animals led to the first clinical application by Hench and co-workers.[18] These developments led to a widespread and continued interest in the anti-inflammatory and immunosuppressive potential of glucocorticoids. The relevant literature has been reviewed repeatedly.[1,20,71-86]

Early investigations led only to modest advancement of our knowledge with regard to the effect of glucocorticoids on immune responses, mainly because neither the immune system nor the mechanism of action of steroid hormones were understood sufficiently for major contributions in this area. Nevertheless it became clear that glucocorticoids affect lymphoid cells and tissues in many ways. Major species differences were also recognized, namely the mouse, rat, hamster, and rabbit were found to be steroid sensitive, whereas the guinea pig, monkey, and man were shown to be steroid resistant. The lymphoid cells of steroid sensitive species are easily lysed by glucocorticoids and antibody production is inhibited by these agents. Lymphoid cells of resistant species are not lysed easily by steroids, and it is difficult to demonstrate inhibition of circulating antibody production by these hormones. Differences were also recognized within the same species. Lymphoid cells of different origin, (e.g., thymus derived, bursa derived, and bone marrow derived) showed differences in responses to steroids. It was also noted that lymphocyte activation by mitogens or specific antigen was affected by steroids even in the absence of lysis.[78] With the identification of T and B lymphocytes and their subsets, the clarification of cell interactions during immune reactions, and our increasing understanding of steroid hormone action, it became possible during the past decade to analyze the mechanism of action of glucocorticoid hormones on the immune system.

1. Glucocorticoid Receptors in Lymphoid Tissue

Physiological responses to glucocorticoid hormones are mediated through specific intracellular receptors that are present in most mammalian tissues.[87] Loss of the receptor is associated with a loss of steroid response. Steroids penetrate the cell membrane readily where they are bound to specific cytoplasmic receptors. The hormone receptor complexes then become activated and are translocated to the nucleus where they are bound to the genome. Increased RNA synthesis will follow with transcription of specific mRNAs. The mRNAs are then transported to the cytoplasm where they initiate protein synthesis.[80,88] Glucocorticoid receptors and steroid sensitivity in normal and neoplastic human lymphoid tissue has been reviewed recently by Homo-Delarche.[89] It is clear that the cells residing in the bone marrow, thymus, spleen and lymph node, and peripheral leukocytes all have glucocorticoid receptors. Receptor studies on human lymphoid tissue are summarized in Table 1.

It appears from Table 1 that bone marrow cells and macrophages have the highest density of glucocorticoid receptors, whereas peripheral blood lymphocytes, T and B cells, and even polymorphonuclear leukocytes appear to have roughly the same number of receptors ranging from 3000 to 7000 per cell. This does not mean, however, that certain subpopulations of lymphoid cells would not differ in their receptor content. For instance, Distelhorst and Benutto[90] reported that peripheral blood T cells isolated on nylon wool had a mean of 4000 receptors per cell, whereas T cells isolated by the E rosette technique had almost twice as many (7 to 10,000). On the other hand Ozaki et al.[91] did not find a difference in the number of receptors between T cells having Fcγ receptors and those without such receptors. Stimulation of human peripheral blood lymphocytes with Con A resulted in a striking increase in the number of receptor sites per cell and the cells remained sensitive to glucocorticoids.[92] Similarly, the number of receptor sites in human T lymphocytes increased to tenfold 24 hr after stimulation by PHA or exposure to conditioned tissue culture medium.[93]

The number and affinity of glucocorticoid receptors in thymocytes were found to be identical in fetal, newborn, and adult CBA mice. Steroid hormone induced inhibition of ^{3}H-uridine incorporation by fetal and adult thymocytes were also similar.[94] The glucocorticoid receptor activity in normal infant thymocyte was found to be 2146 ± 726 sites per cell with a dissociation constant of 14 nM. Treatment with a partially purified thymic factor, thymosin fraction 5, reduced the glucocorticoid binding activity of human infant thymocytes and also increased their resistance to the cytolytic effect of dexamethasone.[95]

The concentrations of glucocorticoid receptors were lower in cytosols from liver and thymus of female than of male rats. Adrx increased receptor concentrations in the cytoplasm from the liver and thymus. The sex difference of glucocorticoid receptors disappeared after Adrx or hypophysectomy. Ovariectomy led to an increase of thymic but not of liver receptors. Ovariectomized rats responded to Adrx as did intact males. It was suggested that these sex-related receptor changes were probably due to the influence of the ovary on plasma corticosterone concentrations.[96]

After the unilateral immunization of Adrx male rats, a 50% increase in glucocorti-

Table 1

GLUCOCORTICOID RECEPTORS IN HUMAN LEUKOCYTES AND LYMPHOID CELLS AS REVEALED BY WHOLE CELL ASSAY

Cell type	Ligand used	No. of receptors per cell ± S.E.	Dissociation constant (Kd × M)	Ref.
Bone marrow	^{3}H-dexamethasone	13,923	$\approx 1 \times 10^{-8}$	114
Thymocytes		3,100	$3—5 \times 10^{-8}$	115
Thymocytes		2,146 ± 726	1.4×10^{-8}	95
Peripheral blood lymphocytes		2,700	5.5×10^{-9}	117
		3,151 ± 726	7.1×10^{-9}	92
		4.850 ± 1,340	1.2×10^{-8}	100
		4,850 ± 1,340		118
		7.069 ± 682	1.0×10^{-9}	119
		6,617 ± 979	4.8×10^{-9}	99
PB — T cells		3,130 ± 1,316	3.5×10^{-9}	120
PB — non T		2,892 ± 1,068	4.0×10^{-9}	120
PB — T + null		3,600 − 6,000	$5—7 \times 10^{-8}$	116
PB — B cell		3,600 − 6,000	$5—7 \times 10^{-8}$	116
PB — T (NW)		4,000 ± 200	7.6×10^{-9}	90
PB — T (ER)		7,200 ± 400	10.3×10^{-9}	90
PB	^{3}H-prednisolone	3,940 ± 3,640	6.5×10^{-9}	91
PB — B		3.590 ± 1,980	9.2×10^{-9}	91
PB — T		3,130 ± 3,150	9.6×10^{-9}	91
PB — T$_\gamma$		2.840 ± 1,550	7.9×10^{-9}	91
PB — T nonγ		4,200 ± 2,070	11.2×10^{-9}	91
PB — PMN		3,330 ± 2,390	7.1×10^{-9}	91
PB — MC		5,350 ± 3,640	12.5×10^{-9}	91
Alveolar Mf		9,790 ± 4,050	9.0×10^{-9}	91
PB — PMN	^{3}H-dexamethasone	4,900	1.0×10^{-8}	113
PB — MN		4,720	1.0×10^{-8}	113
PB — MC		9,000	7.7×10^{-9}	111

Note: B = bone marrow derived lymphocyte; MC = monocyte; Mf = macrophage; MN = mononuclear; null = lymphocyte without T or B cell markers; PB = peripheral blood; PMN = polymorphonuclear cell or granulocyte; T = thymus derived lymphocyte; T (ER) = E rosette separated T cells; T (NW) = nylon wool separated T cells; T$_\gamma$ = cells with Fc receptors for IgG.

coid receptor sites per cell was demonstrated in lymphocyte suspensions of homolateral lymph nodes over those from contralateral nonimmunized nodes. In spite of the increase in receptors, the cells from the homolateral and contralateral nodes were equally sensitive to the inhibitory effects of dexamethasone as determined by measurements of RNA and DNA synthesis or by in vitro cell survival.[97]

Seven normal volunteers were given four doses of dexamethasone (4 mg orally every 6 hr) and glucocorticoid receptor levels of peripheral blood lymphocytes were determined at various times after treatment. Six volunteers showed a decrease in receptor number after glucocorticoid administration (median maximum decrease 2046 sites/cell), which occurred rapidly, reaching a nadir within 30 hr after treatment. The return of receptor number to base line was gradual, requiring 3 to 17 days.[98] The administration to healthy subjects of 1 mg dexamethasone, or 5 mg of prednisone, or 37.5 mg of cortisone acetate resulted in 30% decrease in binding sites after 1 week of treatment, with no change in binding affinity. This diminished number persisted for 1 week after discontinuation of glucocorticoid treatment. Lymphocytes from hospitalized patients taking 40 to 60 mg of dexamethasone daily demonstrated a similar change in the number of binding sites. If binding assays were carried out at 37°C, the same degree of decrease in binding sites was observed after dexamethasone administration, and there was a twofold increase in binding affinity.[99] Kontula et al.[100] found no significant difference in cellular content of glucocorticoid receptors among healthy controls, ten patients with Cushing's syndrome, and three patients with Addison's disease. Receptor affinity was also similar. However, in a patient with hypercortisolism (due to an adrenal adenoma with only slight clinical signs) there was a 70% decrease of receptors. Receptor content lymphocytes from two patients with anorexia nervosa was also below normal.

The number and affinity of glucocorticoid receptors in peripheral blood mononuclear leukocytes of men and women did not differ, it didn't change in subjects ranging in age from 18 to 53 years, and no diurnal or seasonal variations were found. On the other hand, cells from five pregnant women in the last trimester showed decreased receptor affinity and increased receptor number. No changes in receptor number or affinity were found in three patients with Cushing's disease, four prednisone treated asthmatics, or in six patients with untreated thyrotoxicosis.[101]

Theophylline was shown in vitro to enhance the rate of binding of cortisone to cytosol receptors of human leukocytes and to increase its affinity for the steroid.[102] Mitogen stimulated human peripheral lymphocytes and rat lymph node cells were separated by unit gravity sedimentation into populations of G_0, G_1, S, and post-S phase cells. A two- to threefold increase in glucocorticoid receptor sites per cell in the S and post-S phase cells over those in G_0 and G_1 was found with both nonstimulated rat lymph node cell suspension and Con A stimulated human peripheral lymphocytes, indicating that the formation of new glucocorticoid receptors takes place near the S phase.[103]

Residual thymocytes 48 hr after in vivo hydrocortisone treatment were partly sensitive to steroid as demostrated by uridine incorporation and exhibited low steroid as demonstrated by uridine incorporation and exhibited low steroid binding.[94] The number of glucocorticoid receptors was lower in mouse splenic T cell enriched fractions compared with the fractions depleted of T lymphocytes.[104]

It is interesting to note that there are strain differences in these receptor counts. The B10A mouse strain has significantly higher glucocorticoid receptor levels than the B10 strain.[105] These strains differ only within the H-2 gene complex, which influences immune reactions.

Steroid hormone cytoplasmic receptor complexes were compared from rat liver, thymus, and prostate in their capacity to bind to nuclei from liver, prostate, thymus, spleen, and kidney. Two types of receptor complexes were found in cytosols of liver and prostate; one binds to nuclei from kidney, spleen, thymus, liver, and prostate, and the other binds only to nuclei of liver and prostate. This latter type of receptor complex was not observed in the cytosol from thymus.[106] Cytosol receptors from goat polymorphonuclear and mononuclear leukocytes had similar binding affinities for dexamethasone.[107]

Comparative studies of glucocorticoid sensitivity and receptors in lymphoid tissues of chicken, mouse, and rat revealed no direct correlation between glucocorticoid sensitivity and either binding capacity or affinity of receptor for hormones. Furthermore, the surviving cells of chicken lymphoid tissues after in vivo treatment with high doses of hydrocortisone contained an amount of dexamethasone receptor sites similar to that of the whole population.[108] Calcium ions at 25°C increased significantly the inactivation rate of steroid-free receptor in chick thymus cytosol, but only slightly influenced it in the case of receptors from bursa of Fabricius or from rat thymus cytosol. Calcium ion strongly decreased the binding of cytosol hormone-receptor complex to isolated nuclei or DNA cellulose. The mechanism of calcium action on glucocorticoid receptors is probably due to the activation of some proteolytic enzymes.[109] Glucocorticoid receptors and response of the corticosensitive mouse and corticoresistant guinea pig were compared. A 20-fold difference in receptor affinity was found between the two species, and the concentrations of dexamethasone necessary for half maximal inhibition of thymidine incorporation closely approximated the half maximum values of glucocorticoid receptor occupancy.[110] Glucocorticoid binding was measured at resident and thioglycollate elicited mouse peritoneal macrophages, rabbit alveolar macrophages, and human monocytes. These cells contained approximately 4 to 10×10^3 high affinity receptor sites with a K_d of 2 to 8 nM dexamethasone. Cortisol, corticosterone, and progesterone competed with dexamethasone for binding, whereas estradiol, dihydrotestosterone, and 11-epicortisol competed very little.[111] Plasma cortisol levels and urinary free cortisol excretion are higher in New World monkeys than in Old World primates and prosimians. However, New World monkeys do not show pathological signs of excess cortisol because of end-organ resistance. The hypothalamic-pituitary-adrenal axis is resistant to suppression by dexamethasone. Although the number of glucocorticoid receptors in circulating mononuclear leukocytes was the same in Old and New World species, binding affinity for dexamethasone was markedly decreased in New World monkeys. Therefore, the resistance of these species to the action of cortisols is due to the decreased binding affinity of the glucocorticoid receptors.[112-120]

2. The Effect of Glucocorticoids on Embryonic Development of the Immune System

Glucocorticoids influence the embryonic development of the hemo- and lymphopoietic system. Liver erythropoietic cells obtained from 15- or 16-day-old rat fetuses were found to bound dexamethasone first by the cytosol, which was translocated rapidly to the nucleus after incubation at 37°C. Thus, glucocorticoid receptors are present in erythropoietic cells of fetal rat liver.[121]

Fetal liver erythroid progenitor cells from mice formed a reduced number of colonies when cultured for 9 days in the presence of dexamethasone. Corticosterone, cortisol, prednisone, and 9α-fluorocortisol had a similar effect, whereas 11α-cortisol and tetrahydrocortisol and progesterone did not influence erythroid colony formation. The formation of erythroid colonies was also reduced when the cells were incubated with the inhibitory steroid hormones for 1 hr, washed, and cultured in plasma clots.[122]

Ritter[123] studied the effect of corticosterone on embryonic mouse thymus development in vitro. *Physiological* levels of corticosterone enhanced the expression of Thy-1.2 antigen whereas higher concentrations had an inhibitory effect, appearing to kill selectively small lymphocytes while leaving large and medium lymphocytes intact. Daily injections of 2.5 and 5 μg of dexamethasone into pregnant mice from the 8th gestational day until delivery led either to a wasting appearance and death of offspring within 1 week or to retardation of growth without any wasting appearance. The surviving animals had an impaired antibody response and cytotoxic T cell activity. Histologically the lymphoid organs, thyroid, and adrenals showed atrophy, and serum thyroxin levels were significantly reduced. Thus, intrauterine exposure of the fetus to dexamethasone can disrupt the normal development and function of endocrine and immune organs that leads to early death or retardation of growth after birth.[124]

3. The Effect of Glucocorticoids on Hemo- and Lymphopoiesis

Treatment of adult mice with cortisol decreased the frequency of mature B lymphocytes in the bone marrow, whereas B progenitors were not affected. Treatment of bone marrow graft recipients with cortisol impaired the generation of mature B cells from primitive progenitor cells. The differentiation of B cells into antibody secreting cells was less dramatically affected by cortisol.[125] The injection of a single well tolerated dose of hydrocortisone acetate to mice left the bone marrow relatively unaffected, but severe and prolonged cell depletion was observed in the thymus, spleen, mesenteric, inguinal and popliteal lymph nodes.[126] Similarly, hydrocortisone injection in young rats caused an increase in the proliferative response of bone marrow cells but led to the disintegration of the thymus gland.[127] Chronic corticosteroid administration to guinea pigs (seven daily doses) induced a lymphocytopenia in the circulation and reduced bone marrow lymphocyte content and marrow lymphocyte production.[128] Further experiments indicated that this corticosteroid induced lymphocytopenia was the result of sequestration of long-lived lymphocytes into the marrow.[129] The injection of dexamethasone phosphate i.p. in doses of 5, 20, and 200 μg/mouse induced a fall in the number of stem cells in peripheral blood that was followed by a rise.[130]

The proliferation of marrow erythroid progenitors in two infants with Diamond-Blackfan syndrome was studied before and during prednisone treatment. Patient one had a brisk erythropoietic response to prednisone and the anemia improved, whereas patient two was steriod-unresponsive. Apparently, this syndrome is heterogenous and in one form the insensitivity of stem cells to erythropoietin can be corrected with prednisone, whereas in the other form prednisone is ineffective.[131]

In mice, corticosteroids enhanced the return of granulopoiesis after myelotoxic chemotherapy with cyclophophamide. Apparently, corticosteriods are able to alter the proliferative state of granulopoietic progenitor cells.[132] Granulopoietic progenitor cells of mice were found to be less inhibited by physiologic concentrations of dexamethasone and cortisone than early erthyrocyte progenitors.[133] Interleukin 1 blocked the inhibitory effect of dexamethasone on granulocyte/macrophage colony formation in response to colony-stimulating factor.[134]

Physiological and therapeutic levels of hydrocortisone (10^{-7} to $10^{-5}M$) stimulated the formation of granulocyte/macrophage colonies in cultures of normal human bone marrow. Physiological concentrations of progesterone were without effect.[135] Others also found that hydrocortisone stimulated the formation of human neutrophil containing colonies in vitro and inhibited macrophage colony formation. There was a significant increase in neutrophil colonies when the cells were preincubated with hydrocortisone for 24 hr. Delayed addition of hydrocortisone to the cultures was less effective. Hydrocortisone also increased the number of neutrophil colonies when the cultured bone marrow was depleted of T lymphocytes and phagocytes.[136]

4. The Effect of Glucocorticoids on the Thymus

The influence of glucocorticoids on the thymus has been studied extensively in the mouse, to a lesser extent in rats and man, and occasionally in other species. Nevertheless, it appears that glucocorticoids affect the thymus in all vertebrates since there are reports to this effect in chicken,[137] in turtle and frog,[138] and even in the rainbow trout.[139] Although glucocorticoids and sex hormones appear to influence directly hormone production by thymic epithelial cells,[140,141] this aspect of thymus physiology has not been elucidated to date.

a. Mouse

Initial studies in mice revealed that after glucocorticoid treatment the profoundly involuted thymus actually contained more cells capable of responding to PHA, pokeweed mitogen, and to antigenic stimuli. The frequency of such cortisone resistant immunocompetent cells in the thymus was estimated to be 2 to 6%, and it was suggested on the basis of studies with thymus grafts bearing the T6 marker that these cells have undergone thymic processing, but have not yet been released from the thymus.[142-145]

Mice having H-2^a histocompatibility antigens were more sensitive to hydrocortisone induced thymus atrophy than mice belonging to other major histocompatibility complex (MHC) type. The genes determining susceptibility were mapped between the I and D regions. Mice with d or q alleles in this region are sensitive, while those that have b or k are resistant.[146]

Steroid administered to normal mice significantly decreased the level of circulating thymic hormone, but high doses were necessary (over 2 mg of hydrocortisone hemisuccinate per mouse) and the reduction was only 50 to 70%.[147]

Cortisone sensitive thymic lymphocytes are located in the cortex, whereas resistant cells are found in the medulla.[148] Cortisone resistant thymocytes appear to express receptors for C3,[149] and the Qa-1 antigen. Terminal deoxynucleotidyl transferase is a marker for the sensitive cortical cells.[150] Furthermore, cortisone resistant thymocytes are deficient in helper T cells, suggesting that this T cell subset is more sensitive to corticosteriods than the killer/suppressor variety.[151] Cortisone resistant cells are heterogeneous with regards to their density, electrophoretic mobility, DNA synthesis, and response to PHA.[152]

Kinetic studies indicated that the initial increase of intrathymic cytotoxic T lymphocyte precursors after in vivo hydrocortisone administration is followed at 6 to 8 days by a phase of rapid decrease. The frequency of cytotoxic cells returns to normal level by 28 days post treatment.[153,154] Morphologically the effect of corticosteroids on sensitive thymocytes is characterized by widespread chromatin condensation, increased incidence of degenerative mitochondria, and a decreased electrophoretic mobility. This is followed by the ingestion of such degenerated cells by thymic phagocytic cells beginning 2 hr after hydrocortisone injection and continuing up to 8 hr.[155-157]

Thymocytes from Adrx BALB/c male mice were separated with the aid of peanut agglutinin (PNA) into corticosenstive PNA+ cells and corticoresistant PNA- cells. Glucocorticoid receptor profiles of these two populations did not differ in affinity or cellular concentration, or in cytoplasmic and nuclear compartmentalization. On two-dimensional gel electrophoresis, PNA+ and PNA- thymocytes showed patterns of incorporation of ^{35}S-methionine into protein that differed in at least 12 spots as revealed by autoradiography. After exposure to dexamethasone both PNA+ and PNA- cells showed substantial overlapping changes in protein synthetic profiles.[158] Killing of mouse thymocytes by glucocorticoids requires RNA and protein synthesis and an extensive fragmentation of nuclear DNA into oligonucleosomal subunits. This fragmentation is the result of the action of an endonuclease that is found in the nuclei of thymocytes and some other cells, and requires calcium and magnesium ions for its activation. If isolated, fresh thymocyte nuclei are incubated with these ions and up to 77% of their DNA is cleaved within 90 min. Therefore, it is not the endonuclease itself that is induced by glucocorticoids, but rather some protein, which is necessary for its activation. This protein may be part of a system for transplanting calcium into the nucleus. The endonuclease is inhibited by zinc, which also prevents thymocyte death. Mature T cells also contain the endonuclease but lack the glucocorticoid inducible mechanism for activation, and thus they are glucocorticoid resistant.[159]

Thymocytes that resist glucocorticoids in vivo are quite sensitive to its toxic effect in vitro.[150,160] It has been suggested that the thymus may produce factor(s) in vivo that protect the medullary subpopulation from glucocorticoid-induced lysis. Indeed, it was observed by others that thymic humoral factor increased the resistance of murine thymocytes to hydrocortisone.[161] Human thymic factor had a similar effect on murine thymocytes.[162]

Glucocorticoids (cortisone and hydrocortisone) caused a prolonged decrease by 80 to 90% of thymidine kinase (TK) activity of both thymus and spleen. Heparin injected 6 hr before glucocorticoid treatment inhibited the decreasing effect of cortisone, but not that of hydrocortisone on TK activity in the thymus, and fully inhibited the effect of both hormones on the enzyme activity in the spleen. The combined use of heparin and cortisone increased the splenic TK activity above the control value on the 2nd day after treatment.[163] Heparin injected i.p. 3 hr prior to steroid administration inhibited

Table 2
CHARACTERISTICS OF GLUCOCORTICOID SENSITIVE AND RESISTANT MURINE THYMOCYTES

Properties	Sensitive	Resistant	Ref.
Location	Thymic cortex	Thymic medulla	148
Frequency	94—98%	2—6%	142,143,169
Morphology	Smaller	Larger	158
Immunocompetence	No	Yes	144
Response to mitogens	No	Yes	142,143,169
Markers	High Thy 1, terminal Deoxynucleotidyl Transferase, PNA⁺	Low Thy 1, Qa-1, C3 Receptor, PNA⁻	149,150,151

Note: Thy 1 = thymocyte and T cell specific antigen, Qa-1 = surface antigen, PNA⁺ = receptor is present for peanut agglutinine, PNA⁻ = no receptor for PNA, C3 = third component of complement.

the suppressive effect of cortisone, but not hydrocortisone, on DNA synthesis in the thymus. Heparin was ineffective if injected by another route. It was suggested that peritoneal cells (macrophages) are involved in the influence of heparin on glucocorticoid action.[164]

Concanvalin A (con A) induced activation of mouse thymus cells is extremely sensitive to the inhibitory effect of hydrocortisone. This inhibitory effect can be abrogated by interleukin 2 but not by interleukin 1.[165] Treatment of PNA⁻ thymocytes with dexamethasone for 24 hr in vitro eliminated their subsequent capacity to function as helper cells in primary antibody responses, to respond to mitogens or to alloantigenic cells, or to generate killer T cells. Exposure of such thymocytes to macrophage supernatants containing interleukin 1 restored their capacity to function as helper cells, but reactivity to mitogens, alloantigens, and the ability to develop killer cells was not restored by such supernatants.[166] Treatment of hydrocortisone-suppressed mice with thymosin facilitates recovery from immunosuppression as revealed by Con A responsiveness of lymphoid cells.[167]

Equal numbers of thymus and spleen cells from mice treated with hydrocortisone exhibited an increased stimulation of DNA synthesis in response to PHA, Con A, and pokeweed mitogen (PWM) whereas the response to LPS was not affected.[168,169] Some characteristics of glucocorticoid sensitive and resistant murine thymocytes are summarized in Table 2.

b. Rat

In rats, glucocorticoids induce thymocyte degeneration in a specific and dose-dependent fashion that is characterized by the progressive apprearence of pyknotic cells with increased nuclear fragility. A sharp but transient increase in buoyant density can be observed, and more than 80% of the chromatin in affected cells is low molecular weight. This is the result of endonuclease activity.[170,171] Although the administration of dexamethasone to Adrx and castrated rats caused a marked increase in the acid protease activity in the cytosol of whole thymus or thymic lymphocytes, the minimun hormone dose required for half-maximal thymolytic effect was much lower (0.05 mg/kg) than the dose required for half-maximal effect on the protease (0.3 mg/kg). Furthermore, in vitro exposure of isolated thymocytes to dexamethasone failed to affect the acid protease activity in the cytosol, but produced marked time dependent cytolytic response. Therefore, glucocorticoid-induced cytolysis in rat thymic lymphocytes is not mediated by a direct effect of the hormone on the endogenous protease.[172] Treatment of rat thymocytes in vitro with dexamethasone induced a 50% stimulation of RNA degradation within 4 hr of steroid treatment. This RNA degradation was glucocorticoid specific and dependent on the concentration of the hormone employed. It was hypothesized that RNA degradation contributed to the lethal effect of the hormone on lymphoid cells.[173]

Newly synthesized proteins labeled with ^{35}S-methionine were studied in glucocorticoid sensitive and resistant rat thymocytes by two-dimensional gel electrophoresis. Of the proteins, 18 were different between these two cell populations, 13 increased in the resistant state, and 5 decreased. One major change was the appearance of a new protein with a molecular weight of 36,000 daltons in resistant rat thymocytes. This protein migrated to the same position on the gels as the protein found in corticosteroid resistant P1798 mouse lymphosarcoma cells. Thus, the presence of one or more proteins may confer glucocorticoid resistance on rat thymocytes.[174]

Treatment of rats with progesterone or cortexolone potentiated the thymolytic effect of cortisol, but had no effect on TA induced thymus involution. In vitro progesterone and cortexolone behaved as partial agonist-antagonist when tested alone or in combination with cortisol, but were inactive in combination with TA. These results indicate that the effect of progesterone and cortexolone depends on the nature of the glucocorticoid used.[175]

c. Man

Thymic precursor cells (prothymocytes) were isolated from human fetal thymic tissues after depletion of the E-rosetting thymocytes on Ficoll-Hypaque gradient. The prothymocytes were larger, showed different nuclear chromatin pattern, lacked the E-rosetting and natural attachment capacities, and did not bind the lectin PNA. These human prothymocytes were highly sensitive to the cytolytic effect of hydrocortisone in vitro, whereas the thymocytes were resistant.[176-178] The capacity of dexamethasone to inhibit human peripheral blood lymphocyte mitogenesis was inversely correlated with the PHA concentration used. However, dexamethasone inhibited thymocyte mitogenesis completely, irrespective of PHA concentrations. T cells purified from peripheral blood behaved as thymocytes with regard to the dexamethasone inhibitory pattern. The addition of macrophages or interleukin 1 was effective in removing the inhibitory effect of dexamethasone on T cells purified from blood, but not from thymocytes. Therefore, the higher sensitivity of thymocyte mitogenesis to glucocorticoids in comparison to peripheral blood lymphocytes cannot be explained by differences in macrophage content, but rather, it is an intrinsic property of less mature T cells.[179]

5. The Effect of Glucocorticoids on Leukocyte Distribution and Recirculation
a. Mouse

In mice a clear circadian rhythm in the number of peripheral blood and spleen lymphocytes was demonstrated. Peripheral blood lymphocytes were low during the light phase, which is the least active period in this nocturnal species, and it was high at night. The number of T and B lymphocytes varied in parallel with the total lymphocyte counts. In mice conditioned under both normal and reversed lighting, the lymphocyte counts started to decrease with the increase of plasma corticosterone levels in the early dark phase and reached a low in the dark phase, which is known to be a period of high corticosterone levels. A clear circadian rhythm in the number of lymphocytes was lost in Adrx mice. Administration of prednisolone at physiologic concentrations to the Adrx mice produced a reversible depression of circulating lymphocytes appearing early after drug administration.[180]

The administration of glucocorticoids to mice resulted in a rapid decrease of circulating monocytes within 3 to 6 hr, the duration being dependent on the nature and dose of the compound used. The water soluble dexamethasone sodium phosphate was only briefly active (less than 12 hr), but hydrocortisone acetate, which formed a subcutaneous depot, reduced the number of monocytes for more than 2 weeks. Cortisol did not affect the number of macrophages already present in the peritoneal cavity, but the transit of monocytes from the circulation into the peritoneal cavity was arrested. During an inflammatory response, both the number of monocytes in the peripheral blood and the increase in the peritoneal cavity are suppressed by cortisol. No lytic action of glucocorticoids on the mononuclear phagocytes could be demonstrated.[181]

Treatment of ^{51}Cr-labeled peritoneal cells in vitro with cortisol resulted in greatly increased migration of cells to the recipient's spleen after i.p. injection. A similar effect was produced if steroid hormone was administered to the recipient after cell injection. In this case, cortisol increased the number of cells accumulating in the spleen, whereas transport of labeled cells to other areas was unaffected. Treatment of donors with cortisol reduced the numbers of peritoneal cells harvested from each donor, but such cells were found to distribute normally in untreated syngeneic recipients. From these results the existence of cortisol-sensitive and cortisol-resistant subpopulations of peritoneal cells was predicted.[182]

Cortisol acetate rapidly reduced bone marrow promonocytes to about 65% over a period of 96 hr. However, the mitotic activity of promonocytes was not decreased, and the production of monocytes was only moderately diminished to about 80% of normal. After in vivo labeling with ^{3}H-thymidine, the monocyte labeling indices were initially significantly higher in cortisol treated mice. Therefore, a decreased production of monocytes in the bone marrow cannot account for the prolonged monocytopenia after cortisol administration. However, cortisol interferes with the release of newly-formed monocytes from the bone marrow.[183]

A single dose of dexamethasone, which caused a short and severe monocytopenia, did not influence the number of pulmonary macrophage. In vivo labeling studies showed that the monocytes disappeared temporarily from the circulation, but did not enter the pulmonary tissue in any significant numbers. A depot of cortisol acetate caused severe monocytopenia and a decrease of pulmonary macrophage population to about two thirds, which persisted for up to 144 hr. Labeling studies showed a reduced influx of monocytes into the lung. It was calculated that 48 hr after cortisol administration the monocyte influx was 14% of normal, the local production of macrophages 7% of normal, the pulmonary macrophage eflux was 12% of normal, and the mean turnover time was five and a half times longer than normal. Therefore, the maintenance of the reduced pulmonary macrophage population at 48 hr postcortisol depended on a reduced eflux.[184] Cortisol acetate treatment induced eosinopenia in mice that was independent of the thymus.[185]

b. Rat

In rats given four daily doses of 25 mg of cortisol acetate, blood lymphocytes and monocytes were greatly reduced, while the numbers of circulating granulocytes showed a marked increase. Granulocytes continued to rise during 3 days following treatment and constituted 98% of the circulating WBC at that time. Acute inflammatory exudate was induced by injecting latex particles i.p. following the final dose of cortisol. The migration of lymphocytes and monocytes into the inflammatory exudate was reduced by cortisol. The granulocytic population of the inflammatory exudate was also suppressed, even when there was a fourfold elevation of granulocytes in the blood. Pretreatment with cortisol did not affect the ability of individual cells to phagocytose latex particles.[186]

The recirculation of radioactively labeled thoracic duct lymphocytes was investigated in syngeneic recipients, which had been given a continuous i.v. infusion of prednisolone at 1 mg/hr for 15 to 18 hr previously. The most prominent effect of prednisolone was to retard recirculating lymphocytes within the bone marrow, spleen, and lymph nodes. Lymphocyte traffic was almost completely eliminated by prednisolone, but the lymphocytes were not killed. Prednisolone impaired the influx of lymphocytes from the blood into lymph nodes. Previous antigenic stimulation prevented this inhibition. It took a longer time for lymphocytes to cross the walls of high endothelial venules in the lymph nodes of prednisolone treated rats. Finally, prednisolone increased the rate at which lymphocytes entered the bone marrow from the blood by crossing sinusoidal endothelium.[187]

The influence of corticosteroids on lymphocyte recirculation has been compared in the corticosteroid-sensitive rat with the corticosteroid-resistant guinea pig. A single high glucocorticoid dose induced a rapid depression of lymphocyte level in both normal and thymectomized animals of both species. Recovery occurred within 1 day, and the returning cell population showed the same size distribution and label index profile as before treatment. Thus, the main effect of a single steroid dose appeared to be a trapping of lymphocytes from the circulation in some tissues, which was more pronounced in the sensitive rat. Both B and T lymphocytes were affected, and corticosteroid induced depression was independent of thymic function. The same course of events was observed in normal rats after stress, but not in thymectomized rats.[188] Rats had the same lymphocyte cell size distribution before, during, and after corticosteroid treatment. Thymectomy did not influence these parameters. Similarly, both intact and thymectomized guinea pigs kept the same size distribution during the different phases of corticosteroid treatment. These findings support the identity of the original, with the returning lymphocyte population, and are compatible with the hypothesis that lymphocyte trapping and redistribution is the major effect of a single corticosteroid dose in both the rat and the guinea pig.[189] Subsequent studies with ^{3}H-thymidine labeled lymphocytes in rats revealed that the original lymphocyte population had a higher percentage of labeled small lymphocytes (50%) in comparison to the population returning after a high corticosteroid dose (35%). This decrease of small lymphocytes in the returning cell population may indicate a minor lymphocytolytic effect of corticosteroid on circulating lymphocytes.[190]

Cortisol sodium succinate was found to inhibit in a dose-dependent fashion the random and direct migration of rat spleen and human peripheral blood T lymphocyte in vitro. Rat splenic B lymphocytes were more sensitive to cortisol induced inhibition than were T lymphocytes.[191]

c. Guinea Pig

The administration to guinea pigs, of either cortisol sodium succinate (100 mg/kg single dose), or cortisone acetate (100 mg/kg subcutaneously for 7 days), caused a marked increase in the numbers of alveolar macrophages recovered from the lungs 4 and 24 hr after the last injection. Both corticosteroid treatments caused similar levels of peripheral blood lymphocytopenia and monocytopenia in the same time intervals.[192]

d. Man

Systemically administered glucocorticoids (Solu-Medrol, 100 mg) to five subjects caused a marked decrease in the percentage of E-rosette-forming T cells within 6 hr after injection, the effect being maximum at 24 hr, but recovering by 48 hr. The absolute number of lymphocytes was not modified during the time of observation.[147] The effect of cortisol on lymphocyte kinetics was studied in nine normal volunteers, employing ^{51}Cr-labeled autologous lymphocytes. One hour after infusion, 21.8 ± 3.2% of the labeled lymphocytes remained in circulation. Cortisol (400 mg), administered i.v. 24 hr after infusion, caused a profound lymphocytopenia, which was maximal at 4 hr and returned to normal by 24 hr after drug application. Concomitant with the lympho-cytopenia, there was a dramatic increase in lymphocyte specific activity (cpm/10^6 lymphocytes), but the total lymphocyte associated radioactivity remained unchanged in the circulation, indicating that corticosteroid administration depleted the unlabeled recirculating cells. When the lymphocyte counts returned to normal following cortisol, the specific activity also returned to normal. Therefore, cortisol caused a transient lymphocytopenia by preferential depletion of the recirculating portion of intravascular lymphocyte pool.[193] Eight subjects all developed lymphocytosis, with predominant effect on B cells, after a treadmill exercise at 8 mi/hr for 10 min. When the same exercise was repeated 5 hr after receiving 60 mg of prednisone, the lymphocytosis of both T and B cells was suppressed. When this experiment was repeated 2 hr after receiving prednisone only, lymphocytosis of the T subpopulation was suppressed.[194]

Circadian rhythms of human T, B, K, and null cells were studied in the peripheral blood in relation to changes in plasma cortisol levels. T and B cell showed covariation with a peak at night and a depression during the day, whereas null and K cells showed an inverted rhythm with a decrease during the night and an increase during the day. Changes in plasma cortisol levels were inversely related to T and B cells variations.[195] The inverse relationship of lymphocyte levels and plasma cortisol concentrations, observed in healthy individuals, was lacking in patients with adrenal insufficiency. Administration of replacement doses of cortisol to these patients caused a dose-dependent lowering of lymphocyte levels. There was a significant increase in numbers of lymphocytes in healthy adults during the day, with the proportion of E-rosette-forming lymphocytes being constant. These observations suggest that endogenous cortisol is an important factor in the regulation of lymphocyte recirculation (Figure 1).[196]

The effect of systemically administered glucocorticoids on various subsets of lymphocytes have been investigated by several laboratories. Normal subjects given 60 mg of prednisone orally at 8:00 a.m. developed a transient lymphopenia by 2:00 p.m. E-rosette-forming T lymphocytes decreased by 56 to 69%, whereas Fc-receptor-bearing lymphocytes increased by 21 to 45%. In all cases the absolute numbers of T cells and Fc-receptor-bearing cells were decreased. The density distribution of lymphocytes did not change after prednisone treatment.[197]

Others observed that oral administration of prednisolone induced a T lymphocyto-penia in the peripheral blood that affected OKT4+ lymphocytes more than OKT8+ cells, resulting in a slight decrease in the ratio OKT4/OKT8. The proliferative responses of peripheral blood lymphocytes were not affected after a single dose of 10 mg of prednisolone, but 30 or 60 mg doses decreased proliferative responses. In vitro experiments revealed that prednisolone causes a temporary depletion from the peripheral blood of highly reactive T lymphocytes and that any effect of prednisolone on nonstimulated lymphocytes is reversible.[198] T lymphocytes bearing receptors for IgM were selectively depleted from the circulation by the administration of glucocorticoids, whereas T cells with receptors for IgG were relatively resistant to the lymphopenic effect of these hormones. This differential effect could not be explained on the basis of receptor content, since both cell types had similar quantities of receptors with similar binding affinities.[199]

After an i.v. injection of 200 mg of cortisol to five normal subjects, the mean blood granulocyte pool increased from 79 to 138×10^7 cells per kilogram of body weight. Cortisol injection resulted in a mean decrease in blood granulocyte egress of 74% and in cell inflow of 450%. The rate of granulocyte migration from the blood to an inflammatory exudate was also reduced after the administration of cortisol by 75%, as revealed by the skin window technique.[200] An infant with chronic benign neutropenia responded to stress-induced rise in plasma cortisol with a pronounced rise in peripheral neutrophil count. Studies with radioactively labeled neutrophils following stress-in-

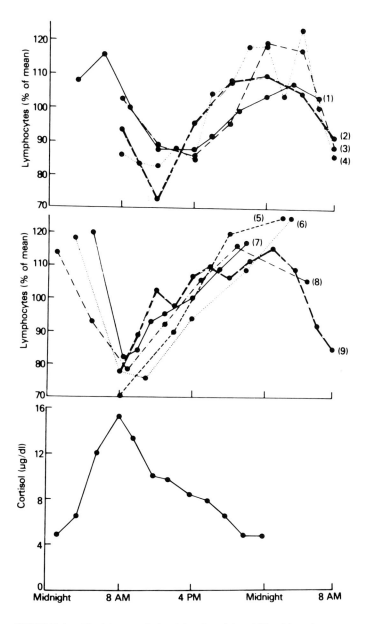

FIGURE 1. The inverse relationship of peripheral blood lymphocytes and cortisol. This figure is constructed from data of nine independent studies for lymphocyte changes and from five studies for the mean cortisol changes.[196]

duced neutrophilia, or during and following cortisol stimulation, revealed that neutrophils were removed from the circulation at a normal rate, whereas the release of neutrophils from the bone marrow was increased.[201]

6. The Effect of Glucocorticoids on T Lymphocytes
a. Mouse
Corticosteroid treatment of SJL mice produced a marked decrease in the number of viable lymphocytes 48 hr later in the thymus, spleen, and lymph node, with no change

in the peripheral blood. The most marked change noted was the dose-related increase in the Lyt-2 population of T lymphocytes in all the lymphoid organs examined.[202] Other investigations revealed that the B cell content of the spleen decreased more rapidly than did the T cell content after single i.p. injections of cortisol acetate. The in vitro reactivities to the B cell mitogens, LPS and PPD, were strongly depressed by cortisol injection, whereas the reactivity to the T cell mitogens, Con A and PHA, remained relatively unchanged.[203] However, physiological concentrations of glucocorticoids (10^{-8} to 10^{-7} M) inhibited in vitro the reaction of mouse lymphoid cells to Con A.[204] Furthermore, in vitro treatment with pharmacological concentrations (10^{-6} M) of dexamethasone reduced drastically the production of T cell growth factor (IL-2) by murine T cells, but failed to interfere with the mitogenic activity of IL-2 on T cell blasts.[205]

Cortisol treatment of mice inhibited T cell function in humoral immunity, while the cells responsible for the initiation of GVHR showed resistance.[206,207] However, the generation of cytotoxic T cells by the i.v. injection of parental spleen cells into lethally irradiated F_1 hybrid mice was markedly impaired by the treatment of cell donors with cortisol. Treatment with antithymocyte serum (ATS) resulted in an almost complete loss of such activity. The mixing of spleen cells from cortisol treated parental donors with the spleen cells from ATS-treated parental donors before injection to F_1 recipients resulted in a synergistic amplification of the cytotoxic response. Treatment of either spleen cell population with anti-Thy-1 serum abolished the synergism completely. It was concluded that corticosteroid-resistant T cells acted in this system as precursors of cytotoxic lymphocytes, whereas ATS resistant T cells were amplifying (helper) cells.[208] A single, relatively large dose of cortisol, given to mice at the time of priming with carrier antigen, eliminated carrier specific helper T cell activity. A significant amount of helper activity was also eliminated if cortisol was given after such T cells had been generated. However, under the same experimental conditions, suppressor and amplifier T cell activities were unaffected.[209] Dexamethasone, in doses equivalent to elevated physiologic concentrations, abolished the activity of antigen primed suppressor T cells, whereas antigen primed helper T cell function was resistant to even pharmacologic concentrations of dexamethasone. This apparent steroid resistance of the helper T cell population was found to be mediated by products of activated macrophages.[210] Subsequent studies revealed that the function of carrier primed, antigen-specific helper T cells were unaffected by dexamethasone, while carrier primed helper cells that do not recognize antigen were inactivated by pharmacologic concentrations of this steroid.[211]

The effector function of splenic cytotoxic T lymphocytes, obtained after i.p. immunization with allogeneic cells, was not inhibited by acute exposure to glucocorticoids, but preincubation of cytotoxic cells for several hours with subnanomolar concentrations of several different glucocorticoids caused marked inhibition. The relative inhibitory potency of steroids tested correlated with their activity in glucocorticoid receptor binding assays and with their anti-inflammatory potency in man. The inhibitory effects of low concentrations (10^{-10} to 10^{-9} M) of dexamethasone were reversed by human or mouse interleukin-2 containing supernatants, but not by IL-1 containing supernatants. The inhibitory effect of high concentrations (10^{-8} to 10^{-7} M) of dexamethasone could not be reversed even by very high concentrations of mouse IL-2. It was suggested that glucocorticoids may act in the system on IL-2 production and also directly on the cytotoxic cells.[212]

A new lymphokine, called glucosteroid response modifying factor (GRMF) has been described by Fairchild et al.[213] This mediator is secreted by mouse spleen cells after stimulation with Con A and also by a murine T cell hybridoma. GRMF blocks glucocorticoid suppression of helper T cell function and the growth of granulocyte/macrophage progenitor cells in vitro.

b. Rat

Cortisol caused a dose-dependent depression of blood lymphocyte response to PHA, but enhanced the response of spleen cells when the steroid was added after the mitogen into the culture. An inverse relationship between blood and splenic lymphocyte responses to PHA was observed after a single dose of cortisol to rats. Blood lymphocytes from rats treated with multiple doses of cortisol had enhanced response to PHA. Serum collected within 5 min of injection from single dose treated rats depressed normal rat blood lymphocyte responses, whereas serum obtained from rats after multiple doses of cortisol enhanced blood lymphocyte responses to PHA. The primary antibody response to sheep erythrocytes was not affected by near toxic doses of cortisol.[214] Con A responsive T cells were found to be resistant to the effects of a single oral dose of dexamethasone, while PHA responsive cells showed a dose-dependent suppression at dose levels of 0.35 and 1 mg/kg. Dexamethasone did not alter serum antibody production against sheep erythrocytes at dose levels that produced a significant depression of the PHA response.[215]

Rat lymphocytes express receptors for IgE and produce IgE binding factors after incubation with homologous IgE. Pretreatment with 1 to 5 μM dexamethasone inhibits the expression of Fc receptors on both B and T lymphocytes. T cells activated with Con A, in the presence of IgE, produce IgE-potentiating factor, which binds to lentil lectin and enhances selectively the IgE response. Pretreatment of such Con A activated T cells with dexamethasone, before incubation with IgE, alters the nature of IgE-binding factor formed by the cells. It fails to bind to lentil lectin and suppresses selectively the IgE response. Similar alteration of IgE-binding factor is observed in vivo, after the treatment of rats infected with *Nippostrongylus brasiliensis,* with a single dose of 0.2 mg dexamethasone. Glucocorticoid treatment prevents the glycosylation of IgE-binding factor and thereby changes its biological activity from enhancing to suppressive.[216]

c. Man

(i) In Vivo Observations

Patients with bronchial asthma exhibited a decreased lymphocyte transformation response to PHA after the administration of ACTH, which was inversely related to serum cortisol levels.[217] Lymphocytes, obtained from normal volunteers 4 hr after the i.v. injection of 1 mg/kg methylprednisolone (MP), were significantly less responsive in vitro to PHA and Con A. A significant decrease in the level of circulating T lymphocytes at the time of sampling may have contributed to the decrease of responsiveness. However, plasma obtained 1 hr after MP injection suppressed the in vitro response of normal autologous lymphocytes as well, indicating an additional direct corticosteroid effect on lymphocytes.[218] MP, administered i.v., depleted circulatory lymphocytes and reduced markedly the proliferative response of residual cells to PHA and Con A, 4 to 8 hr after the injection. The addition of MP in vitro to the residual cells further inhibited cell proliferation, indicating that these cells were not steroid resistant.[219] The in vitro response of peripheral lymphocytes to PHA, Con A, and PPD from children exposed in utero to short-term or long-term glucocorticoid therapy was found to be normal 3 to 7 years after delivery.[220]

Immunoglobulin production of PWM-stimulated peripheral lymphocytes, obtained from normal volunteers before, and 4 hr after i.v. administration of MP, was studied. Unfractionated lymphocytes showed a consistent decrease in immunoglobulin and total protein synthesis after glucocorticoid treatment. Purified B lymphocytes from corticosteroid treated donors showed a markedly diminished immunoglobulin response to normal T lymphocytes. IgE, IgM, and IgA production were equally affected. Purified T lymphocytes from steroid treated donors were capable of providing normal help for B cells in immunoglobulin production. Suppressor T cell activity was absent, however, as observed with normal T lymphocytes at high T-to-B cell ratios. Therefore, B cell responsiveness is diminished, suppressor T lymphocyte activity is removed, and helper T lymphocyte function is unaffected by systemic treatment with glucocorticoids.[221]

Lymphocytes from approximately 10% of normal people did not respond in vitro to PWM stimulation, which was due to the presence of naturally occurring suppressor cells. The administration of hydrocortisone to such individuals abrogated the function of natural suppressor cells and converted normal nonresponder peripheral blood cells to responder status. However, 4 hr after hydrocortisone administration, at the time of maximal lymphocytopenia, suppressor cells remaining in the circulation could still be activated by Con A. Furthermore, unstimulated cells obtained 4 hr after treatment, markedly enhanced PFC responses, when co-cultured with fresh autologous cells. This enhancement was independent of monocyte depletion, or changes in B cell numbers, and most likely reflected kinetic changes of immunoregulatory cell populations in the circulation.[222] Con A inducible suppressor cell activity was found to be grossly impaired in transplant recipients under corticosteroid therapy.[223]

Normal adult human subjects showed considerable variation in their sensitivity to cortisol induced depression of lymphocyte responsiveness to mitogens. This was not related to the relative numbers of helper/inducer (determined by OKT4 monoclonal antibodies) and suppressor/killer (identified by OKT8 monoclonal antibody) T cell subpopulations.[224] Lymphocytes from patients with allergies and asthma were resistant to glucocorticoids.[225] Histamine inhibited mitogen induced proliferation of human lymphocytes and, when given to patients in addition to MP, or used in vitro in combination with MP, a further inhibition of PHA and Con A responses compared to the steroid effect alone could be demonstrated.[226]

Peripheral blood from patients suffering from acute infectious mononucleosis, but not from convalescent patients, suppressed the PWM induced Ig response of normal human lymphocytes in allogeneic co-cultures. This suppressor cell activity was removed by treatment with anti-T cell antiserum and complement, as well as by the addition of 10^{-5} M cortisol, to the cell cultures.[227]

Patients with open-angle glaucoma have increased prevalence of HLA-B12 and B7 antigens and are more responsive to glucocorticoids, when compared with normal individuals. Lymphocytes from both ocular normotensive and ocular hypertensive individuals with HLA-B12 required significantly lower concentrations of prednisolone to inhibit PHA induced transformation.[228] Mitogen stimulated lymphocytes from healthy elderly individuals were significantly less sensitive to inhibition by cortisol than lymphocytes of healthy young controls.[229]

(ii) In Vitro Experiments

Suprapharmacological amounts (10^{-2} M/mℓ) of cortisol and MP lysed human mononuclear cells in vitro, whereas dexamethasone had no lytic effect, as revealed both by ^{51}Cr-release and electron microscopy.[230] Immuno-activated T lymphocytes are readily lysed by upper *physiological* and pharmacological concentrations of cortisol. This lysis of the sensitive population was specifically induced by glucocorticoids, but not by other steroid hormones.[178] Cortisol, at 0.01 to 10 μg/mℓ concentrations, inhibited the stimulation of peripheral blood lymphocytes by PHA in vitro.[231] Glucocorticoids were maximally effective in inhibiting the PHA response, when added to cultures 1 hr before the mitogen. If added 6 hr after PHA, their effect was minimal.[225] MP inhibited colony formation by PHA stimulated human blood lymphocytes at very low concentrations. The inhibition was exerted at an early stage and it was due to the lack of production of a soluble factor by accessory cells.[232] Cortisol reduced the number of cells entering the G_1 phase after PHA stimulation. Preincubation of the cells with cortisol potentiated greatly this inhibitory effect.[233]

Corticosteroid binding globulin (transcortin) did not influence the PHA response of human lymphocytes, if stripped of cortisol.[234] When transcortin was added to cortisol, the suppressive effect on the PHA response decreased in proportion to the decrease in the protein free cortisol concentration.[235]

Cortisol, at 1 $\mu g/m\ell$ concentration, depressed the PWM response of lymphocytes in vertical tube cultures if the cells were harvested at 48 hr, but not in similar cultures incubated for 3, 4, or 5 days. In this culture system 10 $\mu g/m\ell$ hormone depressed the level of response in most experiments. By contrast, ^{3}H-thymidine incorporation was enhanced in horizontal PWM cultures by 0.1 and 1 $\mu g/m\ell$ of cortisol, and 10 $\mu g/m\ell$ caused stimulation, or return to the normal level. The depressed thymidine uptake in vertical cultures was thought to be due to a combination of enhanced toxicity of cortisol in deep cultures and loss of incorporated thymidine due to increased cellular fragility.[231]

The addition of cortisol to PWM-stimulated cultures from nonresponders (having natural suppressor cells) reconstituted the response in two of three individuals. Furthermore, the addition of cortisol to allogeneic co-cultures of nonresponder and responder lymphocytes abolished the inhibitory effect of the naturally occurring suppressor cells on the Ig secretion by responder cells. The induction, but not the function, of Con A activated suppressor cells was sensitive to pharmacologic levels of cortisol. The effect of cortisol on naturally occurring suppressor cell function, or on the generation of suppressor cells by Con A, did not involve cell lysis but rather was reversible, requiring the continued presence of cortisol in the culture.[236]

Con A induced suppressor cells, inhibiting PWM-stimulated PFC, were found to be radiation sensitive, but corticosteroid resistant, whereas those suppressing allogeneic cell mediated lympholysis were both radiation and corticosteroid resistant.[237]

Suppressor cells generated from normal human lymphocytes by stimulation with Con A are very sensitive to pharmacological concentrations of dexamethasone.[238] Cortisol, depending on its concentration and time of addition to the culture system, either enhances or diminishes the generation of Con A activated suppressor cells and their suppressor effect on the proliferative responses of fresh lymphocytes. At high cortisol concentrations (10^{-5} M), the generation of suppressor cells was inhibited significantly. When the hormone was added to the second culture only, it enhanced significantly the suppressive effect of Con A preactivated cells at 10^{-6} M concentration. Continuous presence of cortisol in both cultures yielded varying results.[239]

The addition of supernatants from Con A activated human spleen cells to PWM stimulated human spleen cells and peripheral blood lymphocytes suppressed profoundly the polyclonal immunoglobulin synthesis. In contrast, when cortisol (10^{-5} M) was added together with Con A supernatants to PWM-stimulated cells, there was no significant suppression of immunoglobulin synthesis. Thus, cortisol was able to block the suppressive effect of a soluble suppressor factor secreted by Con A activated human spleen cells.[240] The inhibition of Con A activation in cortisol treated (0.1 to 10 $\mu g/m\ell$) cultures was inversely related to the percent of monocytes present. Separated monocytes preincubated with cortisol (1 or 10 $\mu g/m\ell$) and cultured with fresh T cells, as well as cortisol treated T cells cultured with fresh monocytes, showed significantly reduced responses. IL-1, induced by LPS stimulation of monocytes, was blocked in its ability to stimulate Con A induced T cell proliferation by cortisol, if present during the assay for IL-1. Thus, cortisol interferes with both monocytes and T cells during its inhibition of mitogenic reactions.[241]

It has been observed in several laboratories that glucocorticoids inhibit the production of IL-2 by helper T lymphocytes. This inhibition is the result of direct action on IL-2 producing T cells, as well as the inhibition of IL-1 production by adherent cells. Glucocorticoids do not interfere with the process by which resting T cells acquire responsiveness to IL-2.[242-245] The secretion of some other lymphokines by human T cells, such as the leukocyte and neutrophil migration inhibitory factors and the Fc receptor augmenting factor, are also inhibited by glucocorticoids.[246-249]

Human T cells, activated in mixed lymphocyte cultures, were found to be sensitive to the lytic effect of MP and cortisol. Freshly separated blood lymphocytes and PHA activated blasts were resistant. In addition, the activated T lymphocytes isolated from the synovial fluid of arthritic patients were also glucocorticoid sensitive, whereas the blood lymphocytes of the same patients were resistant. The glucocorticoid sensitivity was not accompanied by elevation of cytoplasmic steroid receptor numbers.[177]

Concentrations of MP, sufficient to inhibit both the cellular proliferation and generation of cytotoxic lymphocytes in mixed lymphocyte cultures (MLC), appear to enhance the induction of suppressor cells at approximately 1 μg/mℓ concentration. Furthermore, the presence of low concentration of MP, not sufficient to inhibit proliferation of MLC, potentiated the inhibiting effect of suppressor cells on cellular proliferation. The inhibition, observed by the joint effect of MP and suppressor cells, was equivalent to that seen using five times as many suppressor cells alone.[250] Concentrations of MP as low as 0.01 μg/mℓ were highly effective in inhibiting the generation of cytotoxic memory cells when placed into human MLC during the first 5 days of priming. The generation of cytotoxic lymphocytes was also inhibited, if the steroid was added along with the restimulating cells on day 10, although the degree of inhibition was not as great as when steroids were added at the beginning. Therefore, an important aspect of the immunosuppressive role of steroids is the prevention of the generation of specific memory cells following exposure to alloantigens.[251]

In human MLC, low doses of MP strongly inhibited the generation of secondary proliferative and cytotoxic cells. However, lymphocytes primed in the presence of MP were able to respond to the original stimulus in a primary fashion when restimulated. In contrast, as much as 10 μg/mℓ of MP, which is well above clinical levels, had no inhibitory effect on the induction of suppressor cells in these cultures. Therefore, glucocorticoids prevent priming of specific cytotoxic T cells without inhibiting the induction of suppressor lymphocytes in secondary allogeneic cultures.[252,253]

In low density cultures, dexamethasone enhanced the spontaneous induction of cells bearing Fc receptors for IgM, whereas no effect on the induction of cells bearing receptors for IgG was found.[254] Cortisol was reported to interfere with the interaction of human lymphocytes with measles virus infected cells.[255]

d. Other Species

The production of macrophage mitogenic factor (MMF) by guinea pig lymphocytes was decreased in the presence of physiological concentrations of glucocorticoids (2 $\times$ 10^{-5} M of triamcinolone inhibited by 50%). The inhibition was concentration dependent, glucocorticoid specific, and reversed by the corticosteroid antagonist, cortexolone. On the other hand, pharmacological concentrations of glucocorticoids were necessary for the inhibition of macrophage proliferation induced by MMF. Therefore, the major mechanism of glucocorticoid mediated anti-inflammatory action occurs at the level of MMF producing lymphocyte, rather than at the effector macrophage.[256] At pharmacological levels, glucocorticoids inhibited two antigen-induced functions of guinea pig lymphocytes, in vitro proliferation and lymphokine synthesis. The production of macrophage chemotactic factor (MCF) and macrophage inhibition factor (MIF) were decreased in the presence of cortisol. The steroid hormone blocked also the action of MIF on macrophages, but did not interfere with the action of MCF on macrophages.[257,258] The effect of glucocorticoids on T lymphocytes is summarized in Table 3.

Table 3
THE EFFECT OF GLUCOCORTICOIDS ON T LYMPHOCYTES

Species	Hormone	Dose/concentration	Biological effect	Ref.
Mouse			*In vivo*	
	Hydrocortisone	62.5—500 mg/kg	Increase of Lyt-2 cells	202
	Hydrocortisone acetate	2.5 mg i.p.	Inhibition of T_h for antibody response	207
	Hydrocortisone acetate	50—250 mg/kg	Depletion of T_h for T_k induction	208
	Hydrocortisone sodium succinate	1 mg/mouse i.p.	Depletion of antigen specific T_k, no effect on other type of T_h and T_k cells	209
			In vitro	
	Dexamethasone	$ID_{50} = 10^{-9}$ M	Inhibition of Con A response	204
	Dexamethasone	10^{-5}—10^{-8} M	Antigen-primed T, abolished, T_h resistant	210
	Dexamethasone	10^{-6} M	Antigen-specific T_{h1} resistant, T_{h2} sensitive	211
	Several glucocorticoids	10^{-9}—10^{-10} M	Inhibition of mature T_k by preincubation	212
	Dexamethasone	10^{-6} M	Reduction of TCGF (IL-2) production	205
Rat			*In vivo*	
	Hydrocortisone sodium succinate	100 mg/kg i.v. or i.p.	Depression of blood lymphocyte response to PHA	214
	Methylprednisolone sodium succinate	20 mg/kg i.v. or i.p.	Depression of blood lymphocyte response to PHA	214
	Dexamethasone	0.35—100 mg/kg p. os	Suppression of PHA but not Con A response	215
			In vitro	
	Hydrocortisone	10^{-3}—10^{-8} M	Inhibition of chemotactic migration	191
	Dexamethasone	$1 \times 5 \times 10^{-6}$ M	Conversion of IgE binding potentiating factor to suppressor factor	216
Man			*In vivo*	
	Prednisolone	2.5—15 mg/day	Inhibition of lymphocyte response to PHA	217
	Methylprednisolone sodium succinate	1 mg/kg i.v.	Inhibition of peripheral lymphocyte response to Con A and PHA	218,219

Table 3 (continued)
THE EFFECT OF GLUCOCORTICOIDS ON T LYMPHOCYTES

Species	Hormone	Dose/concentration	Biological effect	Ref.
	Methylprednisolone	48.5 mg i.v.	Inhibition of T_s	221
	Hydrocortisone sodium succinate	400 mg i.v.	Inhibition of T_s	222
	Prednisolone	0.25 mg/kg	Inhibition of T_s	223
	Methylprednisolone	500 mg i.v.	Inhibition of IL-2 production	243
		In vitro		
	Hydrocortisone	0.03—14.7 μg/mℓ	Inhibition of PHA-induced lymphocyte stimulation	233
	Methylprednisolone	10^{-6}—10^{-10} M	Inhibition of colony formation by PHA-stimulated human blood lymphocytes	232
	Dexamethasone	10^{-7}—10^{-9} M	Inhibition of T_μ	199
	Methylprednisolone	0.06—1.0 mg/mℓ	Lytic effect on MLC activated T cells	177
	Hydrocortisone	0.06—1.0 mg/mℓ	Lytic effect on MLC activated T cells	177
	Hydrocortisone	0.1—100 μg/mℓ	Inhibition of Mf-T cell cooperation	253
	Methylprednisolone	0.1—100 μg/mℓ	Inhibition of Mf-T cell cooperation	253
	Hydrocortisone	10^{-5} M	Inhibition of natural suppressor cell	236
	Hydrocortisone	10^{-5} M	Inhibition of induction but not the function of Con A activated suppressor cells	236
	Dexamethasone	10^{-4}—10^{-6} M	Enhancement of induction of T_μ	254
	Hydrocortisone	10^{-5} M	Abrogation of IL-2 production	244
	Hydrocortisone	2-1000 μg/mℓ	Abrogation of IL-2 production	242
	Methylprednisolone	0.3 and 2.5 μg/mℓ	Abrogation of IL-2 production	243
	Dexamethasone	10^{-6}—10^{-7} M	Abrogation of IL-2 production	245
	Methylprednisolone	10—100 ng/mℓ	Inhibition of LIF production by T cells	246
	Methylprednisolone	10^{-7} M	Inhibition of NIF production by T cells	248
	Dexamethasone	2×10^{-7} M	Inhibition of FRAF production by T cells	249
	Triamcinolone			
Guinea pig	Cortisol	2×10^{-7} M	Inhibition of FRAF production by T cells	249
	Hydrocortisone	1—100 μg/mℓ	Inhibition of MIF, CTF production by T cells	258

Note: Con A = concanavalin A; CTF = macrophage chemotactic factor; FRAF = Fc receptor augmenting factor; ID_{50} = effective dose/concentration exerting 50% inhibition in biological response; IL-2 = interleukin 2; IM = infectious mononucleosis; LIF = leukocyte migration inhibitory factor; Lyt-2 = T cell specific surface alloantigen in the mouse; Mf = macrophage; MIF = macrophage migration inhibitory factor; MLC = mixed lymphocyte culture; NIF = neutrophil migration inhibitory factor; PHA = phytohemagglutinine; TCGF = T cell growth factor; T_h = helper T cells; T_{h1} = antigen specific helper cells; T_{h2} = helper T cells; T_k = killer T cells; T_m = memory T cells; T_s = suppressor T cells; T_μ = T cells with Fc receptors for IgM.

7. The Effect of Glucocorticoids on B Lymphocytes

a. Mouse and Rat

The cellular composition of the spleen of CBA mice was investigated 2 days after a single i.p. injection of cortisol acetate in doses ranging from 31 to 750 mg/kg of body weight. The B cell content decreased more rapidly than did the T cell content, and larger lymphocytes were removed preferentially. The in vitro reactivity to the B cell mitogens, LPS and PPD, was strongly depressed.[203,259] Spleen cells responsive for another B cell mitogen, Nocardia water soluble mitogen, were also shown to be sensitive to in vivo treatment with cortisol.[260,261] IgM, IgG, and IgA secreting cells were studied in the spleen, mesenteric lymph nodes, and bone marrow, after a single injection of dexamethasone (16 to 144 mg/kg body weight) to BALB/c mice. The number of Ig secreting cells were markedly reduced in the spleen and lymph nodes within 1 day, but were hardly affected in the bone marrow. The decrease was immediately followed by a recovery and an overshoot, especially in lymph nodes, after the highest doses given. Two weeks after the initial decrease a second decrease was found. When mice were treated daily for 1 week, initially a recovery pattern occurred in spleen and lymph nodes. This was less dose-dependent, and the overshoot reaction was followed by a second period of subnormal numbers of Ig secreting cells, which lasted at least for 1 week. The most important effect of daily treatment was a long lasting decrease of the number of IgG secreting cells, starting 1 week after withdrawal of treatment, which led to a severely decreased serum IgG level.[262]

Serum globulin and IgG levels in rats, treated neonatally with 1 mg of cortisol acetate, increased slowly during development and were significantly lower than controls up to 30 days. Animals with the most severe immunological deficit began to runt on day 12, with marked mortality. Cortisol treatment did not influence the absorption of IgG from the gastrointestinal tract. Severe deficits were demonstrated, however, in the ability of treated rats to synthesize antibody, when immunized with a T-dependent antigen.[263]

The redistribution of mouse lymphocyte surface immunoglobulin (capping) induced by anti-Ig antibody, or by sheep erythrocyte antigen, was inhibited reversibly by cortisol succinate (2×10^{-4} M). Cholesterol and progesterone also inhibited capping, suggesting that the effect was mediated through changes in the physical properties of the cell membrane, rather than by hormonal action.[264]

b. Man

After the administration of a single dose of glucocorticoids, the spontaneous Ig production in the peripheral blood by B cells was enhanced, as measured by an in vitro PFC-assay. PWM induced PFC response was suppressed 4 to 5 hr after a single in vivo pharmacologic dose of corticosteroid and recovery was complete by 24 hr. After a 5-day regimen of corticosteroids, the suppressed PFC response did not recover up to 60 hr, even though the T lymphocyte profile returned to normal by 36 hr.[265]

Immunoglobulin producing human lymphoid cells were inhibited, in a dose-dependent fashion, by high concentrations of prednisolone (10 to 100 μg/ml), and there was no correlation between the length of drug treatment and reduction in the percentage of Ig producing cells.[266] Physiologic and pharmacologically attainable concentrations of cortisol enhanced markedly the PWM-induced PFC response of normal human peripheral blood B lymphocytes in vitro. Cortisol was effective only if added within the first 24 hr to the cultures. Suprapharmacologic concentrations (10^{-3} M) inhibited early B cell activation. Late states of antibody production were resistant to suppression by even these high concentrations. Cortisol did not replace the T cell requirement of PWM-induced Ig secretion.[267] A similar enhancement of PWM-stimulated IgG synthesis was observed with 10^{-2} M prednisolone at various T:B ratios. Addition of prednisolone to cultures of autologous and allogeneic mixtures of T and B lymphocytes resulted in enhancement of PWM-stimulated IgG synthesis. This was independent of T:B ratio and occurred with purified B lymphocytes that contained monocytes. Pretreatment of purified B lymphocytes plus monocytes, but not purified T lymphocytes, with prednisolone enhanced PWM-induced IgG synthesis in reconstituted mixtures of T and B lymphocytes. Thus, glucocorticoid induced enhancement of PWM-stimulated IgG synthesis by human mononuclear cells is independent of T lymphocyte regulation.[268]

A marked enhancement of immunoglobulin secretion was observed in unstimulated cultures of human peripheral blood mononuclear cells in the presence of cortisol, when compared to cultures without hormone. This augmented response occurred only when the cultures were performed in fetal calf serum and not in human serum. No enhancement of Ig secretion by cortisol was seen in cultures maximally stimulated with PWM, regardless of the serum used.[269] The addition of 0.1 mM to 10 nM cortisol to human lymphocytes in culture, in the absence of other mitogens, resulted in the dramatic induction of immunoglobulin production, with responses comparable to those in similar cultures stimulated with PWM. Stimulation was seen first after 48 hr and peaked at 8 to 10 days of culture. IgG, IgA, and IgM were induced by glucocorticoids, but not estrogens or androgens. Cultures depleted of either T cells or monocytes did not produce immunoglobulin when stimulated with glucocorticoids, and proliferation of B cells or T cells could not be detected by ³H-thymidine incorporation or by total cell recovery.[270]

To determine the cellular target for glucocorticoid induced immunoglobulin secretion in culture, separated populations of T cells and non T cells were preincubated with corticosteroids and then recombined. No immunoglobulin was produced in any of the preincubation experiments. However, supernatants from 3-day cultures of unstimulated, as well as glucocorticoid treated, peripheral blood mononuclear cells contained a T cell replacing factor that permitted T-depleted mononuclear cells to produce immunoglobulin upon corticosteroid stimulation. Both the factor and glucocorticoids were necessary for the induction of Ig synthesis. The production of this lymphokine required the presence of T cells and adherent cells in culture, and it was not present in supernatants of cultures stimulated with PWM, PHA, Con A, or alloantigens. This steroid dependent T cell replacing factor was unable to replace helper T cells for PWM-induced immunoglobulin production and required the presence of adherent cells in the T cell depleted responder population. It was inactivated by trypsin treatment heating to 56°C, freezing, lyophilization, or storage at 4°C for more than 3 weeks.[271] The effect of glucocorticoids on B lymphocytes is summarized in Table 4.

8. The Effect of Glucocorticoids on Monocytes and Macrophages
a. Mice

Mice treated with oral prednisolone for 2 days had normal clearance of *Staphylococcus aureus* from the lungs after aerosol exposure. However, mice treated for 2 weeks or more had delayed clearance 6 and 22 hr after aerosol exposure, and clearance returned to normal by 2 weeks after therapy.[272]

Hepatic uptake and glomerular deposition of i.v. administered human serum albumin-anti-human serum albumin immune complexes were examined in mice after cortisone administration. An initial rapid disappearance of complexes from the circulation of control mice, which was caused by increased vascular permeability, was absent in cortisone treated animals. The half-life of complexes containing more than two antigen and antibody molecules was prolonged from 1.93 hr in control mice to 4.71 hr in cortisone treated mice, whereas the half-life of small complexes was unchanged (11.4 vs. 12.04 hr). The quantity of complexes located in the liver at 1, 2, and 4 hr was not significantly different in the two groups. The persistence of large circulating complexes

Table 4
THE EFFECT OF GLUCOCORTICOIDS ON B LYMPHOCYTES

Species	Hormone	Dose/concentration	Biological effect	Ref.
Mouse				
		In vivo		
	Hydrocortisone	62 mg/kg	Depressed reactivity of spleen cells to LPS, PPD, and NWSM	203
	Hydrocortisone acetate	5 mg/mouse i.p.	Depressed reactivity of spleen cells to LPS, PPD, and NWSM	261
	Dexamethasone sodium phosphatase	16—144 mg/kg i.p.	Decrease of IgG secreting cells	262
		In vitro		
	Hydrocortisone	2×10^{-4} M	Inhibition of capping	264
		In vivo (neonatal)		
Rat	Cortisol acetate	1 mg/pup s.c. at birth	Severe humoral immunodeficiency	263

Table 4 (continued)

THE EFFECT OF GLUCOCORTICOIDS ON B LYMPHOCYTES

Species	Hormone	Dose/concentration	Biological effect	Ref.
Man		In vivo		
	Prednisolone	60—80 mg single dose p. os	Enhanced spontaneous Ig production	265
	Prednisolone	20 mg every 6 hr for 5 days, orally	Suppressed Ig secretion	265
		In vitro		
	Hydrocortisone sodium succinate	10^{-5} M	Enhancement of PWM induced PFC formation	267
	Prednisolone	10^{-6} M	Enhancement of PWM induced PFC formation	268
	Hydrocortisone sodium succinate	10^{-5}—10^{-9} M	Enhancement of spontaneous Ig production if cultured in fetal calf serum	269,270
	Dexamethasone	10^{-9} M		
	Prednisolone	10^{-6} M	Induction of steroid dependent T cell replacing factor that stimulated Ig secretion	271
	Dexamethasone	10^{-6} M		

Note: LPS = lipopolysaccharide from Gram-negative bacteria; PPD = purified protein derivative from *Myobacterium tuberculosis*; NWSM = *Nocardia*-derived water soluble mitogen; PWM = pokeweed mitogen.

was associated with enhanced and prolonged glomerular deposition of complexes in cortisone treated mice.[273]

Spleen and thymus cells from cortisone treated mice were unable to generate allo-reactive cytotoxic T cells when cultured with semi-allogeneic spleen cells or allogeneic tumor cells. This was due to a defect in accessory cell function, which could be corrected by the addition of irradiated peritoneal macrophages.[274] The antibody response to thymus dependent antigen was markedly suppressed in cortisone treated animals, but the response to thymus independent antigens was preserved. The relative independence of the immune response to thymus independent antigens of radioresistant cortisone sensitive accessory cells may explain this difference.[275]

Reduction of plasma corticosterone levels through feedback, Adrx, or by the injection of the corticosteroid synthesis inhibitor, aminoglutethimide phosphate, produced a parallel augmentation in monocyte numbers and delayed hypersensitive responses. The antibody response was also affected after immunization with supraoptimal doses of antigens.[276]

In vitro experiments revealed that the exposure of thioglycollate-induced mouse peritoneal macrophages to glucocorticoid hormones up to 96 hr induced a progressive, dose related, inhibition of cell growth and protein synthesis. Net glucose uptake, lactate production, and carbon dioxide (CO_2) production were also decreased in a dose related manner, which was specific to steroids with glucocorticoid action. Half maximal inhibition occurred at about 10^{-9} M for dexamethasone.[277] Dexamethasone phosphate influences the degradation of hemoglobin iron by macrophages and increases the release of iron suitable for reutilization.[278] Corticosteroids inhibit the expression of surface Ia antigen by peritoneal macrophages, both in vitro and in vivo, reduce the production of IL-1, and inhibit antigen presentation for T cell proliferation. The concentrations of cortisol and prednisone that inhibited Ia expression by 50% ranged from 2 to 5×10^{-8} M.[279]

Normal mouse macrophages are rendered cytotoxic by treatment with a lymphokine (arming factor) produced in MLC between skin graft recipients and donor spleen cells. Corticosteroids administered in vivo or in vitro depressed macrophage arming by interfering with the capacity of the normal macrophage to respond.[280] Glucocorticoids, at near *physiologic* concentrations, and their synthetic derivatives, markedly inhibited the cytotoxic activity of interferon treated macrophages for MBL-2 leukemia cells, even when applied after the macrophages have reached full morphologic activation. Macrophages from mice stressed by physical restraints were also inhibited.[281] Finally, a number of investigators established that glucocorticoid treatment interferes with the phagocytosis and intracellular killing of numerous, but by no means all, pathogenic and nonpathogenic microorganisms.[282-287]

Accessory cells stimulated by bacterial LPS, peptidoglycan, or lipoprotein, elaborate a GRMF, which is capable of interfering with the suppressive effect of dexamethasone on the humoral immune response in vitro. The target of GRMF is the helper T cell.[288] Furthermore, mice injected with LPS have in their serum a glucocorticoid antagonizing factor (GAF), which inhibits the glucocorticoid induced synthesis of the hepatic gluconeogenic enzyme, phosphoenolpyruvate carboxykinase. Macrophages are the major source of GAF in endotoxemic mice. GAF is remarkably similar to tumor necrosis factor, which can also be induced by LPS injections.[289]

b. Rat

Irradiated rat peritoneal macrophages secreted markedly more IL-1 in vitro when pretreated with *carrageenan*. Exposure of cultures of either carrageenan treated or untreated macrophages to cortisol (10^{-4} to 10^{-6} M) induced a dose-dependent inhibition of IL-1 secretions.[290]

c. Guinea Pig

Neither in vitro cortisol (1 and 10 μg/ml), nor cortisol administration in vivo, had any effect on either PHA induced or antibody dependent cellular cytotoxicity of alveolar macrophages against SRBC targets. However, after treatment with a depot preparation of cortisone acetate, a marked decrease in cytotoxic effector function of alveolar macrophages was observed. The suppressed killer cell function could be overcome by increasing the density of antibody and PHA on target cells.[192]

Topical or systemic administration of betamethasone-dipropionate or betamethasone-valerate caused a marked decrease in the density of epidermal Langerhans cells, which correlated with the concentration and known vasoconstrictive potency of the glucocorticoids administered.[291]

The administration of cortisone acetate to guinea pigs inhibited significantly the biosynthesis of complement factor C2 and C4 by alveolar macrophages. After 1 week of treatment, local complement synthesis was inhibited by approximately 80%, although serum levels were normal.[292]

The clumping of guinea pig bronchoalveolar macrophages by preformed macrophage aggregation factor was completely inhibited by 10^{-4} M cortisol 21-hemisuccinate. The inhibited macrophages remained viable.[293] Cortisol and dexamethasone, at pharmacological concentrations, blocked the response of macrophages to MIF. Cortisol influenced neither antigen processing by macrophages, nor the ability of antigen stimulated lymphocytes to produce MIF.[257,258] The response of guinea pig macrophages to the lymphokine, MMF, was inhibited by pharmacological concentrations (4×10^{-7} M) of triamcinolone acetonide (TA). At supraoptimal dilutions of MMF, glucocorticoids caused a twofold potentiation of macrophage proliferation. This potentiation was concentration dependent, glucocorticoid specific, and reversed by glucocorticoid antagonists.[256]

d. Man

Human monocytes which had differentiated to macrophages during 8 days in culture without steroids were not influenced by cortisol in the engulfment or the digestion step of phagocytosis. Continuous exposure to cortisol during differentiation resulted in a dose-dependent inhibition of the transformation of monocytes to macrophages.[294] Cortisol succinate, at 2.5 μM concentration, altered markedly monocyte to macrophage differentiation, as revealed by the inhibition of development of tumoricidal activity, protein synthesis, acid phosphatase, and 5′-nucleotidase. The development of lysosomes and of membrane bound electron lucent vacuoles was also inhibited, as was ³H-uridine incorporation. Dexamethasone inhibited the development of tumoricidal activity at tenfold lower concentrations than did cortisol.[295]

Betamethasone inhibited significantly the binding of immunoglobulin coated O Rh⁺ red cells to human fetal macrophages.[296] Monocytes of normal women expressed significantly greater numbers of Fc γ receptors than did similar cells from man. Monocyte Fc γ receptors were increased in patients of both sexes with autoimmune hemolytic anemia. Glucocorticoid treatment was associated with a dose-dependent decrease in monocyte Fc γ receptor number, both in normal volunteers and in patients.[297]

Monocyte chemotaxis, random migration, and bactericidal activity was reduced markedly by cortisol succinate at 16 μg/ml concentration. MP succinate and unesterified cortisol produced similar impairment of monocyte chemotaxis, while two drugs which were unmodified, and therefore do not enter cells, cortisol phosphate and cortisone acetate, had no effect on chemotaxis.[298] The chemotactic activity of monocytes from each of 16 normal subjects was suppressed by prednisolone at 25 ng/ml, maximum suppression occurring at 100 ng/ml (48%). In contrast, monocytes isolated from ten patients receiving corticosteroid therapy showed no significant suppression of chemotactic activity when exposed to the above concentrations of prednisolone, even though the monocytes responded normally to a chemotactic stimulus.[299]

The production of IL-1 by human cells of the monocyte-macrophage lineage was inhibited by glucocorticoids.[243,244] The presentation of viral or bacterial soluble antigen by monocytes to autologous T lymphocytes was inhibited by relatively high concentrations (greater than 10 μg/mℓ) of MP, but not by cortisol. MP also inhibited antigen presentation by umbilical vein and endothelial cells.[253]

Cultures of human monocytes exposed to cortisol produced a factor that stimulates the migration of polymorphonuclear cells in vitro. Steroid treated lymphocytes did not produce this factor.[300] The effect of glucocorticoids on monocytes and macrophages is summarized in Table 5.

9. The Effect of Glucocorticoids on Killer and Natural Killer Cells
a. Mouse and Rat

Antibody dependent cell mediated cytotoxicity (ADCC) was examined in mice and rats after treatment with cortisone acetate, using both chicken erythrocytes and the mouse lymphoma cell line AKR.A as target cells. The AKR.A assay detects lymphoid effector cells only, whereas a wide variety of effector cells will lyse chicken erythrocytes in the presence of antibody. The lymphoid K cells in rat spleen and blood were unaffected by corticosteroid treatment sufficient to cause lymphopenia, whereas splenic anti-chicken-erythrocyte cytotoxicity of whole and phagocyte free spleen cells were suppressed the most by cortisone. This may have been in part attributable to the redistribution of effector cells, since the cytotoxic capacity of nonphagocytic bone marrow cells was increased by 70% when the activity in the spleen was 25% of normal.[301]

In mice, NK cells and cells that mediate F_1 antiparent response differ in their sensitivity to cortisol acetate. NK cell activity decreases dramatically after in vivo drug administration, whereas the induction of specific F_1 antiparent or anti-allogeneic cytotoxicity and hybrid resistance to parental marrow grafts is not impaired.[302] Cortisol acetate given to mice by two daily i.p. injections (2.5 or 3.75 mg each) caused a significant but transient reduction of splenic NK cell activity against YAC-1 lymphoma targets. This effect was not dependent on the thymus, since splenic NK activity decreased in congenitally athymic mice after cortisol treatment. The cortisol induced decrease of cytotoxic activity could be partially restored in vitro by removing a subpopulation of cells adherent to, or phagocytic for, carbonyl iron particles. However, the suppressor cells could not be removed by depleting the cell population adherent to Sephadex® columns, or to plastic. The suppressor cells were radioresistant and elaborated a soluble suppressor factor.[303]

A model system for culturing NK cells has been established by Cox and co-workers.[304] In this system the NK activity of spleen cells of several inbred strains of mice was suppressed by treatment with dexamethasone. Suppression was time-dependent, requiring at least 5 hr for maximal suppression, and dose-dependent at pharmacologic concentrations.

b. Man

Eleven normal adults were given intravenously 400 mg of cortisol, and NK and ADCC activity was examined in the peripheral blood. NK activity was measured on Molt-4 and ADCC activity on antibody-sensitized RL male target cells. Four hours after cortisol treatment, both NK and ADCC activities were significantly but transiently increased.[305] Five normal volunteers received 300 mg of cortisol i.v. and the NK activity of their peripheral blood lymphocyte was studied using K562 cells as targets. The activity of NK cells increased significantly at 4 hr, decreased at 24 hr, and returned to normal at 48 hr after drug administration. Parallel variations were found in the fraction of lymphocytes bearing Fc receptors for IgG. Neither NK activity, nor the

Table 5

THE EFFECT OF GLUCOCORTICOIDS ON MONOCYTES AND MACROPHAGES

Species	Hormone	Dose/concentration	Biological effect	Ref.
Mouse		**In vivo**		
	Prednisolone	15 mg/kg/day p. os	Delayed clearance of *S. aureus* from lungs	272
	Cortisone	300 mg/kg s.c.	Inhibition of cell mediated immunity due to accessory cell deficiency	274
	Cortisone acetate	5—10 mg/mouse	Inhibition of humoral immunity due to accessory cell deficiency	275
	Hydrocortisone } Methylprednisolone	1—10 mg/mouse	Suppression of macrophage arming	280
		In vitro		
	Dexamethasone	$ID_{50} = 10^{-9}\ M$	Reduced glucose uptake, lactate production, CO_2 production	277
	Hydrocortisone } Prednisone	$ID_{50} = 2-5 \times 10^{-8}\ M$	Inhibition of Ia antigen expression	279
	Dexamethasone	0.2 mg/ml	Increased release of iron	278
	Hydrocortisone } Methylprednisolone	0.01—0.1 µg/ml	Suppression of arming by lymphokine	280
	Glucocorticoids	$10^{-7}-10^{-9}\ M$	Inhibition of cytotoxicity by interferon treated macrophages	281
	Hydrocortisone } Dexamethasone	$\left\{\begin{array}{l}25-100\ \mu g/ml \\ 2 \times 10^{-4}-10^{-8}\ M \\ 10^{-6}-10^{-9}\ M \\ ID_{50} = 2 \times 10^{-8}\ M\end{array}\right\}$	Decrease of phagocytosis and intracellular killing of certain microorganisms	282 283 285 287
Rat		**In vitro**		
	Hydrocortisone	$10^{-4}-10^{-6}\ M$	Inhibition of carrageenan-induced IL-1 secretion	290

83

Species		Drug	Dose/Concentration	Effect	Ref.
Guinea pig	*In vivo*	Cortisone acetate	100 mg s.c. for 7 days	Decrease of ADCC by alveolar Mf	192
		Bethamethasone	0.1—0.5% solution for topical treatment	Decrease in number of epidermal Langerhans cells	291
		Cortisone acetate	100 mg/kg s.c. daily for 7 days	Inhibited biosynthesis of C2 and C4	292
	In vitro	Hydrocortisone	10^{-4}—10^{-6} M	Inhibition of Mf aggregation due to macrophage aggregation factor	293
		Hydrocortisone	1—10 µg/mℓ	Blockage of migration inhibitory factor action on Mf	258
		Dexamethasone	1 µg/mℓ		257
		Triamcinolone acetonide	$ID_{50} = 3 \times 10^{-8}$ M	Inhibition of response to Mf mitogenic factor	256
		Dexamethasone	10^{-6} M		
		Prednisolone	10^{-6} M		
Man	*In vitro*	Cortisol	1 mg/mℓ, 2.5×10^{-6} M	Inhibition of monocyte to macrophage differentiation	294,295
		Bethamethasone	1.5 µg/mℓ	Inhibition of Fc receptors	296
		Hydrocortisone }	16 µg/mℓ	Inhibition of chemotaxis, random migration, and bactericidal activity	298
		Prednisolone	25—100 ng/mℓ		299
		Hydrocortisone	10^{-5} M	Inhibition of IL-1 production	244
		Methylprednisolone	0.3 and 2.5 µg/mℓ	Inhibition of IL-1 production	243
		Hydrocortisone	0.1—100 µg/mℓ	Inhibition of antigen presentation	253
		Hydrocortisone	10 µg/mℓ	Induction of PMN migration stimulating factor	300

Note: ADCC = antibody dependent cellular cytotoxicity; Ia = I region coded surface antigen; ID_{50} = dose/concentration exerting 50% inhibition; IL-1 = interleukin 1; PMN = polymorphonuclear.

number of Fc receptor positive cells, was influenced by cortisol treatment, when the results were related to blood volume. In vitro preincubation of NK cells with cortisol for 24 hr had no effect on viability, expression of surface markers, or cytotoxicity. Therefore, NK cells are cortisol resistant, at least under the conditions studied. The variations observed after in vivo administration of cortisol seemed to be due to a reversible redistribution of NK effectors.[306] The activity of NK cells from peripheral blood of six female patients with lupus erythematosus, which were not on corticosteroid therapy, was compared with 15 age-matched corticosteroid treated female patients. Cytotoxic activity was significantly suppressed in the steroid treated group, especially in patients on high dose corticosteroid. However, there was no close correlation between the daily doses of steroids, when cytotoxic activity was determined before and during corticosteroid therapy in the same patients.[307]

NK cell activity of human peripheral blood lymphocytes, as measured by the lysis of K562 cells, was inhibited transiently and reversibly by dexamethasone treatment in vitro.[308] In vitro treatment of human peripheral blood leukocytes for 18 to 24 hr with *physiological* concentrations of glucocorticoids resulted in a marked decrease (up to 90%) of NK activity. The effect was both time- and dose-dependent and was specific for glucocorticoids. Viabilities of corticosteroid treated and untreated cultures were similar. Mixing experiments did not demonstrate the involvement of suppressor cells in the inhibition. Inducers of interferon and purified human leukocyte interferon subtype A enhanced NK activity in the presence of glucocorticoids, although this enhancement was lower when compared to the one produced in steroid free cultures.[309]

Effector cells mediating ADCC and NK cytotoxicity in humans could not be separated in vitro by a variety of procedures. However, the administration of dexamethasone to cell donors caused a relative increase in ADCC but a profound decrease in NK activity. In vitro dexamethasone treatment in pharmacologic and suprapharmacologic concentrations caused no change in ADCC but significantly decreased NK activity.[310] The treatment of human lymphocytes with prednisolone inhibited significantly both the NK activity (7.5×10^{-3} to 1×10^{-5} M) and ADCC activity (7.5×10^{-3} to 1×10^{-4} M), when added directly to the mixture of effector and target cells. Preincubation of lymphocytes with prednisolone for 24 hr suppressed significantly NK activity at concentrations ranging from 10^{-4} to 10^{-6} M. Inhibition was dose-dependent and was observed as early as 1 hr of incubation, at various effector target cell ratios and with several targets. Prednisolone also inhibited NK and ADCC activities of purified T cells, non T cells, and NK-enriched effector cells. In target binding assays, prednisolone decreased the binding capacity of effector cells in a dose-dependent manner. Prednisolone induced inhibition could be reversed by the incubation of lymphocytes for 1 hr with interferon or IL-2. The inhibition of cytotoxicity by prednisolone was not due to direct toxicity to the effector cells.[311] The effect of glucocorticoids on killer and NK cells is summarized in Table 6.

10. The Effect of Glucocorticoids on Granulocytes and Mast Cells
a. Mouse

Pretreatment of mouse mast cells with dexamethasone (10^{-7} to 10^{-6} M), during overnight sensitization with mouse IgE antibodies, resulted in inhibition of antigen induced histamine release and degranulation. This inhibition was time-dependent, reaching a maximum after approximately 16 hr. The addition of dexamethasone to sensitized mast cells immediately before antigen challenge was ineffective. Dexamethasone bound to specific cytoplasmic receptors of mast cells and did not affect the binding of IgE to mast cells or intracellular cAMP levels. Dexamethasone inhibited the antigen induced phospholipid methylation and calcium ion uptake, but failed to affect histamine release by the calcium ionophore A23187.[312]

Table 6
THE EFFECT OF GLUCOCORTICOIDS ON KILLER AND NATURAL KILLER CELLS

Species	Hormone	Dose/concentration	Biological effect	Ref.
Mouse		*In vivo*		
	Cortisone acetate	500 mg/kg s.c.	Splenic K cells depressed by 25%, bone marrow K cells increased by 70%	301
	Hydrocortisone acetate	2.5 mg/mouse i.p.	NK cells sharply decreased, F_1 resistance to parental marrow unaffected	302
	Hydrocortisone acetate	2.5 or 3.75 mg/mouse i.p.	Substantial transient reduction of splenic NK due to suppressor cells	303
		In vitro		
	Dexamethasone	10^{-7}—10^{-11} M	Suppression of NK cells in spleen cultures	304
Man		*In vivo*		
	Hydrocortisone	400 mg i.v.	NK and ADCC increased at 4 hr	305
	Hydrocortisone	300 mg i.v.	Increase of NK at 4 hr, decrease at 24 hr, return to normal at 48 hr	306
		In vitro		
	Dexamethasone	12 mg p. os	Decrease of NK, increase of ADCC effector cells	310
	Dexamethasone	100—200 $\mu g/m\ell$	Reversible inhibition of NK	308
	Glucocorticoids	10^{-6}—10^{-7} M	Decrease of NK activity, interferon A reversed suppression	309
	Prednisolone	7.5×10^{-3}—10^{-5} M	{ Inhibition of NK, reversed by IL-2 / Inhibition of ADCC, reversed by IL-2	311 / 311

Note: K cells = killer cells active in antibody dependent cellular cytotoxicity; NK = natural killer cells; F_1 = first generation after crossing two inbred strains; ADCC = antibody dependent cellular cytotoxicity.

b. Rat

A single dose of cortisone, given to rats, led to the destruction of mast cells, which was followed by regeneration in the lymphatic organs. However, depletion of mature cells was evident even after 5 days. Prolonged treatment caused a similar destruction, but regeneration was slow.[313] Mast cells from rats, injected i.m. with dexamethasone for 4 days, had unaffected β adrenergic receptor function, but exhibited an impaired ability to release mediators. This was shown by sensitization with IgE antibodies and challenge with the specific antigens, or by exposure to the calcium ionophore A23187.[314] Rats were treated with cortisol (0.4 to 400 μg), MP (0.5 to 500 μg), or dexamethasone (7.6 μg) daily for 3 days. The late phase reaction to the intradermal injection of anti-IgE (capable of inducing mast cells degranulation), or of isolated mast cell granules, was then investigated. Corticosteroids prevented the development of late phase inflammatory response in the skin, which in controls was characterized by polymorphonuclear infiltrates at 2 to 8 hr, followed by mononuclear cell infiltrates at 24 to 48 hr.[315]

Rat peritoneal mast cells release substantial amounts of type E prostaglandin when stimulated in vitro by fetal calf serum or incubated in the presence of arachidonic acid. Hydrocortisone did not affect such prostaglandin release.[316]

A single dose of cortisol, given to rats aged 5 to 6 months, led to a sharp decrease of eosinophils in the spleen, due primarily to the reduction of mature eosinophils. At the same time there was a relative increase in the number of proliferating eosinophil precursor cells. Long-term administration of cortisol resulted in an inhibition of mitotic activity of these eosinophil precursors. There was no indication that the peripheral eosinopenia caused by cortisol treatment could be due to the migration of eosinophils to the spleen and/or splenic destruction of eosinophils. Mature eosinophils were also decreased in the bone marrow. During repeated injections, there was a continued proliferation of eosinophil precursor cells, but mitotic activity was reduced.[317,318] Others found that cortisol induced a migration of eosinophil leukocytes from blood to lymphoid organs such as the spleen, lymph nodes, and thymus, but not to other tissues.[319]

c. Man

After the intradermal injection to human subjects of anti-IgE antiserum, a dual cutaneous allergic reaction occurs. It is characterized by an early wheel- and flare-response and a late allergic response due to infiltration of the site by polymorphonuclear and mononuclear cells. Corticosteroid failed to inhibit the early inflammatory response, but it did inhibit the late allergic response.[320] In vitro exposure of human basophils to glucocorticoids inhibits the IgE mediated histamine release. The order of potency of various glucocorticoid preparations was TA > dexamethasone > betamethasone > prednisolone > hydrocortisone. Histamine release induced by formyl methionine containing peptide (f-met-leu-phe), or by the calcium ionophore A23187, or by phorbol diester, was not inhibited by dexamethasone. Dexamethasone did not consistently alter the total, or occupied, basophil IgE Fc receptor numbers.[321,322]

Human eosinophils contained $10.8 \pm 3 \times 10^{-3}$ high affinity receptor sites per cell, with a dissociation constant of 15.3 ± 0.6 nM as revealed in ^{3}H-dexamethasone binding assays. Cortisol was capable of competing with ^{3}H-dexamethasone in the binding reaction, whereas progesterone, estradiol, estriol, and testosterone were less effective. Glucocorticoid binding in neutrophils had a K_d of 17.7 ± 0.8 nM dexamethasone with $11.0 \pm 0.8 \times 10^3$ highly specific sites per cell.[323] The incubation of human peripheral blood eosinophils in vitro with cortisol, or MP, resulted in a dose-dependent inhibition of chemotaxis. The minimal effective concentration was 0.1 mg/mℓ for both drugs. Using leading-front chemotaxis techniques, significant inhibition was detected at 1μg/mℓ cortisol. Eosinophils, incubated and washed free of corticosteroids, responded normally to chemo-attractants, indicating that the inhibitory effect was reversible. Eosinophils, isolated from donors receiving 40 mg of prednisone orally for 4 days, showed normal chemotactic responses, but eosinophils from donors receiving a 300 mg bolus of hydrocortisone exhibited a reduced chemotactic response. Eosinophil adherence to nylon wool columns was also reduced transiently following in vivo corticosteroid administration.[324]

Granulocytes, isolated from the blood of patients treated with a high dose of MP, or by alternate day prednisone, exhibited a decreased adherence to plastic surfaces, which was of transient nature.[325,326] Neutrophils from ten patients receiving prednisone, dexamethasone, or cortisol sodium succinate were found capable of normal phagocytosis of latex particles. The reduction of nitroblue tetrazolium was impaired in cells of such patients. Normal neutrophils, treated in vitro with 5 μg/mℓ of cortisol, exhibited normal latex phagocytosis. Impaired nitroblue tetrazolium reduction occurred only at 20 times higher drug concentration.[327]

The exposure of highly purified polymorphonuclear leukocytes to cortisol in vitro augmented the isoproterenol induced increase of cAMP content and inhibited enzyme release.[328] Preincubation of human neutrophils with isoproterenol for 3 hr resulted in an 86% reduction of subsequent isoproterenol stimulated cAMP accumulation in the cells. This phenomenon was associated with a 40% reduction in the number of β-adrenergic receptors, and the remaining receptors appeared to be relatively uncoupled from adenylate cyclase. When cortisol was added to the desensitizing incubations (combined treatment), a significant attenuation in the desensitization process was observed, as revealed by increased cAMP levels in the cells. Although this combined treatment did not influence the decline in receptor number, it did prevent the uncoupling of the receptors. Prednisolone was similar to cortisol in attenuating isoproterenol-induced uncoupling.[329]

Cortisol sodium succinate inhibited the adherence of IgG-coated erythrocytes to human peripheral blood neutrophil monolayers in a dose-dependent and reversible manner. This effect was demonstrable even when cortisol was added at the same time as erythrocytes, though it was unable to displace bound erythrocytes. Therefore, cortisol can interfere with the availability of neutrophil Fc receptors for binding.[330] A significant increase in the sphingomyelin content of human polymorphonuclear leukocytes was observed after incubation with dexamethasone (8×10^{-9} to 8×10^{-5} M) for 2 hr, together with an increase in sphingomyelinase content.[331] Lysosomal enzyme discharge from human neutrophils by immobilized, heat aggregated IgG was inhibited by MP sodium succinate, triamcinolone acetonide hemisuccinate, paramethasone acetate, and cortisol sodium succinate. These glucocorticoids also inhibited zymosan-induced release of β-glucuronidase from neutrophils that had been pretreated with cytochalasin B in order to prevent the onset of phagocytosis. Mineralocorticoids were ineffective in this respect. None of the glucocorticoids tested elicited any significant effects on neutrophil adherence or lysosomal enzyme activities.[332] Pretreatment of human neutrophils with corticosteroid inhibited the induction of elastase by LPS.[333]

Aggregation of neutrophils, induced in vitro by zymosan-activated plasma, was inhibited by MP and cortisol at concentrations comparable to plasma levels achieved with large bolus (30 mg/kg i.v.) therapy, advocated in shock states. Dexamethasone had little effect. Polymorphonuclear aggregation and embolization in mesenteric vessels of rats, given intra-arterial infusions of zymosan-activated plasma, was also prevented by pretreatment with 30 mg/kg of MP.[334] Cortisol, MP, and dexamethasone treatment of human granulocytes inhibited the interaction of the synthetic chemotaxin, f-methionine-leucine-phenylalanine, with its specific receptor. Receptor number was unaffected, but a decrease in association rate was observed. Furthermore, aggregated granulocytes were found to disaggregate upon addition of corticosteroids. The order of the potency was MP > cortisol > dexamethasone, with MP concentration of 2 to 3 mg/mℓ being required for disaggregation.[335] LPS inhibits the chemotactic response of neutrophils to C5a, but has no effect on chemotaxis toward bacteria derived factors. MP $(5 \times 10^{-5}\ M)$, cortisol $(4.5 \times 10^{-4}\ M)$, and dexamethasone $(1.25 \times 10^{-5}\ M)$ interfered effectively with this LPS effect. Thus, the inhibition of human neutrophil chemotaxis by endotoxin can be antagonized by glucocorticoids.[336]

The attachment and ingestion of IgE-C3d complexes by human neutrophils was decreased by cortisol treatment $(5 \times 10^{-5}\ M)$. Cortisol primarily affected the binding capacity of Fc and C3d receptors.[337] Cortisol, at high concentrations (0.5 to 2 mg/mℓ), reduced the phagocytosis of *Staphylococcus aureus* and the production of lactate by human neutrophils. Bactericidal activity and production of CO_2 from glucose in phagocytosing leukocytes was not influenced by these cortisol concentrations.[338]

Cortisol sodium succinate inhibited in vitro the ADCC of human neutrophil cells. Inhibition was dose-dependent and reversible. Cortisol, added after the binding between effector and target cells, was still inhibitory, suggesting that the drug interferes in a later step that takes place after effector target interactions. MP and dexamethasone had a similar effect.[339] The effects of glucocorticoids on granulocytes and mast cells are summarized in Table 7.

11. The Effect of Glucocorticoids on Platelets
a. Man

Human platelets metabolize cortisol to 20 β-hydrocortisol and tetra-hydrocortisol.[340] Furthermore, cortisol inhibits platelet aggregation in vitro by inhibiting platelet phospholipase A_2. This inhibition occurs at greater concentrations than what is usually achieved in clinical practice. In patients with collagen and hematological diseases treated with prednisone, the bleeding time, capillary fragility, threshold ADP concentrations for secondary platelet aggregation, and platelet adhesiveness were unchanged by 2 days and 6 weeks of treatment. Initial high platelet counts were not affected at 2 days of treatment, but fell significantly below normal values after 6 weeks of treatment. Initial high levels of factor VIII related antigen did not increase significantly following 2 days of treatment, but after 6 weeks a significant increase was detected. In patients of this category, a 2-week treatment with commonly used doses of prednisone did not significantly affect platelet function.[341,342]

12. Glucocorticoids and the Immune Response
a. Mouse

The serum concentrations of IgE, IgA, and IgM were reduced in mice receiving cortisol acetate. Turnover studies, using ^{131}I-labeled IgG2a, demonstrated that high dose corticosteroid increased the catabolic rate. This was not due to excess loss in the urine or stool, but rather reflected an increase in endogenous catabolism.[343] Mice given cortisone acetate (4 to 5 mg/kg) near the time of sheep red cell antigen injection, exhibited depressed IgG and IgM antibody formation.[344] Mice, treated with 5 mg cortisone acetate 1 day prior to the injection of SRBC, showed more than 95% suppression of splenic PFC, but the anti-SRBC hemolytic titer in the blood was not affected. PFC in the bone marrow of cortisone treated mice increased to more than ten times their number compared with control animals.[345] IgM and IgG antibodies in serum and PFC in the thymus, spleen, femoral marrow, popliteal-, thoracic-, and mesenteric lymph nodes of mice, given a single injection of cortisol acetate, were examined at various times after primary immunization with SRBC. There was a close correlation between suppression of serum antibody and the splenic PFC response, and a few PFC could be detected elsewhere.[346]

Daily injections of mice with dexamethasone, starting 1 day before immunization

Table 7

THE EFFECT OF GLUCOCORTICOIDS ON GRANULOCYTES AND MAST CELLS

Species	Hormone	Dose/concentration	Cell type	Biological effect	Ref.
Mouse	Dexamethasone	In vitro 10^{-7}—10^{-6} M	Ma	Inhibition of antigen-induced histamine release	312
	Hydrocortisone acetate	In vivo 2 mg/mouse s.c.	Eo	Eosinopenia	185
Rat		In vivo			
	Cortisone acetate	10—50 mg/kg i.m.	Ma	Destruction, inhibited regeneration	313
	Dexamethasone	100 μg/rat i.m. for 4 days	Ma	Inhibition of mediator release	314
	Cortisol	5 mg/rat single or every 6 hr for 3 days	Eo	Eosinopenia due to destruction and altered distribution	317 318
	Hydrocortisone sodium succinate	50 mg/kg i.v.	Eo	Eosinopenia due to destruction and altered distribution	319
Man		In vitro			
	Glucocorticoids	$ID_{50} \cong 10^{-7}$—10^{-9} M	Ba	Inhibition of IgE-dependent mediator release	321,322
		In vivo/vitro			
	Hydrocortisone	1 μg—2 mg/mℓ	Eo	Concentration, dose dependent and reversible inhibition of chemotaxis	324
	Hydrocortisone Prednisone	300 mg bolus i.v. 40 mg orally			

Table 7 (continued)
THE EFFECT OF GLUCOCORTICOIDS ON GRANULOCYTES AND MAST CELLS

Species	Hormone	Dose/concentration	Cell Type	Biological effect	Ref.
		In vivo			
	Cortisol	200 mg i.v.	Ne	Granulocytosis	200
	Hydrocortisone	100 mg i.v.	Ne	Granulocytosis	201
	Prednisone	30—125 mg/day			
	Dexamethasone	16 mg/day			
	Prednisone	30—125 mg/day	Ne	Impaired reduction of nitroblue tetrazolium	327
	Dexamethasone	16 mg/day			
	Hydrocortisone sodium succinate	30—125 mg/day			
	Hydrocortisone	2.7×10^{-6} M	Ne	Modulation of β-adrenergic receptor	329
	Hydrocortisone	2×10^{-4} M	Ne	Inhibition of FcR-IgG interactions	330
	Hydrocortisone	5×10^{-5} M	Ne	Inhibition of FcR-IgG and C3b-receptor interactions	337
	Methylprednisolone Hydrocortisone Dexamethasone	0.2—3 mg/mℓ	Ne	Inhibition of chemotactic receptor — chemoattractant (f — methionine — leucine — phenylaline) interaction	335
	Dexamethasone	8×10^{-9}—8×10^{-5} M	Ne	Increase in sphingomyelin and sphyngomyelinase content	331
	Glucocorticoids	10^{-5}—10^{-9} M	Ne	Inhibition of LPS induced elastase accumulation	333
	Methylprednisolone Triamcinolone Paramethasone	10^{-6} M	Ne	Inhibition of lysosomal enzyme discharge triggered by immobilized aggregated IgG or by zymosan	332
	Hydrocortisone	$ID_{50} = 10^{-5}$ M			
	Methylprednisolone	5×10^{-5} M			
	Hydrocortisone	4.5×10^{-5} M	Ne	Inhibition of chemotaxis elicited by LPS	336
	Dexamethasone	1.25×10^{-5} M			
	Methylprednisolone	0.25—4.0 mg/mℓ	Ne	Inhibition of aggregation due to zymosan activated plasma	334
	Hydrocortisone	0.25—12.5 mg/mℓ			
	Hydrocortisone	0.5—2 mg/mℓ	Ne	Inhibition of phagocytosis of *S. aureus* and production of lactate	338

Note: B = basophilic; C3b = split product of the 3rd complement component; Eo = eosinophilic; FcR = Fc receptor; ID_{50} = drug concentration exerting 50% inhibition; LPS = lipopolysaccharide isolated from Gram-negative bacteria; Ma = mast cell; Ne = neutrophilic granulocyte.

with LPS, suppressed the anti-LPS PFC response in the spleen, which was dose related. The bone marrow PFC response showed a dose-dependent enhancement at the same time, reaching the maximum of a 3- to 15-fold increase at 7 days, after daily injections of 16 mg dexamethasone per kilogram body weight. The same effect was found in genetically athymic nude mice, indicating that T cells are not involved.[347] The antibody response of cortisol pretreated mice against thymus dependent and thymus independent antigens was compared with those of normal mice. The antibody response to all antigens tested was significantly reduced by cortisol. Additional experiments performed in vitro suggested that the susceptibility of splenic B cells to cortisol treatment was higher than that of T cells, although the helper T cell function was suppressed significantly. No impairment of macrophage functions by cortisol was observed.[348]

Mice were immunized with human IgG, incorporated into a water-in-oil-in-water emulsion, of which the water-in-oil droplets contained the antigen and, in some groups, dexamethasone phosphate (a water soluble cortisone). Dexamethasone suppressed the antibody response to human IgG when incorporated with the antigen into the emulsion, but had no effect when applied separately. Both IgG and IgM antibodies were affected. When dexamethasone and LPS (a thymus independent antigen) were incorporated into oil droplets and used for immunization, no suppressive effect was observed.[349]

Intraperitoneal injection of BALB/c mice with *Corynebacterium parvum* 3 days prior to injection of SRBC stimulated the IgG PFC response. Simultaneous i.p. injection of cortisol depressed the stimulatory effect of *C. parvum* on IgM PFC, but not the IgG PFC response.[350]

Tolerance, induced in mice by isologous IgG coupled to fluorescein, was maintained for a longer period with cortisone administration, without the induction of tolerance being affected. Antigen binding cells were cortisone resistant in the system and were present in treated animals for a longer period of time than in animals injected with a tolerogen only. Receptor blockage by cortisone was proposed as the mechanism of maintenance of tolerance.[351]

The IgE response in SJL mice showed a diurnal curve which appeared to be determined by normal variations in endogenous corticosteroid levels. Furthermore, the normal IgE pattern could be perturbed by administration of cortisone at the proper time of day.[352]

Heparin, injected subcutaneously in a depot form 2 hr before immunization, restores the antibody response of mice immunosuppressed by cortisol. A similar pretreatment, 3 days before immunization, decreases the PFC count in the spleen. Cortisone administered i.p. or heparin given subcutaneously at about the time of immunization, with suboptimal doses of SRBC, had little or no effect on splenic PFC count and serum antibody levels. However, cortisone and heparin applied jointly exerted a stimulatory effect on the antibody response to SRBC.[353]

Cortisol treatment of mice reduced lymphocyte numbers in the spleen by 88% after 48 hr, but cultures of the remaining cells produced as many PFC in vitro after stimulation with SRBC as did cultures of equal numbers of normal spleen cells. When normal spleen cell cultures were incubated with cortisol for 4 hr prior to the addition of the antigen, PFC responses per culture, and per 10^6 cells, occurred 24 hr later than in controls and averaged, respectively, 27 and 140% of control values. Minimum viable cell numbers were observed in cortisol treated cultures at 3 days, and the cell numbers increased gradually thereafter. The PFC responses were not significantly altered when cultures were treated simultaneously with cortisol and antigen, or if the addition of antigen preceded that of cortisol by more than 4 hr. Suppression was also considerably reduced if fetal calf serum was used when preparing cells for culture.[354] Small amounts of cortisol were found to be necessary for the in vitro production of antibody with primed cell populations in serum free medium.[355]

The production of antibody in vitro by normal and antigen primed mouse spleen cells was suppressed by the addition of cortisol to the cultures. Both normal and antigen activated helper T lymphocytes and accessory cells were inhibited. Spleen cells, cultured overnight in medium containing fetal bovine serum, became highly resistant to the effects of cortisol. Resistance also occurred, when spleen cells were cultured with accessory cells, that previously had been activated with bacterial LPS to produce cell free factors termed *glucocorticosteroid response modifying factors* (GRMF). These factors provided protection against steroid immunosuppression in a dose-dependent fashion leading to the recovery of helper T cell function, which otherwise was suppressed by steroids. Activity of GRMF was also obtained from murine monocyte cell lines.[356,357]

Cortisone treatment of mice bearing allogeneic skin grafts leads to significant prolongation of graft survival.[358] When recipient mice are treated with small doses of cortisol, in combination with inhibitors of prostaglandin synthesis (indomethacine or flufenamate), the mean survival of allogeneic grafts was prolonged from 11.4 days to 20.9 and 23.8 days, respectively.[359]

Cortisone treatment of donors decreased the cell population in the spleen to 21%, the bone marrow to 79%, and the thymus to 6% of normal value, but did not abolish the ability of these cells to induce GVHR. On the contrary, cortisone treated cells were significantly more active when compared with equal numbers of untreated cells.[360]

Topically applied corticosteroids inhibited the induction of contact hypersensitivity reactions in mice by DNCB.[361] Cortisol treatment of mice, 3 days after sensitization with oxazolone, suppressed the manifestation of delayed-type hypersensitivity on the 10th day, but not on the 17th day. The weight of lymph nodes was also significantly decreased both in control and oxazolone sensitized mice. Dexamethasone binding capacity of regional lymph node cells was increased 72 hr after sensitization. High doses of cortisol, given 3 days after sensitization, did not permanently eliminate delayed hypersensitivity to oxazolone, indicating that memory cells survived.[362]

Cortisol, at concentrations of 25 to 150 μg/mℓ, inhibited the cytotoxic effect of specifically sensitized lymphoid cells without preventing their aggregation with the target cells.[363] In MLC containing BALB/c responder and C57BL/6 stimulator splenocytes, DNA synthesis was markedly reduced in the presence of cortisol. The in vitro generation of cytotoxic lymphocytes was also inhibited. Cortisol did not suppress the cytotoxic activity of previously sensitized effector cells.[364]

b. Rat

Rats, treated with a single injection of cortisone during the 1st week of life, developed general wasting, growth retardation, which was associated with a destruction of lymphoid tissue, and immune depression.[365] The rejection of F$_1$ kidney grafts by Lewis rats was delayed by treatment with MP (16 mg/kg/day), in conjunction with enhancing serum.[366]

The sensitization of rat lymphocytes against mouse or rat embryonic fibroblasts in culture was facilitated by 1 μg/mℓ of cortisol or prednisolone. During sensitization, a prolonged decrease in the total number of recoverable lymphocytes was observed. However, the lytic potency of large, transformed lymphocytes was much greater in these treated cultures. The same concentration of glucocorticoid hormones inhibited the cytolytic effect by about 50% without reducing the viability of sensitized lymphocytes. Dose-dependent toxicity to lymphocytes and increasing inhibition of cytolytic effect appeared at higher concentrations of these hormones. Cortisol probably suppressed cytolysis by preventing the primary activation of the cytolytic mechanism. Suppression was most efficient when cortisol was added at the beginning of the cytolytic reaction. The cytolytic mechanism itself appeared to remain intact and could be activated by Con A, despite the presence of cortisol. The influence of cortisol on cytolysis was not modified by vitamin A, an agent that antagonizes the effect of this hormone on lysosome membranes. Cortisol was less effective in suppressing the cytotoxicity of lymphocytes, which had already been sensitized in the presence of cortisol. During sensitization, cortisol enhanced lymphocyte multiplication during the quiescent stage. Once proliferation started, neither cortisol nor the antigen specific sensitizing fibroblasts were necessary. Treatment of lymphocytes with cortisol for 1 hr before their contact with the sensitizing cells was sufficient to augment proliferation during sensitization. These effects of cortisol are not directly related to the degree of lymphocyte elimination. Therefore, in addition to killing unreacted lymphocytes, cortisol facilitates the induction of cell mediated immunity in vitro by enhancing the proliferation of lymphocytes.[367-369]

c. Guinea Pig

The effect of corticosteroids on the in vivo clearance of ^{51}Cr-labeled guinea pig erythrocytes, sensitized with purified rabbit IgG or IgM antibody, was studied. Corticosteroid therapy for 5 days prior to the injection of antibody coated cells was required for a maximal increase in the survival of sensitized erythrocytes.[370]

The established cellular immune response of guinea pigs, previously sensitized to tuberculin, was decreased after chronic cortisone treatment, as revealed by antigen induced MIF and proliferation assays. Although similar levels of lymphocytopenia were induced by acute and chronic glucocorticosteroid treatment, only chronic treatment was associated with depression of certain cell mediated lymphocyte functions.[371] Tuberculin hypersensitivity in guinea pigs was diminished by three daily injections of cortisone, as compared to one injection of ACTH. Fourteen days after treatment with cortisone, or ACTH, there was an opposite trend — the treated animals showed more hypersensitivity than the controls.[372]

In vitro cortisol (10^{-3} M) did not prevent guinea pig lymphocytes from secreting macrophage aggregation factor after exposure to the specific antigen, but did interfere with the response of nonimmune macrophages to this factor.[373]

d. Rabbit

Treatment of rabbits with 10 mg cortisone daily prolonged the survival of skin homografts. The grafts appeared healthy but did not heal into the graft bed, and failed to vascularize when, 2 mg of cortisone was applied to the graft at the time of grafting and on the 3rd and 6th days afterwards. Whenever graft survival was prolonged, there was a significant reduction in the number of immunoblasts in the draining lymph node.[374] Skin grafts were prolonged and spleen weights were reduced in rabbits treated with 1 mg/kg of MP for 5 days with 2 mg/kg on alternate days, or by the combination of these two treatment schedules.[375]

Acute allergic alveolitis, induced in rabbits by inhaled allergens, was inhibited by MP acetate given every 72 hr. This treatment induced a pronounced peripheral lymphopenia, thymic involution, and an almost complete disappearance of bronchial lymphoid tissue. A marked decrease in the total cell count and in the percentage of lymphocytes was noticed in the bronchial alveolar fluid of the treated animals with hypersensitivity pneumonitis. No signs of interstitial or intra-alveolar inflammatory reactions were seen in the lungs of glucocorticoid treated animals 3 weeks after aerosol antigen challenge.[376] Complement and neutrophil mediated immune reactions, induced in rabbits, were inhibited only minimally by cortisol and MP, although protein exudation induced by bradykinin and histamine were inhibited significantly.[377]

Secondary antibody response can be initiated in lymph node organ cultures prepared from immunized rabbits. During the inductive phase (day 0 to 9), in serum-free medium, there was an absolute requirement for *physiological levels* (0.01 to 0.1 μM) of cortisol, corticosterone, or certain related glucocorticoids. Other steroids, such as progesterone, testosterone, and estrogen did not support the antibody response and at 1 to 10 μM levels were inhibitory during the induction phase. This inhibition was partially overcome by cortisol at high, nontoxic levels (1 to 10 μM).[378]

e. Man

The effects of therapeutic doses of prednisone (30 mg/day) on IgG metabolism was studied in eight patients. There was no significant decrease in the measured levels of serum IgG, but in all patients the half-life was shortened and the catabolic rate was increased. The maintenance of normal IgG levels under these conditions must be the result of an increased synthetic rate.[379] Seventeen normal adult male volunteers were given 96 mg of MP daily for 3 to 5 days and compared to 12 untreated controls studied simultaneously. IgG, IgA, and to a lesser extent, IgM levels were decreased significantly in volunteers: the lowest immunoglobulin levels occurring on the 2nd week after a 3-day course and during the 3rd week after a 5-day course of MP. Increase in the rate of plasma clearance of IgG occurred only during the treatment period itself. Three months after drug administration IgG concentrations had turned toward normal but were still somewhat below base line values; so were total γ globulin concentrations. By this time IgM and IgA concentrations were normal.[380,381] Immunoglobulin levels were studied also in asthmatic patients requiring corticosteroid therapy and were compared with patients not receiving corticosteroids. IgG and IgA levels were decreased, IgM was unchanged, and serum IgE was elevated significantly 1 week after initiation of therapy, but returned to base line, or below, at 6 to 8 weeks. Suppression of IgG and IgA levels was prolonged.[382,383] In patients with immune thrombocytopenia, prolonged high dose corticosteroid therapy decreased IgG secretion by bone marrow cells, beginning at 3 weeks after treatment and reaching levels approximately one fourth of pretreatment rates after 6 weeks. Splenic IgG production was not affected. Marrow IgG synthesis in these patients was found to be three to ten times greater than the corresponding splenic production rates and appeared to correlate with serum IgG levels.[384]

Twelve children with asthma, six receiving prednisone therapy, were immunized with keyhole limpet hemocyanin (KLH). Prednisone treatment tended to enhance the primary IgG and IgM antibody response, but had no effect on antibody levels formed after a second injection of KLH.[385] Groups of six patients with classic rheumatoid arthritis, unresponsive to conventional therapy, were given 1 g i.v. doses of MP daily, and the immune response and clinical activity were followed for 16 weeks. Skin test reactivity to recall antigens, such as PPD and histoplasmin, were preserved. The primary antibody response to KLH, and secondary antibody responses to tetanus and typhoid vaccines, were similar in both the prednisolone treated and nontreated groups. Serum gamma globulin concentrations were unchanged.[386]

Plasma samples were obtained from 12 patients on chronic prednisone treatment, following their usual oral dose of prednisone (0.262 to 0.053 mg/kg/day), and following an equivalent amount of prednisone given i.v. The plasma concentrations of prednisone, capable of inhibiting the mixed lymphocyte reaction (MLR) by 50% following the oral and i.v. applications, were 66.3 ± 26.7 and 86.5 ± 30.9 ng/mℓ, respectively; for free prednisone concentrations, the corresponding values were 10.0 ± 5.0 and 12.4 ± 12.6 ng/mℓ.[387] Single oral doses of 10, 15, and 30 mg of prednisone caused a diminution of circulating T cells and monocytes and inhibited significantly the autologous, but not the allogeneic, MLR. These effects were maximal 6 hr after drug administration and disappeared by 24 hr. Autologous MLR reactions were significantly and consistently suppressed 2 hr after drug administration, before reduction in circulating lymphoid cells had occurred. Macrophage enriched stimulating cells were more easily suppressed than responding T cells.[388]

Low concentrations (10^{-7} to 10^{-5} M) of cortisol inhibited profoundly the primary in vitro antibody response of human peripheral blood lymphocytes. The kinetics of the response was not modified. However, cortisol (10^{-5} M) did not prevent the generation of Con A induced suppressor cells for antibody response. Nonspecific immunoglobulin secretion, which was associated with the specific response, was relatively resistant to cortisol.[389] Mitogen stimulated immunoglobulin secretion was augmented by 1 μg/mℓ of cortisol in culture.[390]

The continuous presence of cortisol in culture, curing the generation of cytotoxic T lymphocytes against alloantigens, reduced the total number of killer cells recovered. However, equal numbers of effector lymphocytes, generated in the presence or absence of cortisol, produced equivalent specific lysis. Cortisol or MP failed to influence significantly the killing process.[391] The response of normal human T lymphocytes to autologous irradiated lymphocytes, enriched in B cells, was suppressed completely by the addition to the culture of 4×10^{-7} M cortisol. Even 2 to 8×10^{-8} M cortisol suppressed this autologous MLR by 62 to 84%, whereas it did not affect proliferation in the allogeneic MLC. This marked suppression of autologous MLR, without any suppression of the allogeneic MLR, by *physiological* concentrations of cortisol, suggests a regulatory role of T cell autoreactivity in vivo.[392]

There is a vast amount of literature on the treatment of various immune disorders and inflammatory conditions by a number of synthetic glucocorticoid preparations in patients. It is beyond the scope of this chapter to survey these publications. Instead, the interested reader is referred to recent reviews.[85,86] The effects of glucocorticoids on immune reactions are summarized in Table 8.

f. Other Species

Chicks were treated intramuscularly with 7.5 mg of cortisone acetate, twice a day at hatch, from hatch to 2 days, from hatch to 4 days, and from 7 to 10 days of age. Treatment from hatch to 2 or 4 days suppressed significantly antibody production in all experiments, whereas treatment between 7 and 10 days did not influence the antibody response.[393]

The rejection of renal adenocarcinoma allografts, planted into the anterior eye chamber of northern leopard frogs (*Rana pipiens*), was inhibited by corticosterone (500 μg/20 g) and aldosterone (50 μg/20 g), though the number of circulating small lymphocytes in steroid treated frogs was not significantly different from those of uninjected, or solvent injected frogs.[394]

IV. CATECHOLAMINES AND ACETYLCHOLINE

In a recent textbook of endocrinology, Melmon[395] discusses catecholamines, acetylcholine, serotonin, histamine, and vasoactive polypeptides under the general term autacoids, which is created from the Greek words *autos* meaning self, and *akos* meaning medical agent or remedy. The justification for this new classification is that these substances share common occurrences; often have coordinating interactions under physiologic or pathologic conditions; their direct effect often mimics or complements each other; and drugs that affect the synthesis or function of one often affect the body's response to the others. Autacoids interact simultaneously at multiple levels in the body directly or indirectly and sometimes in combination. Their effects may be additive or antagonistic.

Histamine and serotonin have been discussed briefly as mediators released by basophilic leukocytes and mast cells. Therefore, they are regarded as internal regulatory substances of the immune system rather than neurohormonal regulatory factors. For further information the reader is referred to the key references cited in Chapter 1.

Table 8

THE EFFECT OF GLUCOCORTICOIDS ON IMMUNE REACTIONS

Species	Hormone	Dose/concentration	Reaction	Biological effect	Ref.
Mouse		**In vivo**			
	Hydrocortisone acetate	0.25—5 mg/mouse s.c. daily	HI	Increased catabolism of IgG, IgA, IgM, leading to decreased serum levels	343
	Cortisol acetate	4—500 mgl/kg	HI	Depressed IgG and IgM antibody formation	345
		5 mg/mouse		Suppressed anti SRBC-PFC in spleen, but normal hemolytic titer in blood	346
		10 mg/mouse s.c.		Suppressed IgM and IgG PFC in spleen and serum antibody	
	Dexamethasone	16 mg/kg/day for 7 days	HI	Suppression of anti-LPS PFC in spleen, enhancement in bone marrow	347
	Hydrocortisone acetate	2.5 mg/mouse i.p.	HI	Reduced antibody response to TD and TI antigens	348
	Dexamethasone phosphate	0.25 and 1.0 mg/mouse	HI	Inhibition of antibody response against TD but not TI antigen, if given jointly in water-in-oil emulsion	349
	Hydrocortisone	50 μg/mouse i.p. for 2 consecutive days	HI	Inhibition of the adjuvant effect of *Corynebacterium parvum* on IgM antibodies	350
	Cortisone acetate	5 mg/mouse s.c.	HI	Prolongation of tolerance to TD and TI antigens	351
	Cortisol acetate	2.5 mg/mouse s.c.	HI	Inhibition of anti-SRBC PFC	354
		In vitro			
	Hydrocortisone	0.1 μg/mℓ	HI	Needed for antibody production by primed cells	355
		In vivo			
	Cortisone	0.5 mg/mouse on days 0—14	CMI	Inhibition of skin allograft rejection	358 359
		6—30 mg/kg			
	Glucocorticoids	0.05—0.1% lotion/ cream	DTH	Local inhibition of contact sensitivity	361
	Hydrocortisone acetate	400 mg/kg s.c.	DTH	Delay of DTH manifestation	362

Species	Drug	Route	Dose		Effect	Ref.
	Hydrocortisone	In vitro	25—150 μg/mℓ	CMI	Inhibition of cytotoxic effector cells	363
	Cortisol		1 ng—10 μg/mℓ	CMI	Inhibition of DNA synthesis and the generation of cytotoxic lymphocytes, no suppression of mature cytotoxic cells	364
Rat	Cortisone acetate	In vivo	1.25 mg/pup during 1st wk of life	HI,CMI	Wasting, growth retardation, lymphopenia	365
	Methylprednisolone		16 mg/kg	CMI	Delayed rejection of kidney grafts	366
	Hydrocortisone Prednisolone	In vitro	1 μg/mℓ	CMI	Facilitation of sensitization, inhibition of cytotoxic effector phase	367—69
Guinea pig	Cortisone acetate	In vivo	10—100 mg/kg for 4 days	HI	Decrease the clearance of IgG and IgM coated guinea pig erythrocytes	370
	Hydrocortisone sodium succinate		100 mg/kg single, or daily, for 7 days i.v.	CMI	Lymphopenia, decrease of MIF production after tuberculin challenge	371
	Methylprednisolone sodium succinate Cortisone		25 or 100 mg/kg 1 mg/guinea pig s.c. daily	CMI	Diminished tuberculin hypersensitivity	372
	Cortisol	In vitro	10^{-3} M		Prevention of Mf response to MAF	373

Table 8 (continued)

THE EFFECT OF GLUCOCORTICOIDS ON IMMUNE REACTIONS

Species	Hormone	Dose/concentration	Reaction	Biological effect	Ref.
Rabbit		*In vivo*			
	Cortisone	10 mg/rabbit daily	CMI	Prolongation of skin homograft rejection	374
	Methylprednisolone	1 mg/kg for 5 days	CMI	Prolongation of skin homograft rejection	375
		2 mg/kg, alternate days			376
	Methylprednisolone acetate	1-2 mg/kg every 3 days	CMI	Inhibition of allergic alveolitis	
		In vitro			
	Cortisol Corticosterone	$10^{-7}-10^{-8}\ M$	HI	*Physiological* concentrations are required for the secondary antibody response in serum free medium	378
Man		*In vivo*			
	Prednisone	30 mg/kg	HI	Shortened half life of IgG, increased catabolic rate, increased synthesis	379
	Methylprednisolone	96 mg, 3—5 days	HI	Decrease of circulating τ globulin, IgG, μgA, IgM, increased clearance of IgG	380
	Prednisone	38—54 mg/day	HI	Decrease of IgG production in bone marrow but not in spleen	381
					384

In vitro

| Hydrocortisone | 1 μg/mℓ | HI | Enhanced mitogen induced antibody synthesis | 390 |
| Hydrocortisone | 10^{-7}—10^{-5} M | HI | Inhibition of primary antibody response | 389 |

In vivo

| Prednisone | 0.262—1.053 mg/kg/day | CMI | Plasma inhibits the MLR reaction | 387 |
| Prednisone | 10—30 mg per os | — | Significant reduction of autologous MLR | 388 |

In vitro

| Hydrocortisone, methylprednisolone | 1—10 μg/mℓ | CMI | Reduction of generation of T_k in culture | 391 |
| Hydrocortisone | 2—8×10^{-8} M | — | Reduction of autologous MLR | 392 |

Note: CMI = cell mediated immunity; DTH = delayed-type hypersensitivity — a form of CMI; HI = humoral or antibody mediated immunity; LPS = bacterial lipopolysaccharide; MAF = macrophage aggregating factor; MIF = migration inhibitory factor; MLR = mixed lymphocyte reaction; PFC = plaque-forming (antibody secreting) cells; SRBC = sheep red blood cells; TD = T cell or thymus dependent; TI = T cell independent; T_k = killer T cell.

A. Catecholamines

Epinephrine (or adrenaline), norepinephrine (or noradrenaline), and dopamine are commonly referred to as catecholamines because of their structural relationship and common biosynthetic pathways. Catecholamines are synthesized in the brain, in sympathetic nerve endings, and in some cells of neural crest origin: the adrenal medulla and the organ of Zuckerkandl. Catecholamines have profound effects on smooth muscle, adipose tissue, myocardium, liver, brain, formed elements of the blood, a number of hormone producing organs, and the myometrium. Although the thymus and spleen both have innervation and the lymphoid cells residing in these organs may well be exposed to catecholamines secreted by nerve endings, the cells in the blood are exposed only to circulating catecholamines and are not influenced by the neuronally-derived catecholamines released in other tissues.

The major circulating catecholamine, epinephrine, is produced almost exclusively by the adrenal medulla, whereas norepinephrine originates from sympathetic nerve endings and, to a lesser extent, from the adrenal medulla. Although nerve stimulation is an important regulatory factor of catecholamine synthesis, ACTH is also involved in the normal maintenance of catecholamine synthesis by the adrenal medulla, through the mediation of glucocorticoids.[396,397] Glucocorticoids control tyrosine hydroxylase in the adrenal medulla, which is the rate-limiting enzyme of catecholamine synthesis. Furthermore, when humans or animals are subjected to extraordinary stress, the rate of catecholamine synthesis increases greatly. This is associated with an increase in production of synthesizing enzymes and sometimes may be limited by the availability of substrate for the enzymes. The rate of synthesis is integrated with, but not entirely dependent upon, production of ACTH, corticosteroids, and perhaps other trophic hormones produced by the pituitary. Epinephrine, in turn, stimulates the release of ACTH from the pituitary gland and has a synergistic effect with corticotropin releasing factor.[397-399] At the same time, catecholamines inhibit the release of other pituitary hormones, such as PRL, GH, luteinizing hormone (LH), and follicle stimulating hormone (FSH).[399,400] Therefore, there is a mutual regulatory interaction between catecholamines and pituitary function.

1. Catecholamine Receptors on Lymphoid Cells, Granulocytes, and Platelets

During studies of physiological responses to adrenergic agents, two primary types of adrenergic receptors were distinguished: α-adrenergic receptors, which respond to agonists in the order of potency of epinephrine > norepinephrine >> isoproterenol; and β-adrenergic receptors, which respond in the order of isoproterenol > epinephrine >> norepinephrine. Further subtypes of α_1 and α_2, β_1 and β_2 could be identified with the use of adrenergic radioligands. For instance ^{3}H-prazosin is a ligand specific for α_1 receptors, whereas ^{3}H-yohimbine is α_2 receptor specific. Although no selective ligands exist for β_1 and β_2 receptors, they can be separately identified in competitive binding experiments, using a nonselective radioligand and a relatively selective inhibitor.

The second messengers mediating the various receptor responses are distinct. The β receptors activate adenylate cyclase and thereby increase the cellular levels of cAMP. The α_1-adrenergic receptors elevate intracellular calcium levels and, in many cases, increase physiological hydrolysis, whereas α_2 receptors inhibit adenylate cyclase activity and decrease cellular cAMP levels.[401,402] The β_2-adrenergic receptor isolated from frog erythrocytes was identified as a glycoprotein of 58,000 daltons mol wt.[403]

Fetal mouse thymocytes were compared to young adult thymocytes in relation to their responsiveness to adrenoreceptor agonists and the ability to bind ^{3}H-dihydroalperenolol (^{3}H-DHA), a specific radioligand of the β adrenoreceptor. The rises of cAMP in fetal thymocytes after stimulation with isoproterenol were greater than in adult thymocytes. The number of ^{3}H-DHA binding sites was the same in both fetal and adult thymocytes, but the affinity of binding was less for adult cells than for fetal cells (with K_d values of 8 and 2.2 nM, respectively).[404]

Murine lymphocytes were found to have high affinity β-adrenergic binding sites (K_d = 1 nM), approximately 500 sites per cell.[405] Direct radioligand receptor assay was performed on intact viable murine lymphocytes with the β-adrenoreceptor antagonist, ^{125}I-hydroxybenzyl pindolol (^{125}I-HYP). Competitive inhibition with a number of adrenergic agents indicated the presence of β_2-type receptors. Approximately 3000 binding sites per cell were detected with an average dissociation constant of 0.92 nM. In 24 different inbred mouse strains, there was no significant difference in binding characteristics between lymphocytes from individual mice of either sex, or between T and B enriched lymphocyte populations. Thymocytes carried a lower affinity receptor. The β-adrenoreceptor was shown not to be associated with H-2^k, H-2^d, Ia, Ly-1,-2,-3,-4, or -5, Tla or Thy antigens, as revealed by specific antisera. However, specific antibodies to the Ly-7 antigen did inhibit partially the binding of radioactive tracer.[406]

Dopamine receptors have been detected on mouse B lymphocytes with ^{3}H-spiroperidol (^{3}H-SP) and found to have a dissociation constant of 4.8 ± 0.2 nM. At maximum binding, it was estimated that 60,000 sites are present per cell. All antidopaminergic drugs tested were effective inhibitors of ^{3}H-SP binding. Apomorphine and dopamine were effective inhibitors at μM concentrations, whereas norepinephrine, serotonin, and an antiserotonin drug, methysergide, were inactive.[407] Furthermore, dopamine stimulated phospholipid methylation in mouse B lymphocytes, which was inhibited by dopaminergic antagonists. The presence of L-methionine, which unmasks cryptic dopaminergic receptors, was necessary for this effect.[408]

Rat peritoneal mast cells were shown to have 40,000 ± 14,000 β-adrenergic receptors per cell, with a binding affinity of 1.58± 0.56 nM for ^{3}H-DHA. Competition studies revealed that 83.5% of the receptors are β_2 subtype and 16.5% are β_1. Neither sensitization with specific IgE antibodies nor subsequent challenge with the corresponding antigen altered mast cell β-adrenergic receptor characteristics. Resting mast cells stimulated with adrenergic agonists demonstrated a marked rise in cAMP levels after 15 sec of incubation. However, the same concentrations of these agonists had no effect on IgE mediated mast cell histamine release.[409]

Through the binding of ^{3}H-SP, rat lymphocytes were shown to have dopamine receptors, with a dissociation constant of 1.9 nM.[410]

Rabbit peripheral blood lymphocytes bound ^{125}I-HYP specifically through their β-adrenergic receptors, with a K_d of 0.53 ± 0.18 nM and a binding capacity of 3461 ± 235 sites per cell.[411]

Human peripheral blood lymphocytes were shown to have β-adrenergic receptors by ^{3}H-DHA, 14.8 ± 5.7 × 10^4 binding sites per cell being present.[412] The adrenergic receptor of human lymphocytes was subclassified as β_2 type, using the new radioligand, ^{125}I-cyanopindolol.[413]

The number of β-adrenergic receptors per lymphocyte in normal subjects, drug free asthmatics, and patients taking β stimulants, was 1146 ± 98, 845 ± 114, and 582 ± 47 sites per cell, respectively, as determined by the use of ^{125}I-HYP. The differences in sites per cell were statistically significant among these groups, whereas no significant differences were found in dissociation constants. A 42% decrease in the number of β_2-adrenergic receptors per lymphocytes was found in four normal volunteers after the administration of 6 mg/day of terbutaline for 7 days. There was a significant correlation between the number of β-adrenergic receptors per lymphocyte and the respiratory threshold for acetylcholine, and also in the percentage increase in blood sugar, 20 min after subcutaneous injection of 4 μg/kg epinephrine.[414]

Beta-adrenergic receptors of unfractionated human lymphocytes and of purified subpopulations of T cells (fractions 1 and 2) and B cells were studied with ^{125}I-HYP.

Fractions 1 and 2 of T cells were obtained by filtration through nylon wool columns. Binding sites on unfractionated lymphocytes, purified B cells, and fraction 2 of T cells were similar, numbering 4 to 600 sites per cell with a K_d of 25 nM. No detectable binding was noted by fraction 2 of T cells. T cells obtained by a rosetting technique displayed 200 receptors per cell.[415]

The number of β-adrenergic receptor sites and their affinity on lymphocytes from patients with cystic fibrosis were found to be similar to those of lymphocytes from normal individuals. However, patients' lymphocytes have significantly reduced cAMP response to isoproterenol, which suggests a defect in receptor-adenosine cyclase coupling.[416] Bishopric and co-workers[417] did not find any difference in the number, or the affinity, of β-adrenergic receptors in purified human B and T lymphocytes, as assayed by ³H-DHA. On the other hand, Bidart and co-workers[418] concluded that T cells exhibit a lower number of binding sites than B lymphocytes, as revealed by the ³H-DHA and ³H-SP assays.

Human platelets have α-adrenergic receptors, as revealed by ³H-dihydroergocryptine. Approximately 100 binding sites are present per platelet with a K_d of 3 to 10 nM.[419] Blood platelets isolated from humans, in contrast to those from other mammalian species, aggregate on exposure to epinephrine or norepinephrine; this is mediated by α-adrenergic receptors.[420] This receptor is subject to ligand regulation, as revealed by catecholamine mediated aggregation and release of ¹⁴C-5-hydroxytryptamine. Platelets, incubated with epinephrine for 4 to 5 hr, become refractory to aggregation by a second exposure to this hormone.[421] Catecholamine receptors of leukocytes and platelets are summarized in Table 9.

2. The Biological Effects of Catecholamines on the Immune System
a. Mouse

Basal activities of adenylate cyclase in lymphoid cells and liver were similar in suckling and weaned Ames pituitary dwarf mice and normal litter mates. However, epinephrine (10 μM) failed to stimulate cyclase levels in weaned dwarf mice, whereas significant stimulations of cyclase in thymus (300%) and spleen cells (150%) of normal litter mates was observed. Similar results were obtained with weaned Snell-Bagg dwarf mice, although the lymphoid cell adenylate cyclase responded somewhat better to epinephrine.[422] Mice were immunized with various doses of ovalbumin and the cAMP response of splenic lymphocytes to adrenalin was examined at various times after immunization. An antigen dose of 5 μg increased cAMP in B lymphocytes on the 1st day and the response to epinephrine was reduced somewhat, compared to nonimmunized controls. The cAMP response to epinephrine increased on the 2nd and 3rd day of immunization and gradually returned to normal on later days. Immunization with 50 μg of albumin induced a more marked rise in basic cAMP content of B lymphocytes on the 2nd day after incubation with epinephrine. This elevation decreased on the 3rd day and fell rapidly on later days. Immunization with 1 mg of albumin reduced the increase in cAMP levels, due to epinephrine, on the first 3 days, but the reactivity returned to normal after 5 to 8 days.[423] Thymus cells, prepared from 14-day-old mouse embryos, were incubated in serum-free medium for 90 min at 37°C with catecholamines, histamine, and peptide hormones, and the expression of Thy-1 and TL antigens were studied by antibody and complement mediated cytotoxicity tests. Catecholamines and histamine increased significantly the proportions of Thy-1 and TL positive cells, which could be inhibited by β-adrenergic or H-2 antagonists.[424]

The number of complement receptor rosette forming cells in suspensions of mouse spleen cells was increased by the β-adrenergic stimulant, isoproterenol. The α-receptor stimulant, norepinephrine, inhibited slightly the number of rosette forming cells, whereas epinephrine, which is known to stimulate both α- and β-adrenergic receptors

Table 9
CATECHOLAMINE RECEPTORS OF LEUKOCYTES AND PLATELETS

Species	Cell type	Ligand used	Type	Receptor no./ cell	K_d	Ref.
Mouse	Thymocyte	^{3}H-dihydroalprenolol	β		2.2—8 nM	404
	Spleen cells	^{3}H-dihydroalprenolol	β	500	1.0 nM	405
	Lymphocytes	^{125}I-hydroxybenzylpindolol	β_2	3,000	0.92 nM	406
	B lymphocytes	^{3}H-spiroperidol	δ	60,000	4.8 nM	407
Rat	Mast cell	^{3}H-dihydroalprenolol	β_2	$40 \pm 14 \times 10^3$	1.58 nM	408
	Lymphocytes	^{3}H-spiroperidol	δ		1.9 nM	410
Rabbit	Mononuclear cells	^{125}I-hydroxybenzylpindolol	β	$3,461 \pm 235$	0.53 nM	411
Man	Lymphocytes	^{3}H-dihydroalprenolol	β	$14.8 \pm 5.7 \times 10^3$		412
	Lymphocytes	^{125}Iodocyanopindolol	β_2		57 pM	413
	Lymphocytes	^{125}I-hydroxybenzylpindolol	β	$1,146 \pm 98$		414
	Lymphocytes	^{3}H-dihydroalprenolol	β	969 ± 165		416
	Granulocytes	^{3}H-dihydroalprenolol	β	$1,462 \pm 249$		416
	B,T lymphocytes	^{125}I-hydroxybenzylpindolol	β	4—600	25 nM	415
	B,T lymphocytes	^{3}H-dihydroalprenolol	β	No difference		417
	B,T lymphocytes	^{3}H-dihydroalprenolol	β	T cells lower		418
		^{3}H-spiroperidol	δ	T cells lower		418
	Platelet	^{3}H-dihydroergocryptine	α	100	3—10 nM	419

Note: K_d = dissociation constant; B = bone marrow derived — ; T = thymus derived lymphocyte; α,β = types of adrenergic receptors; δ = dopamnine receptor.

had no effect.[425] The response of murine lymphocytes to LPS was inhibited strongly by norepinephrine in vitro. Similarly, the response to Con A was inhibited by a variety of β-adrenergic agents.[426]

Spleen cells were prepared from mice 6 or 13 days after immunization i.p. with SRBC, and the effect of catecholamines on plaque formation was examined. Beta adrenergic agents inhibited significantly the formation of indirect (IgM) plaques.[427] Mice were given 4 μg of epinephrine i.p. at various intervals before immunization with SRBC. When epinephrine administration was within 24 hr of antigen injection, the immune response was accelerated, as evidenced by the indirect PFC response. Epinephrine treatment 2 days before antigen administration was inhibitory.[428] Mice, treated with extremely low concentrations (2 or 0.2 ng/mouse i.p.) of polyadenylic-uridylic acid (poly A:U), at the time of immunization with SRBC, exhibited an enhanced antibody formation. However, high amounts of isoproterenol inhibited the antibody response and reduced or abolished the stimulatory effects of poly A:U. In vitro, norepinephrine alone enhanced antibody formation, as did isoproterenol. The in vivo effects of isoproterenol, but not the effects of poly A:U, were blocked by propranolol, indicating that these two adenyl cyclase stimulators operate via different cell receptors.[429]

Norepinephrine and the synthetic α-adrenergic agonist, clonidine, strongly suppressed the in vitro induced immune response of murine spleen cells to SRBC. Furthermore, a decrease of norepinephrine was detected in the splenic pulp, just preceding the exponential phase of the immune response to SRBC (days 3 and 4).[430]

Graft rejection and GVH disease was inhibited in mice by serotoninergic and β-adrenergic drugs, in combination with dopaminergic and α-adrenergic blocking agents.[431]

Propranolol and other β-adrenergic blocking agents caused the degranulation of mouse peritoneal mast cells in vitro. Catecholamines failed to cause any degranulation, but isoproterenol protected the mast cells against the degranulation induced by propranolol.[432]

b. Rat

Control rats, and those immunized with thyroglobulin, were given i.p. epinephrine 30 min before sacrifice and the removal of spleen. Lymphocytes from epinephrine injected rats responded to PHA, or to antigen, with a decreased DNA synthesis.[433]

In Adrx rats, various doses of epinephrine induced an eosinophilia, which was dose-dependent. No eosinophilia was observed in splenectomized-adrenalectomized rats after epinephrine treatment. In such animals 200 μg of epinephrine actually evoked eosinopenia. Aqueous adrenocortical extracts antagonized the eosinophilic effect of epinephrine.[434] Epinephrine, given to intact rats, causes eosinopenia, which is dependent on a functional ACTH-adrenocortical axis. Increased levels of glucocorticoids mediate the eosinopenic response.[398]

Low doses of dopaminergic agents (dopa and apomorphine) elevated, while high doses lowered the blood eosinophil count in rats. The response to high doses of dopa was not affected by an inhibitor of dopamine-β-hydroxylase (U 10, 157), but it was prevented by a centrally acting dopa decarboxylase inhibitor (NSD 1015). Thus, the eosinopenia observed was due to the action of dopamine, newly-formed from the precursor. A central site of dopamine action was indicated by the fact that intracerebroventricular injections of L-dopa also produced eosinopenia. The eosinopenic response to apomorphine was antagonized by a dopamine receptor blocking agent, haloperidol. The hypophysis seemed to play a crucial role in the phenomenon observed, since no eosinopenia was produced by dopa in hypophysectomized rats.[435]

Catecholamines inhibited the degranulation of rat mast cells, not by affecting cellular cyclic AMP levels, but rather by the inhibition of transmembrane passage of calcium.[436,437] Propranolol, or other β-adrenergic blocking agents, caused the degranulation of mast cells that could be inhibited by isoproterenol.[432]

c. Guinea Pig

The injection of epinephrine, norepinephrine, or isoproterenol, to guinea pigs caused a rapid release of lymphocytes and granulocytes from the spleen without altering the splenic blood flow. This led to leukocytosis, which could be inhibited by the blocking of adrenergic receptors.[438,439] The catecholamine induced activation of adenylate cyclase in guinea pig macrophages was shown to be regulated by guanine nucleotides.[440]

d. Man

Epinephrine administration to normal human subjects induced leukocytosis, which was maximal 30 min after treatment, but returned to normal by 2 hr. The relative percentages of total T lymphocytes, B lymphocytes, and monocytes did not change after epinephrine administration. However, changes were found in the ratio of T cell subsets, as revealed by monoclonal antibodies. Thus, the T4:T8 ratio was 2.19 before injection, declined to 1.56 at 60 min, then increased to 3.1 at 2 hr postinjection. The percentage of natural killer to killer cells (HNK-1$^+$) increased from a base line of 15.5% before epinephrine injection to 29.6% at 30 min and declined to 11.4% by 2 hr after injection.[441] An augmentation of cytotoxicity by peripheral blood NK cells was also observed within 15 to 30 min after epinephrine administration to normal healthy individuals, which returned to base-line values within 2 hr.[442] Epinephrine administration induced comparable leukocytosis within the first 30 min in three healthy normal, and three healthy splenectomized males, indicating that the contraction of the spleen plays no significant role in this phenomenon. More than one peak was observed during the early lymphocytosis phase. A variable neutrophilia followed with relative lymphopenia.[443] Neither the α-receptor blocking agent, phenoxybenzamine, nor the β-receptor blocking drug, propranolol, produced marked alteration in the pattern of epinephrine induced leukocytosis. However, these two drugs, when given in combination, substantially reduced the subsequent white cell response to epinephrine.[444] Epinephrine and isoprenaline induced eosinophilia within 15 min after administration, which was followed by eosinopenia at 180 min. This later phase was dependent on an intact ACTH-adreno-cortical axis. In patients with tropical pulmonary eosinopenia, only the eosinopenic response could be observed to epinephrine, whereas the subsequent fall of eosinophils at 3 hr was insignificant.[398,445]

Propranolol administration (160 mℓ/day) for 5 days induced a 43% increase of β-adrenergic receptors of peripheral blood lymphocytes in comparison with pretreatment levels. After the withdrawal of propranolol, the density of β-adrenergic receptors did not return to pretreatment level for several days.[446] In patients with chronic congestive heart failure with long-term treatment with the β-adrenergic agonist, pirbuterol, depressed the density of β-adrenergic receptors on lymphocytes significantly, when compared with similar patients, who were not treated with pirbuterol.[447] The treatment of human lymphocytes with isoproterenol in vitro led to a decrease of β-adrenergic receptors and to a loss of β-adrenergic agents, as revealed by the measurements of intracellular cAMP.[448]

In normal subjects, or asthmatic patients, systemic treatment with high doses of cortisol increased lymphocyte responsiveness to catecholamines. Glucocorticoids stimulated cyclic AMP accumulation in lymphocytes from asthmatic and normal control subjects. Cyclic AMP responses were further potentiated when glucocorticoids were applied jointly with either theophylline or prostaglandin E_1.[449,450] Propranolol (10^{-7} to 10^{-5} M), isoproterenol (10^{-10} to 10^{-7} M), epinephrine (10^{-8} M) and aminophylline (10^{-7} to 10^{-5} M), enhanced significantly the Ig synthesis of normal human peripheral blood lymphocytes in vitro. Cortisol, in addition to one of the above agents, could only induce a further enhancement of Ig synthesis, if epinephrine was also present.[451] Isoproterenol stimulated more cAMP in E-rosette-forming T cells than in rosette-depleted cells. Maximal responses occurred at 5 to 12 min, except for the rosette-depleted population, which showed equal response at all incubation times. These results indicate that there is a striking difference between the β-adrenergic response of T and B lymphocytes.[452] Mononuclear cells from peripheral blood of healthy human subjects, treated with epinephrine, showed a significantly reduced response to PHA and PWM, for up to 60 min after drug administration. The response to Con A was reduced at 15 min only. All responses returned to preinjection levels by 120 min postinjection.[453]

Studies with human neutrophil plasma membranes revealed that β-adrenergic receptor-adenylate cyclase uncoupling is associated with amplified GTP activation and altered receptor regulation by GTP.[454] Propranolol (10^{-6} to 10^{-4} M) consistently increased neutrophil motility and caused an inhibition of postphagocytic cell metabolic activity (i.e., hexose monophosphate shunt, nitroblue tetrazolium reduction and protein iodination) without any detectable effect on the ingestion rate of C. albicans. Intracellular cyclic GMP levels were also increased after propranolol treatment. It was suggested that propranolol may stimulate neutrophil motility by increasing cGMP levels, or by decreasing neutrophil superoxide production.[455] The β-adrenergic stimulant, fenoterol (2.7×10^{-5} to 10^{-9} M) suppressed in a dose-dependent manner the production of oxygen radicals by human polymorphonuclear leukocytes and monocytes, as revealed by chemiluminescence. This suppressive effect of fenoterol could be reversed by joint incubation with propranolol. The inhibitory action of fenoterol on macrophages, but not on granulocytes, persisted after preincubation.[456]

Szentivanyi[457] proposed the β-adrenergic theory of allergy and bronchial asthma. He regarded asthma not as an immunological disease, but rather as a unique pattern of bronchial hypersensitivity to a broad spectrum of immunological, cyclic infectious, chemical, and physical stimuli. Disease occurs because of a defective homeostatic regulatory mechanism, due to the reduced functioning of the β-adrenergic system, and this adrenergic imbalance deprives the bronchial system from making its normal regulatory adjustment. This functional imbalance may be inherited or acquired.[457,458]

The immunological release of histamine and slow reactive substance of anaphylaxis (SRS-A) from human lung tissue was enhanced by stimulation with the α-adrenergic agents, epinephrine and norepinephrine, in the presence of propranolol. The observation that cGMP produced an enhancement of immunologic release of mediator, while cAMP was inhibitory, suggested that changes in the level of cyclic nucleotides mediate the adrenergic modulation of release of histamine and SRS-A.[459] Histamine, released from sensitized human leukocytes by antigen, was accompanied by increased histamine formation, both of which were inhibited by β-adrenergic agonists.[460]

Asthmatic subjects, treated with β-adrenergic agents, had significantly lower mean serum IgG levels than asthmatics not on β-adrenergic agents. Corticosteroids had the same effect as β-adrenergic agent, and concomitant usage of both drugs was associated with further reduction of IgG levels. There were no differences between the serum levels of IgA, IgM, IgD, and IgE, and complement components C3 and C4.[461]

Isoproterenol and propranolol were applied to the forearm skin of 15 ectopic subjects by iontophoresis. A significant increase of skin reactivity to antigen was observed in areas pretreated with propranolol and a significant reduction in reactivity followed pretreatment with isoproterenol.[462] Epinephrine, or isoproterenol, administered i.v., inhibited skin reactions to antigen, or histamine, in normal man. Phenylephrine, an α-adrenergic agent, produced no effects. Therefore, the inhibition of immediate hypersensitivity was mediated by β rather than α receptors. Furthermore, this inhibitory effect was not solely due to the prevention of release of inflammatory mediators, since the skin reactions to histamine were also inhibited.[463]

Lymphocytes from patients with bronchial asthma bound less ³H-DHA than those from control individuals, suggesting that a lymphocyte β-adrenergic receptor defect is present among some patients with asthma. The magnitude of receptor abnormality was related to disease severity and the degree of airway obstruction. The possibility that the observed receptor changes are drug related could not be excluded with certainty.[464] In normal subjects, both β-adrenergic receptor number and isoproterenol stimulated cAMP response of lymphocytes decreased during therapy with metaproterenol, theophylline, or concomitant metaproterenol and theophylline. Asthmatic subjects were of two types, one responding to similar treatments by down regulation of receptor number to or near to zero values, and the second group showing resistance to down regulation of receptor number.[465]

Autoantibodies to β-adrenergic receptors were identified in three normal subjects four asthmatic patients, one preallergic individual and one patient with cystic fibrosis. The antibodies were heterogeneous but all inhibited β-adrenergic ligand binding to calf lung receptors and to precipitated, solubilized calf lung β-adrenergic receptors. In addition, α-adrenergic and cholinergic hypersensitivity and β-adrenergic hyposensitivity were detected in these individuals.[466,467]

In platelets, α-adrenergic agonists inhibit prostaglandin E_1 (PGE$_1$) stimulated cAMP production, whereas α-adrenergic antagonists reversed this inhibition. Agonists and antagonists of β-adrenergic receptors had no effect, indicating that the physiological role of the α receptor relates to the regulation of cAMP.[468] Treatment of hypersensitive patients with *dl*- propranolol significantly inhibited platelet thromboxane synthesis and the aggregation of platelets due to thrombin or arachidonic acid. Similar dose-related effects were caused by *d*-propranolol, which has very little β-blocking activity.[469]

e. Other Species

Treatment of rabbits with propranolol (20 mg/kg) enhanced both the passive hem-agglutinating and the IgE response to ovalbumin. Phenoxybenzamine (0.4 to 40 mg/kg) had a similar adjuvant effect, but the response was delayed markedly at high doses.[470] Catecholamines elevated cAMP levels in rabbit alveolar macrophages. Phag-ocytosis was accompanied by an increase of cAMP in macrophages, which preceded or coincided with the onset of other metabolic events. Dibutyryl cAMP, which mimics several actions of cAMP, stimulated oxygen consumption and hexose monophosphate activity in phagocytosing alveolar macrophages, whereas no significant change was observed in resting cells. In polymorphonuclear leukocytes the effect of dibutyryl cAMP was opposite to that seen in alveolar macrophages.[471]

Members of two urodele amphibian species *(Triturus cristatus carnifex* and *Cynops hongkongensis)* and two anuran species *(Rana temporaria* and *Xenopus laevis laevis)* were immunized with sheep or horse erythrocytes. After 8 or 14 days splenic lympho-cytes were removed and antigen binding studies were performed. Stimulation with both α- and β-receptor agonists reduced the number of rosettes formed by *Triturus* and *Cy-nops* lymphocytes, whereas a β agonist increased and an α agonist decreased rosette formation by *Rana* and *Xenopus* splenic lymphocytes. These effects could be blocked by α and β-adrenoreceptor antagonists. Low dose immunization of *Xenopus* with sheep erythrocytes gave a minimum number of rosettes 2 and 8 days after immuniza-tion, which could not be influenced by β-adrenoreceptor stimulation.[472] The effect of catecholamines on leukocytes and platelets is summarized in Table 10.

B. Acetylcholine

Acetylcholine is a neurotransmitter synthesized in nerve cells by the acetylation of choline, with the aid of choline acetyl transferase. Acetylcholine is then transported to nerve endings, facing specific receptors, and is stored in granules. These granules are released by exocytosis, which is triggered by a change in action potential and subse-quent calcium influx. Cholinergic receptors are present in skeletal muscle end-plates, in cells of secretory glands, in ganglion cells of the autonomic nervous system, in smooth muscle, and in some cells of the CNS. Two basic types of receptors can be distinguished: (1) nicotinic, which can be activated by nicotine and inhibited by tubo-curarine and can be detected by the specific ligand, α bungarotoxin; and (2) muscar-inic, which can be stimulated selectively by muscarine and blocked by atropine. Sub-types have been proposed for muscarinic receptors.[395]

Muscarinic cholinergic receptors were demonstrated in murine splenic lymphocytes, using ³H-quinuclidinyl benzilate as a specific muscarinic ligand. Approximately 200 receptors were present per cell, with a dissociation constant of 10^{-9} M. Splenic adherent cells had 400 muscarinic receptor sites.[473] Nicotinic receptors were also demonstrated in extracts of rabbit thymus by the specific binding of ^{125}I-α bungarotoxin. Ligand binding was inhibited by carbamylcholine and D-tubocurarine. Furthermore, antibod-ies prepared from the serum of experimental myasthenic rabbits also identified recep-tor antigenicity in rabbit thymus.[474] Nicotinic receptors were also detected on murine thymic lymphocytes with the aid of specific antibodies.[475]

The cholinergic agent, carbamylcholine, enhanced significantly the early, but not the total, E rosette formation by human peripheral T lymphocytes. This effect could be abolished completely by atropine.[476] Cholinergic agents augmented the cytotoxic effect of rat T lymphocytes. Muscarinic ligands were several orders of magnitude more po-tent than nicotinic agents in altering cytotoxicity.[477] Other studies indicated that cholin-ergic ligands increased PHA-induced transformation, RNA, and protein synthesis in lymphocytes.[478]

The synthesis of the second component of complement by human monocytes was

Table 10
THE EFFECT OF CATECHOLAMINES ON LEUKOCYTES AND PLATELETS

Species	Hormone/drug	Dose/concentration	Biological effect	Ref.
		In vitro		
Mouse				
	Isoproterenol	10^{-5} M	Enhance the expression of Thy-1 and TL by fetal mouse thymocytes	424
	Isoproterenol	5×10^{-5} M	Increase complement receptor rosette forming by mouse spleen cells	425
	Norepinephrine	1×10^{-7} M	Inhibition of LPS response	427
	β-agonists	10^{-3}—10^{-6} M	Inhibition of IgM plaque formation by immune spleen cells	
	Isoproterenol Norepinephrine	10^{-4}—10^{-9} $\mu g/m\ell$ 10^{-2}—10^{-4} $\mu g/m\ell$	Enhance antibody formation	429
	Isoproterenol	1% solution	Protection of peritoneal mast cells against propranolol induced degranulation	432
		In vivo		
	Adrenaline	4 μg/mouse i.p.	Acceleration of anti-SRBC PFC if given within 24 hr of immunization, inhibition, if given 2 days prior to immunization	428
	Isoproterenol	0.2 or 2 ng/mouse i.p. 20 μg/mouse i.p.	Enhanced antibody formation when given with poly A:U Inhibition of antibody formation	429
		In vivo		
Rat				
	Epinephrine bitartarate	1 mg/kg i.m. 30 min. before killing	Decrease of antigen and PHA induced DNA synthesis by primed spleen cells	433
	Epinephrine	0.1 mg/rat i.p. 0.05—0.2 mg/rat s.c.	Eosinopenia in intact rats, eosinophilia in adrenalectomized rats	434

In vitro

Epinephrine, Norepinephrine, Isoproterenol	10^{-5} M	Inhibition of calcium dependent mast cell degranulation by interference with transmembrane passage of Ca^{++}	436, 437

In vivo

Epinephrine	0.2—0.5 mg s.c. / 1.0 mg i.m. / 1.5 mg i.v. / 2.8—18 mg infusion/24 hr	Leukocytosis at 30 min, returning to normal at 2 hr; altered T4:T8 ratio and NK cell cytotoxicity; eosinophilia followed by eosinopenia	441-445, 398

In vitro

Epinephrine	0.2 mg s.c.	Reduction of PWM,PHA, Con A responses	453
Metaproterenol sulfate	40—60 mg/day	Decreased serum IgG levels	461
Terbutaline	13.3—15 mg/day	Decreased serum IgG levels	461
Isoproterenol	1:200 w/v aqueous	Local inhibition of immediate hypersensitivity skin reaction	462
Epinephrine, Isoproterenol	20 µg/mℓ infusion / 4 µg/mℓ infusion	Inhibition of skin reactions produced by antigen or histamine	463
dl-Propranolol, d-Propranolol	640 mg/day / 640 mg/day	Inhibition of platelet aggregation and thromboxane synthesis, not mediated by β receptor	469
Propranolol	10^{-6}—10^{-4} M	Increased neutrophil motility	455
Fenoterol	10^{-5}—2.7×10^{-9} M	Suppression of production of oxygen radicals by PMN and Mf	456
Adrenaline, Noradrenaline, Isoprenaline	10^{-10} M / 10^{-8}—10^{-9} M / 10^{-7}—10^{-8} M	Inhibition of histamine release from leukocytes	460

Note: A = adenine; Con A = concanavalin A; LPS = bacterial lipopolysaccharide; Mf = macrophage; PFC = plaque-forming (antibody secreting) cell; PHA = phytohemagglutinin; PMN = polymorphonuclear (neutrophil) cell; PWM = pokeweed mitogen; SRBC = sheep red blood cell; T4 = helper/inducer subpopulation; T8 = suppressor/killer subpopulation of lymphocytes; Thy-1 = T cell specific antigen; TL = thymus-leukemia antigen; U = uridine.

enhanced by acetylcholine and carbamylcholine. This effect was mediated by the nicotinic receptor.[478]

The immunological release of histamine and SRS-A from human lung tissue was enhanced by acetylcholine and carbachol. Atropine prevented the release. This cholinergic-induced release was not associated with a measurable change in the levels of cAMP, and cGMP was suggested as a possible intracellular mediator.[459] The exposure of isolated rat mast cells to low concentrations of acetylcholine was sufficient to cause histamine release.[479]

The possible relationship between the cholinergic nervous system and allergy was studied in man by stimulating the cholinergically innervated sweat glands with mecholyl (0.1 to 100 μg). The sweat responses of four matched groups (male allergic, female allergic, male control, and female control) were compared after intradermal injection with the cholinergic stimulant. The 45 male and 45 female allergic patients demonstrated statistically significant increases in sweat responses to all concentrations of mecholyl examined, when compared with controls, revealing an increased sensitivity of allergic patients to cholinergic stimulation.[480] The involvement of cholinergic mechanisms in exercise induced anaphylaxis has also been demonstrated.[481]

V. THE INFLUENCE OF THE IMMUNE SYSTEM ON THE ACTH-ADRENOCORTICAL AXIS

By now it should be clear to the reader that glucocorticoids, catecholamines, and possibly also endorphins, have significant influences on a variety of immune phenomena and thus may qualify as physiological regulators of immune reactions. This notion is supported by the facts that: (1) receptors for these hormones are readily detectable in cells of the immune system; (2) that physiological hyper-function (i.e. stress) or hypo-function (i.e., adrenalectomy) of the ACTH-adrenal axis alters immune phenomena; and (3) that physiological concentrations of these hormones, especially glucocorticoids, do in fact influence the function of cells involved in immune reactions, as was shown by a number of investigators cited in this Chapter. On the basis of available evidence, one might suggest that the ACTH-adrenal system represents the suppressor arm of the neurohormonal immunoregulatory network. Such a network can only be functional through a feedback regulatory mechanism which allows for a dynamic and flexible regulation. The evidence for the existence of feedback regulatory signals, which originate from the immune system and which have an influence on the ACTH-adrenal axis, is surveyed here.

In rats, GVHR (runt disease) induces a biphasic pattern of corticosterone secretion. Initially, there was a significant elevation, which decreased to subnormal level on the 2nd day, followed by an increase again to almost twice that of normal, the level declining to normal after 26 days. Plasma corticosterone levels varied between 22.4 and 40.9 μg/100 mℓ, and high levels were generally associated with intense clinical symptoms.[482] Adrenal function was studied in 14-day-old neonatal and adult rats with GVH disease. Diseased animals in both groups displayed a shift from the protein bound to the free corticosterone fraction, with no change in total serum corticosterone titers. Diseased adults had enlarged adrenals. In neonates, no adrenal hypertrophy was evident, but lipid droplets and cholesterol were decreased, which are signs of adrenal hyperactivity. Treatment of affected animals with alloantiserum directed against donor cells halted the disease and elevated the adrenal cholesterol content toward control levels.[483]

Experimental allergic encephalomyelitis was induced in rats by immunization with neural tissue and adjuvants, or by the passive transfer of sensitized lymphocytes. In animals with severe clinical signs and lesions, an extensive thymolysis occurred, which was preceded and accompanied by a striking rise in serum corticosterone. With the remission of clinical signs, serum corticosterone levels declined, and the thymus began to regenerate. Adrx, performed early in remission, led to the disappearance of corticosterone and to relapses of clinical signs. Thymic regeneration was necessary for relapses to occur.[484]

In rats with adjuvant arthritis, a minimization of corticosterone, a 5-day periodicity of cortisol levels, and the absence of 21 acetates of cortisol and corticosterone was observed. Maximum swelling of the joints was observed up to 14 days after the induction of arthritis, which was paralleled by changes in two of the corticosteroids. Corticosterone decreased between days 10 to 17, while cortisol showed a periodicity between days 7 to 22, which was reproducible. The level of cortisol was negligible in normal rats and also in arthritic rats, except during the 7 to 22 day period.[485]

Changes in circulating corticosterone levels were also observed in mice and rats during the humoral immune response. Animals immunized with SRBC or HRBC, or with haemocyanin showed three to five times increases in serum corticosterone levels several days after immunization.[486] A strong decrease was also noted on day 11 after immunization with HRBC. The morning (8-hr) serum corticosterone level was increased in mice on the day of peak PFC response to SRBC, or to the trinitrophenyl hapten. This hormonal change was not observed in SRBC-low responder mice, which did not give a significant PFC response. Control animals, injected with saline, showed a regular circadian pattern: low corticosteroid level at 8 hr, followed by a high level at 16 hr. This rhythm was reversed in SRBC immunized animals on the day of the peak PFC response. The immunization induced corticosterone response could be inhibited by diazepam, which implies that the central hypothalamic-pituitary system is involved.[487]

Turkeys were inoculated with *Pasteurella multocida* and their plasma corticosterone concentration was measured. Corticosterone levels rose in some animals over 40 ng/mℓ, while levels in uninoculated turkeys ranged from 1.8 to 27.2 ng/mℓ. Corticosterone increase was proportional to the severity of the infection that developed. Plasma corticosterone was also found to be a sensitive indicator of an incubating infection of *P. multocida*, since it was already very high in turkeys that were bled 1 day before the onset of disease. In general, the plasma corticosterone concentration was higher in turkeys that either died between 5 and 10 days after inoculation, or were depressed at the end of the experiment on day 10, in comparison to the animals that thrived.[488] Injection of rats with typhoid-paratyphoid vaccine led to the increase of plasma corticosterone. This could be abolished by electrolytic lesions of the medium eminence of the hypothalamus, or by pharmacological blockade of the hypothalamic release of corticotropin releasing factor, using a combination of chlorpromazine, morphine and pentobarbital, or morphine and pentobarbital, dexamethasone and pentobarbital. These results suggest that endotoxins stimulate the adrenal axis by acting through the neuro-elements controlling the release of ACTH.[489]

Although the nature of signal(s) emitted by the immune system towards the ACTH-adrenal axis is largely unknown, several mechanisms may be suggested. Histamine, which is commonly released during immune reactions, causes the release of ACTH and of glucocorticoids, which is mediated by H_1-histamine receptors.[490] The administration of histamine (50 mg/kg) to mice, injected with Con A 24 hr previously, caused a marked decrease in antibody synthesis to SRBC. Nonimmunosuppressive doses of Con A were used. Suppression did not occur if the T-independent antigen, polyvinylpyrrolidone, was used, or if histamine was administered after the antigen. Excess suppressor cell generation was excluded by co-cultivation of treated spleen cells with normal cells. A histamine H_1-receptor agonist, 2-methylhistamine, had the same effect as histamine, whereas dimaprit, a histamine H_2-receptor agonist, was ineffective. Furthermore, both ACTH and corticosterone could mimic the effect of histamine.[491] Lymphokine containing supernatants from Con A stimulated cultures of human peripheral blood leukocytes, or of rat spleen cells, were administered to rats. Such supernatants induced, within 30 min to 2 hr, a severalfold increase in corticosterone blood levels. The glucocorticoid levels after lymphokine injection were of the same magnitude as those observed at the peak of the immune response.[492]

A well characterized lymphokine, which could serve as a messenger between the immune system and the ACTH adrenal axis, is the so-called endogenous pyrogen produced by macrophages. It has been suggested recently that this peptide is identical with IL-1. Recent studies suggest that hyperthermia augments the immune response, and thus may be an important factor in host resistance to infections.[493,494] Both histamine and pyrogens are potent inducers of ACTH release in man and considered as acceptable agents for the testing of ACTH reserve in patients.[495]

Thymic and bursal hormones may also function as feedback signals towards the neuroendocrine system. Clearly, the secretion of other steroid hormones is influenced by thymic and bursal activity. Thus, hydroxy corticosteroid and blood glucose levels were found to be significantly higher than normal in rabbits injected with thymosin, and these elevations were dose-dependent. The hyperglycemic effect was not observed in Adrx rabbits.[496] It was also reported that thymosin fraction 5 elevated ACTH, β-endorphin, and cortisol in a dose- and time-dependent fashion, when administered i.v. to prepubertal cynomolgus monkeys. Synthetic thymosin fraction 5 had no acute effects on pituitary function, suggesting that some other peptides in the preparation were responsible for ACTH-releasing activity. In accordance with these findings, total thymectomy of juvenile macaques was associated with decreases in plasma cortisol, ACTH, and β-endorphin. The authors concluded that the prepubertal primate thymus contains ACTH-releasing activity, which may contribute to a *physiological* immunoregulatory circuit between the developing immunological and pituitary-adrenal systems.[497] Thymic hormones (thymosin fraction 5, thymosin α1, α7, and β4), supernatants from Con A stimulated spleen cells (which were demonstrated to contain lymphokine activity), and partially purified mouse interferon, did not influence the steroid output of rat adrenal fasciculata. Therefore, the steroidogenic response to these peptides observed in vivo may be mediated by the CNS.[498]

Chicken embryos were surgically bursectomized by tail bud ablation at 68 hr of their development. Such bursectomized embryos were grafted with bursa on the chorioallantoic membrane at 9.5 days of incubation. In bursectomized chickens, testosterone production by the testis was increased, whereas corticosterone production by the adrenal glands was diminished, as determined by in vitro experiments. The weight and protein content of the oviduct was markedly decreased. These changes were not observed in bursa grafted animals. Thus, the bursa of Fabricius appears to produce factors that influence steroid secreting glands during embryonic development.[499]

The ACTH-secreting cells of the human anterior pituitary gland were found to have an affinity for human IgA, IgG, and IgM. The binding occurred through the Fc portion of the immunoglobulins, suggesting that ACTH cells bear Fc receptors.[500] The binding of bovine immunoglobulins by the anterior and intermediate lobes of bovine pituitaries was also observed.[501-503]

Some other experiments suggest that certain lymphokines may act directly on the adrenal gland. Infection of hypophysectomized rats with Newcastle disease virus caused an increase in corticosterone. Treatment of the animals with dexamethasone inhibited the virus induced elevation of corticosterone concentration. Spleen cells from virus infected, but not from control, mice showed positive immunofluorescence with antibody to ACTH.[504]

Recently, Blalock[505] suggested that human leukocyte interferon preparations contain immunologically and biologically recognizable endorphin and ACTH-like activities.[506-508] A patient with ectopic ACTH syndrome, and without ACTH-producing tumor, has also been reported. A pseudotumor, containing fat and inflammatory tissue, was removed from this patient, which resulted in normalization of both basal plasma ACTH levels and the feedback response of ACTH to cortisol infusion. The authors suggested that leukocytes in the inflammatory tissue were the source of ectopic ACTH.[86]

In other experiments, septic shock plasma from rabbits caused a 40% noncompetitive inhibition of ACTH-induced steroidogenesis by rat adrenocortical cells. *Escherichia coli* endotoxins did not have any effect.[509] Mouse peritoneal macrophages, stimulated with macrophage activating factor, and LPS, elaborated a factor that interfered profoundly with the steroidogenesis of ACTH-stimulated rabbit adrenocortical cells. Continued exposure of adrenocortical cells to this factor resulted in progressively decreasing response to ACTH. Comparable suppression was exerted by supernatants from LPS treated bone marrow derived macrophages. The suppressive activity was not due to carry over LPS. Suppressive supernatants neither inactivated ACTH, nor did they interfere with the assay of steroids.[510]

REFERENCES

1. Dougherty, T. F., Effect of hormones on lymphatic tissue, *Physiol. Rev.*, 32, 379, 1952.
2. Berthrong, M., Rich, A. R., and Griffith, P. C., Effect of ACTH upon experimental cardiovascular lesions produced by anaphylactic hypersensitivity, *Bull. Johns Hopkins Hosp.*, 86, 131, 1950.
3. Bjørneboe, M., Fischel, E. E., and Stoerk, H. C., The effect of cortisone and adrenocorticotropic hormone on the concentration of circulating antibody, *J. Exp. Med.*, 93, 37, 1951.
4. Malkiel, S. and Hargis, B. J., Effect of ACTH and cortisone on the quantitative precipitin reaction, *J. Immunol.*, 69, 217, 1952.
5. Germuth, F. G., Jr., Oyama, T., and Ottinger, B., The mechanism of action of 17-hydroxy-11-dehydrocorticosterone (compound E) and of the adrenocorticotropic hormone in experimental hypersensitivity in rabbits, *J. Exp. Med.*, 94, 139, 1951.
6. Kass, E. H., Kendrick, M. L., and Finland, M., Effect of corticosterone, hydrocortisone and corticotropin on the production of antibodies in rabbits, *J. Exp. Med.*, 102, 767, 1955.
7. Zimmer, J. A. and Lipton, J. M., Central and peripheral injections of ACTH (1-24) reduce fever in adrenalectomized rabbits, *Peptides*, 2, 413, 1981.
8. Hayes, S. P. and Dougherty, T. F., Effect of ACTH and cortisone on antibody synthesis and rate of disappearance of antigen, *Fed. Proc. Fed. Am. Soc. Exp. Biol.*, 11, 67, 1952.
9. Newsom, S. E. and Darrach, M., The effect of cortisone acetate on the production of circulating hemolytic antibodies in the mouse, *Can. J. Biochem. Physiol.*, 32, 372, 1954.
10. Newsom, S. E. and Darrach, M., The effect of corticotropin and corticosterone on the production of hemolytic antibodies in the mouse, *Can. J. Biochem. Physiol.*, 33, 374, 1955.
11. Medawar, P. P. and Sparrow, E. M., Effect of adrenocortical hormones, adrenocorticotropic hormone and pregnancy on skin transplantation immunity, *J. Endocrinol.*, 14, 240, 1956.
12. Spry, C. J. F., Inhibition of lymphocyte recirculation by stress and corticotropin, *Cell. Immunol.*, 4, 86, 1972.
13. Hayashida, T. and Li, C.-H., Influence of adrenocorticotropic and growth hormone on antibody formation, *J. Exp. Med.*, 105, 93, 1957.
14. Berczi, I., Nagy, E., Kovacs, K., and Horvath, E., Regulation of humoral immunity in rats by pituitary hormones, *Acta Endocrinol.*, 98, 506, 1981.
15. Berczi, I., Nagy, E., Asa, S. L., and Kovacs, K., Pituitary hormones and contact sensitivity in rats, *Allergy*, 38, 325, 1983.
16. Berczi, I., Nagy, E., Asa, S. L., and Kovacs, K., The influence of pituitary hormones on adjuvant arthritis, *Arthritis Rheum.*, 27, 682, 1984.
17. Nagy, E., Berczi, I., Wren, G. E., Asa, S. L., and Kovacs, K., Immunomodulation by bromocriptine, *Immunopharmacology*, 6, 231, 1983.
18. Hench, P. S., Kendall, E. C., Slocumb, C. H., and Polley, H. F., Effect of hormone of adrenal cortex (17-hydroxy-11-dehydrocorticosterone; compound E) and of pituitary adrenocorticotropic hormone on rheumatoid arthritis; preliminary report, *Ann. Rheum. Dis.*, 8, 97, 1949.
19. Kass, E. H. and Finland, M., Adrenocortical hormones in infection and immunity, *Ann. Rev. Microbiol.*, 7, 361, 1953.
20. Germuth, F. G., Role of adrenocortical steroids in infection, immunity and hypersensitivity, *Pharmacol. Rev.*, 8, 1, 1956.

21. Mirick, G. W., The effects of ACTH and cortisone on antibodies in human beings, *Bull. Johns Hopkins Hosp.*, 88, 332, 1951.
22. Larson, D. L. and Tomlinson, L. J., Quantitative antibody studies in man. I. The effect of adrenal insufficiency and of cortisone on the level of circulating antibodies, *J. Clin. Invest.*, 30, 1451, 1951.
23. Havens, W. P., Jr., Shaffer, J. M., and Hopke, C. J., Jr., The capacity of patients with chronic hepatic disease to produce antibody, and the effect of ACTH and cortisone on this function, *J. Clin. Invest.*, 30, 647, 1951.
24. Gardner, F. H., McElfresh, A. E., Harris, J. W., and Diamond, L. K., The effect of adrenocorticotropic hormone (ACTH) in idiopathic acquired hemolytic anemia as related to the hemolytic mechanisms, *J. Lab. Clin. Med.*, 37, 444, 1951.
25. Dameshek, W., Rosenthal, M. C., and Schwartz, L. I., The treatment of acquired hemolytic anemia with ACTH, *N. Engl. J. Med.*, 244, 117, 1950.
26. Carey, R. A., Harvey, A. M., Howard, J. E., and Wagley, P. F., The effect of adrenocorticotropic hormone (ACTH) and cortisone on drug hypersensitivity reactions, *Bull. Johns Hopkins Hosp.*, 87, 354, 1950.
27. Germuth, F. G., Jr., The mechanism of action of cortisone in experimental hypersensitivity. II. Hypersensitivity of the serum sickness type, *J. Exp. Med.*, 98, 1, 1953.
28. Leith, W., Graham, M. J., and Burrage, W. S., The effect of ACTH on the immediate skin reaction and passive transfer test in man, *J. Allergy*, 22, 99, 1951.
29. Loveless, M. H., The influence of ACTH on the sensitizing and immunizing antibodies in inhalant allergy, *Bull. N.Y. Acad. Med.*, 27, 495, 1951.
30. Rich, A. R., Berthrong, M., and Bennett, I. L., Jr., The effect of cortisone upon the experimental cardiovascular and renal lesions produced by anaphylactic hypersensitivity, *Bull. Johns Hopkins Hosp.*, 87, 549, 1950.
31. Stollerman, G. H., Rubin, S. J., and Plotz, C. M., Effect of cortisone on passively induced skin hypersensitivity in man, *Proc. Soc. Exp. Biol. Med.*, 76, 261, 1951.
32. Lurie, M. B., Zappasodi, P., Dannenberg, A. M., Jr., and Cardona-Lynch, E., Constitutional factors in resistance to infection: the effect of cortisone and ACTH on the pathogenesis of tuberculosis, *Ann. N.Y. Acad. Sci.*, 56, 779, 1953.
33. Osgood, C. K. and Favour, C. B., Effect of adrenocorticotropic hormone on inflammation due to tuberculin hypersensitivity and turpentine and on circulating antibody levels, *J. Exp. Med.*, 94, 415, 1951.
34. Sparrow, E. M., Effect of cortisone alcohol and ACTH on skin homografts in guinea pigs, *J. Endocrinol.*, 11, 57, 1954.
35. Roth, J. A. and Kaeberle, M. L., Suppression of neutrophil and lymphocyte function induced by a vaccinal strain of bovine viral diarrhea virus with and without the administration of ACTH, *Am. J. Vet Res.*, 44, 2366, 1983.
36. Davison, T. F. and Flack, I. H., Changes in the peripheral blood leucocyte populations following an injection of corticotrophin in the immature chicken, *Res. Vet. Sci.*, 30, 79, 1981.
37. Mehrishi, J. N. and Mills, I. H., Opiate receptors on lymphocytes and platelets in man, *Clin. Immunol. Immunopathol.*, 27, 240, 1983.
38. McDonough, R. J., Madden, J. J., Falek, A., Shafer, D. A., Pline, M., Gordon, D., Bokos, P., Kuehnle, J. C., and Mendelson, J., Alteration of T and null lymphocyte frequencies in the peripheral blood of human opiate addicts: in vivo evidence for opiate receptor sites on T lymphocytes, *J. Immunol.*, 125, 2539, 1980.
39. Wybran, J., Appelboom, T., Famaey, J.-P., and Govaerts, A., Suggestive evidence for receptors for morphine and methionine-enkephalin on normal human blood T lymphocytes, *J. Immunol.*, 123, 1068, 1979.
40. Miller, G. C., Murgo, A. J., and Plotnikoff, N. P., Enkephalins — enhancement of active T-cell rosettes from lymphoma patients, *Clin. Immunol. Immunopathol.*, 26, 446, 1983.
41. Maravelias, C. P. and Coutselinis, A. S., Suppressive effects of morphine on human blood lymphocytes: an *in vitro* study, *IRCS Med. Sci. Biochem.*, 12, 106, 1984.
42. McCain, H. W., Lamster, I. B., Bozzone, J. M., and Grbic, J. T., β-Endorphin modulates human immune activity via non-opiate receptor mechanisms, *Life Sci.*, 31, 1619, 1982.
43. Gilman, S. C., Schwartz, J. M., Milner, R. J., Bloom, F. E., and Feldman, J. D., Beta-endorphin enhances lymphocyte proliferative responses, *Proc. Natl. Acad. Sci. U.S.A. Biol. Sci.*, 79, 4226, 1982.
44. Plotnikoff, N. P. and Miller, G. C., Enkephalins as immunomodulators, *Int. J. Immunopharmacol.*, 5, 437, 1983.
45. Mathews, P. M., Froelich, C. J., Sibbitt, W. L., Jr., and Bankhurst, A. D., Enhancement of natural cytotoxicity by β-endorphin, *J. Immunol.*, 130, 1658, 1983.

46. Shavit, Y., Lewis, J. W., Terman, G. W., Gale, R. P., and Liebeskind, J. C., Opioid peptides mediate the suppressive effect of stress on natural killer cell cytotoxicity, *Science*, 223, 188, 1984.

47. Van Epps, D. E. and Saland, L., β-Endorphin and met-enkephalin stimulate human peripheral blood mononuclear cell chemotaxis, *J. Immunol.*, 132, 3046, 1984.

48. Yamasaki, Y., Shimamura, O., Kizu, A., Nakagawa, M., and Ijichi, H., IgE-mediated ^{14}C-serotonin release from rat mast cells modulated by morphine and endorphins, *Life Sci.*, 31, 471, 1982.

49. Schweigerer, L., Bhakdi, S., and Teschemacher, H., Specific non-opiate binding sites for human β-endorphin on the terminal complex of human complement, *Nature (London)*, 296, 572, 1982.

50. Castellanos, R. C., Leizerovitz, R., Kaiser, N., Galili, N., Polliack, A., Korkesh, A., and Galili, U., Prothymocytes in postirradiation regenerating rat thymuses: a model for studying early stages in T cell differentiation, *J. Immunol.*, 130, 121, 1983.

51. Van Kijk, H. and Jacobse-Geels, H. E. L., Evidence for the involvement of corticosterone in the ontogeny of the cellular immune apparatus of the mouse, *Immunology*, 35, 637, 1978.

52. Emeson, E. E., Weintraub, F. M., and Likhite, V., Effects of adrenalectomy and glucocorticosteroid therapy on bone marrow T cells. Effect on T cell traffic and graft-versus-host (GVH) reactivity, *Immunopharmacology*, 4, 311, 1982.

53. Calvano, S. E., Mark, D. A., Good, R. A., and Femandes, G., In vitro assessment of immune function in adrenalectomized rats, *Immunopharmacology*, 4, 291, 1982.

54. Treloar, O. L., Hormonal regulation of rapid eosinopenia in the rat. I, *Lab. Anim. Sci.*, 27, 635, 1977.

55. Keller, S. E., Weiss, J. M., Schleifer, S. J., Miller, N. E., and Stein, M., Stress-induced suppression of immunity in adrenalectomized rats, *Science*, 221, 1301, 1983.

56. Morales, A., Jolali, S., and Garvie, W. H. H., Enhancement of lymphocyte production by adrenocortical inhibition, *J. Surg. Res.*, 13, 47, 1972.

57. Blecha, F., Kelley, K. W., and Satterlee, D. G., Adrenal involvement in the expression of delayed-type hypersensitivity to SRBC and contact sensitivity to DNFB in stressed mice, *Proc. Soc. Exp. Biol. Med.*, 169, 247, 1982.

58. Graff, R. J., Lappé, M. A., and Snell, G. D., The influence of the gonads and adrenal glands on the immune response to skin grafts, *Transplantation*, 7, 105, 1969.

59. Kieffer, J. D. and Ketchel, M. M., Effects of adrenalectomy and antigenic stimulation on spleen weight in mice, *Transplantation*, 11, 45, 1971.

60. Heim, L. R., Yunis, E. J., and Good, R. A., Pathogenesis of graft-versus-host reaction. II. Influence of thymectomy and adrenalectomy on lymphoid tissue pathology; delineation of nonthymus-dependent lymphoid elements, *Int. Arch. Allergy Appl. Immunol.*, 42, 565, 1972.

61. Heim, L. R., Good, R. A., and Martinez, C., Influence of adrenalectomy on homologous disease, *Proc. Soc. Exp. Biol. Med.*, 122, 107, 1966.

62. Levine, S., Wenk, E. J., Muldoon, T. N., and Cohen, S. G., Enhancement of experimental allergic encephalomyelitis by adrenalectomy, *Proc. Soc. Exp. Biol. Med.*, 111, 383, 1962.

63. Levine, S., Wenk, E. J., Muldoon, T. N., and Cohen, S. G., Passive transfer of allergic encephalomyelitis: acceleration by adrenalectomy, *Proc. Soc. Exp. Biol. Med.*, 121, 301, 1966.

64. Levine, S. and Sowinski, R., The role of the adrenal in relapses of experimental allergic encephalomyelitis, *Proc. Soc. Exp. Biol. Med.*, 149, 1032, 1975.

65. Meacock, S. C. R. and Marsden, C. H., The effects of adjuvants and stress on the production of IgE antibody in rats, *Int. Arch. Allergy Appl. Immunol.*, 45, 136, 1973.

66. Klausen, B., Hougen, H.-P., and Rygaard, J., Induction of plaque-forming cell response in adrenalectomized nude rats using thymosin fraction 5, *Acta Pathol. Microbiol. Immunol. C*, 90, 283, 1982.

67. Besedovsky, H. O., del Rey, A., and Sorkin, E., Antigenic competition between horse and sheep red blood cells as a hormone-dependent phenomenon, *Clin. Exp. Immunol.*, 37, 106, 1979.

68. Selye, H., A syndrome produced by diverse nocuous agents, *Nature (London)*, 138, 32, 1936.

69. Carriere, G., Morel, J., and Gineste, P.-J., Modifications histo-physiologiques du thymus du rat albinos sous l'influence de la folliculine et de la progestine et de l'hormone gonadotrope ou antelobine, *C. R. Soc. Biol.*, 126, 44, 1937.

70. Ingle, D. J., Atrophy of the thymus in normal and hypophysectomized rats following administration of cortin, *Proc. Soc. Exp. Biol. Med.*, 38, 443, 1938.

71. Gordon, A. S., Some aspects of hormonal influences upon leukocytes, *Ann. N.Y. Acad. Sci.*, 59, 907, 1955.

72. White, L., Effects of steroids on aspects of the metabolism and functions of the lymphocyte. A hypothesis of the cellular mechanisms in antibody formation and related immune phenomena, *Ann. N.Y. Acad. Sci.*, 73, 79, 1958.

73. McMaster, P. D. and Franzl, R. E., The effects of adrenocortical steroids upon antibody formation, *Metabolism*, 10, 990, 1961.

74. Dougherty, T. F., Berliner, M. L., and Berliner, D. L., Hormonal control of lymphocyte production and destruction, *Prog. Hematol.*, 3, 155, 1962.

75. Dougherty, T. F., Berliner, M. L., Schneebeli, G., and Berliner, D. L., Hormonal control of lymphatic structure and function, *Ann. N.Y. Acad. Sci.*, 113, 825, 1963.

76. White, A. and Monkman, M. H., Effect of glucocorticoids on thymocytes in vitro, *Adv. Enzyme Regul.*, 5, 317, 1967.

77. Vernon-Roberts, B., The effects of steroid hormones on macrophage activity, *Int. Rev. Cytol.*, 25, 131, 1969.

78. Claman, H. N., Corticosteroids and lymphoid cells, *N. Engl. J. Med.*, 287, 388, 1972.

79. Claman, H. N., How corticosteroids work, *J. Allergy Clin. Immunol.*, 55, 145, 1975.

80. Baxter, J. D. and Harris, A. W., Mechanism of glucocorticoid action: general features, with reference to steroid-mediated immunosuppression, *Transplant. Proc.*, 75, 55, 1975.

81. Fauci, A. S., Mechanisms of the immunosuppressive and anti-inflammatory effects of glucocorticoids, *J. Immunopharmacol.* 1, 1, 1978.

82. Munck, A., Crabtree, G. R., and Smith, K. A., Effects and receptors of glucocorticoids in rat thymus cells and human peripheral lymphocytes, *J. Toxicol. Environ. Health*, 4, 409, 1978.

83. Crabtree, G. R., Gillis, S., Smith, K. A., and Munck, A., Glucocorticoids and immune responses, *Arthritis Rheum.*, 22, 1246, 1979.

84. Beck, J. S. and Browning, M. C. K., Immunosuppression with glucocorticoids: a possible immunological explanation for interpatient variation in sensitivity — discussion paper, *J. R. Soc. Med.*, 76, 473, 1983.

85. Kehrl, J. H. and Fauci, A. S., The clinical use of glucocorticoids, *Ann. Allergy*, 50, 2, 1983.

86. Dupont, A. G., Somers, G., Van Steirteghem, A. C., Warson, F., and Vanhaelst, L., Ectopic adrenocorticotropin production: disappearance after removal of inflammatory tissue, *J. Clin. Endocrinol. Metab.*, 58, 654, 1984.

87. Ballard, P. L., Baxter, J. D., Higgins, S. J., Rousseau, G. G., and Tomkins, G. M., General presence of glucocorticoid receptors in mammalian tissues, *Endocrinology*, 94, 998, 1974.

88. Chan, L. and O'Malley, B. W., Steroid hormone action: recent advances, *Ann. Intern. Med.*, 89, 694, 1978.

89. Homo-Delarche, F., Glucocorticoid receptors and steroid sensitivity in normal and neoplastic human lymphoid tissues — a review, *Cancer Res.*, 44, 431, 1984.

90. Distelhorst, C. W. and Benutto, B. M., Glucocorticoid receptor content of T lymphocytes: evidence for heterogeneity, *J. Immunol.*, 126, 1630, 1981.

91. Ozaki, T., Yasuoka, S., Nakayama, T., and Tsubura, E., Glucocorticoid receptors in human alveolar macrophages and peripheral blood cells, *Clin. Exp. Immunol.*, 47, 505, 1982.

92. Smith, K. A., Crabtree, G. R., Kennedy, S. J., and Munck, A. U., Glucocorticoid receptors and glucocorticoid sensitivity of mitogen stimulated and unstimulated human lymphocytes, *Nature (London)*, 267, 523, 1977.

93. Bonnard, G. D. and Lippman, M. E., Induction of glucocorticoid hormone receptors in human cultured T cells, *Schweiz. Med. Wochenschr.*, 108, 1603, 1978.

94. Duval, D., Dardenne, M., Dausse, J. P., and Homo, F., Glucocorticoid receptors in corticosensitive and corticoresistant thymocyte subpopulations. II. Studies with hydrocortisone-treated mice, *Biochim. Biophys. Acta*, 496, 312, 1977.

95. Ma, D. D. F., Ho, A. H., and Hoffbrand, A. V., Effect of thymosin on glucocorticoid receptor activity and glucocorticoid sensitivity of human thymocytes, *Clin. Exp. Immunol.*, 55, 273, 1984.

96. Endres, D. B., Milholland, R. J., and Rosen, F., Sex differences in the concentrations of glucocorticoid receptors in rat liver and thymus, *J. Endocrinol.*, 80, 21, 1979.

97. Crabtree, G. R., Munck, A., and Smith, K. A., Glucocorticoids and lymphocytes. I. Increased glucocorticoid receptor levels in antigen-stimulated lymphocytes, *J. Immunol.*, 124, 2430, 1980.

98. Shipman, G. F., Bloomfield, C. D., Gajl-Peczalska, K. J., Munck, A. U., and Smith, K. A., Glucocorticoids and lymphocytes. III. Effects of glucocorticoid administration on lymphocyte glucocorticoid receptors, *Blood*, 61, 1086, 1983.

99. Schlechte, J. A., Ginsberg, B. H., and Sherman, B. M., Regulation of the glucocorticoid receptor in human lymphocytes, *J. Steroid Biochem.*, 16, 69, 1982.

100. Kontula, K., Pelkonen, R., Andersson, L. C., and Sivula, A., Glucocorticoid receptors in adrenocorticoid disorders, *J. Clin. Endocrinol. Metab.*, 51, 654, 1980.

101. Junker, K., Glucocorticoid receptors of human mononuclear leukocytes in vitro, *J. Clin. Endocrinol. Metab.*, 57, 506, 1983.

102. Ploc, I. and Felt, V., Effect of theophylline of binding of cortisol to cytosolic receptors of human leukocytes, *Endokrinologie*, 76, 189, 1980.

103. Crabtree, G. R., Munck, A., and Smith, K. A., Glucocorticoids and lymphocytes. II. Cell cycle-dependent changes in glucocorticoid receptor content, *J. Immunol.*, 125, 13, 1980.

104. Duval, D., Homo, F., Fournier, C., and Dausse, J. P., Glucocorticoid receptors in mouse spleen cell subpopulations, *Cell. Immunol.*, 46, 1, 1979.
105. Gupta, C. and Goldman, A., H-2 histocompatibility region: influence on the murine glucocorticoid receptor and its response, *Science*, 216, 994, 1982.
106. Murakami, N., Yoshida, A., and Ichii, S., Studies on the nuclear binding of steroid hormone-receptor complex; binding of liver and thymus dexamethasone-receptor complex and prostate dihydrotestosterone-receptor complex to nuclei from various tissues, *Endocrinol. Jpn.*, 26, 75, 1979.
107. Murakami, T., Brandon, D., Rodbard, D., Loriaux, D. L., and Lipsett, M. B., Glucocorticoid receptor in polymorphonuclear leukocytes: a simple method for leukocyte glucocorticoid receptor characterization, *J. Steroid Biochem.*, 10, 475, 1979.
108. Náray, A., Aranyi, P., and Quiroga, V., Comparative study of glucocorticoid sensitivity and receptors in lymphoid tissues, *J. Steroid Biochem.*, 13, 415, 1980.
109. Náray, A., The effect of a Ca^{2+}-activated protease on the glucocorticoid receptor of lymphoid tissues, *J. Steroid Biochem.*, 14, 71, 1981.
110. Kraft, N., Hodgson, A. J., and Funder, J. W., Glucocorticoid receptor and effector mechanisms: comparison of the corticosensitive mouse with the corticoresistant guinea pig, *Endocrinology*, 104, 344, 1979.
111. Werb, Z., Foley, R., and Munck, A., Interaction of glucocorticoids with macrophages. Identification of glucocorticoid receptors in monocytes and macrophages, *J. Exp. Med.*, 147, 1684, 1978.
112. Chrousos, G. P., Renquist, D., Brandon, D., Eil, C., Pugeat, M., Vigersky, R., Cutler, G. B., Loriaux, D. L., and Lipsett, M. B., Glucocorticoid hormone resistance during primate evolution receptor-mediated mechanisms, *Proc. Natl. Acad. Sci. U.S.A. Biol. Sci.*, 79, 2036, 1982.
113. Kontula, K., Myllylä, G., and Anderson, L. C., Glucocorticoid receptors in human polymorphonuclear and mononuclear leucocytes. Concentrations and binding characteristics, *Scand. J. Haematol.*, 27, 145, 1981.
114. Costlow, M. E., Pui, C.-H., and Dahl, G. V., Glucocorticoid receptors in childhood acute lymphocyte leukemia, *Cancer Res.*, 42, 4801, 1982.
115. Homo, F. and Duval, D., Human thymus cells: effects of glucocorticoids *in vitro*, *J. Clin. Lab. Immunol.*, 2, 329, 1979.
116. Homo, F., Duval, D., Thierry, C., and Serrou, B., Human lymphocyte subpopulations: effect of glucocorticoids *in vitro*, *J. Steroid Biochem.*, 10, 609, 1979.
117. Neifeld, J. P., Lippman, M. E., and Torney, D. C., Steroid hormone receptors in normal human lymphocytes, *J. Biol. Chem.*, 252, 2972, 1977.
118. Ho, A. D., Hunstein, W., and Schmid, W., Glucocorticoid receptors and sensitivity in leukemias, *Blut*, 42, 183, 1981.
119. Nanni, P., Nicoletti, G., Prodi, G., Galli, M. C., DeGiovanni, C., Grilli, S., Lollini, P.-L., Gobbi, M., Cavo, M., and Tura, S., Glucocorticoid receptor and in vitro sensitivity to steroid hormones in human lymphoproliferative diseases and myeloid leukemia, *Cancer*, 49, 623, 1982.
120. Lippman, M. and Barr, R., Glucocorticoid receptors in purified subpopulations of human peripheral blood lymphocytes, *J. Immunol.*, 118, 1977, 1977.
121. Mayeux, P., Billat, C., Felix, J. M., and Jacquot, R., Evidence for glucocorticosteroid receptors in the erythroid cell line of fetal rat liver, *J. Endocrinol.*, 96, 311, 1983.
122. Leung, P. and Gidari, A. S., Glucocorticoids inhibit the growth of murine fetal liver erythroid burst-forming cells, *Endocrinology*, 111, 1121, 1982.
123. Ritter, M. A., Embryonic mouse thymocyte development. Enhancing effect of corticosterone at physiological levels, *Immunology*, 33, 241, 1977.
124. Eishi, Y., Hirokawa, K., and Hatakeyama, S., Long-lasting impairment of immune and endocrine systems of off-spring induced by injection of dexamethasone into pregnant mice, *Clin. Immunol. Immunopathol.*, 26, 335, 1983.
125. Bennett, M., Hemopoietic environment necessary for an early stage in differentiation of antibody-forming cells. Effect of cortisol, *J. Cell. Physiol.*, 76, 197, 1970.
126. Dracott, B. N. and Smith, C. E. T., Hydrocortisone and the antibody response in mice. I. Correlations between serum cortisol levels and cell numbers in thymus, spleen, marrow and lymph nodes, *Immunology*, 38, 429, 1979.
127. Johnell, O. and Hulth, A., The response of bone marrow cells, thymocytes and osteoclasts to hydrocortisone, *Br. J. Exp. Pathol.*, 61, 411, 1980.
128. Brahim, F., Marrow lymphocyte production during chronic hydrocortisone administration, *J. Reticuloendothel. Soc.*, 23, 111, 1978.
129. Brahim, F. and Bahadue, G., Influx of long-lived lymphocytes into guinea pig marrow during hydrocortisone administrations, *J. Reticuloendothel. Soc.*, 25, 297, 1979.
130. Romashko, O. O., Adyushkin, A. I., and Lebedev, V. G., Effect of the degree of glucocorticoid saturation on peripheral blood CFUs levels, *Bull. Exp. Biol. Med.*, 93, 312, 1982.

131. Chan, H. S. L., Saunders, E. F., and Freedman, M. H., Diamond-Blackfan syndrome. I. Erythropoiesis in prednisone responsive and resistant disease, *Pediatr. Res.,* 16, 474, 1982.
132. Joyce, R. A. and Chervenick, P. A., Corticosteroid effect on granulopoiesis in mice after cyclophosphamide, *J. Clin. Invest.,* 60, 277, 1977.
133. Zalman, F., Maloney, M. A., and Patt, H. M., Differential response of early erythropoietic and granulopoietic progenitors to dexamethasone and cortisone, *J. Exp. Med.,* 149, 67, 1979.
134. Mishell, R. I., Lee, D. A., Grabstein, K. H., and Lachman, L. B., Prevention of the in vitro myelosuppressive effects of glucocorticosteroids by interleukin 1 (IL 1), *J. Immunol.,* 128, 1614, 1982.
135. Barr, R. D., Koekebakker, M., and Milner, R. A., Hydrocortisone — a possible physiological regulator of human granulopoiesis, *Scand. J. Haematol.,* 31, 31, 1983.
136. Suda, T., Miura, Y., Ijima, H., Ozawa, K., Motoyoshi, K., and Takaku, F., The effect of hydrocortisone on human granulopoiesis in vitro with cytochemical analysis of colonies, *Exp. Hematol.,* 11, 114, 1983.
137. Zucker, R., Jauker, U., and Droege, W., Cellular composition of the chicken thymus: effects of neonatal bursectomy and hydrocortisone treatment, *Eur. J. Immunol.,* 3, 812, 1973.
138. Zapata, A., Garrido, E., Laceta, J., and Gomariz, R. P., Relationships between neuroendocrine and immune systems in amphibians and reptiles, *Dev. Comp. Immunol.,* 7, 771, 1983.
139. Chilmonczyk, S., Rainbow trout lymphoid organs: cellular effects of corticosteroids and anti-thymocyte serum, *Dev. Comp. Immunol.,* 6, 271, 1982.
140. Stimson, W. H. and Crilly, P. J., Effects of steroids on the secretion of immunoregulatory factors by thymic epithelial cell cultures, *Immunology,* 44, 401, 1981.
141. Homo, F., Russo-Marie, F., and Papiernik, M., Prostaglandin secretion by human thymic epithelium: in vitro effects of steroids, *Prostaglandins,* 22, 377, 1981.
142. Elliott, E. V., Wallis, V., and Davies, A. J. S., Origin of PHA-responsive cells in the mouse thymus after treatment of the animal with hydrocortisone, *Nature (London) New Biol.,* 234, 77, 1971.
143. Jacobson, H. and Blomgren, H., Changes of the PHA-responding pool of cells in the thymus after cortisone or X-ray treatment of mice. Evidence for an inverse relation between the production of cortical and medullary thymocytes, *Cell. Immunol.,* 4, 93, 1972.
144. Vischer, T. L., Effect of hydrocortisone on the reactivity of thymus and spleen cells of mice to in vitro stimulation, *Immunology,* 23, 777, 1972.
145. Ackerman, A. and Eidinger, D., Further studies of thymus-bone marrow cell synergism in cutaneous manifestations of delayed hypersensitivity to methylated human serum albumin. The effect of cortisone acetate, *Immunology,* 24, 813, 1973.
146. Tyan, M. L., Genetic control of hydrocortisone-induced thymus atrophy, *Immunogenetics,* 8, 177, 1979.
147. Bach, J.-F., Duval, D., Dardenne, M., Salomon, J.-C., Tursz, T., and Fournier, C., The effects of steroids on T cells, *Transplant. Proc.,* 7, 25, 1975.
148. Weismann, J. L., Thymus maturation: studies on the origin of cortisone-resistant thymic lymphocytes, *J. Exp. Med.,* 137, 504, 1973.
149. Walia, A. S., Andersson, B., Fuson, E. W., and Lamon, E. W., The enrichment of thymocytes bearing C3 receptors following cortisone involution, *Cell. Immunol.,* 43, 167, 1979.
150. Triglia, D. and Rothenberg, E., "Mature" thymocytes are not glucocorticoid-resistant in vitro, *J. Immunol.,* 127, 64, 1981.
151. Lutz, C. T., The generation of cytolytic activity in mixed leukocyte cultures: cortisone-resistant thymocytes are deficient in helper T lymphocytes, *J. Immunol.,* 127, 1156, 1981.
152. Dumont, F. and Sabolovic, D., Heterogeneity of the hydrocortisone-resistant cell subpopulation in the mouse thymus, *Biomedicine,* 19, 257, 1973.
153. Doherty, P. C. and Korngold, R., Effects of cyclophosphamide and cortisone on the virus-immune response characteristics of thymocytes and the early reconstitution profiles of P → Fl chimeras, *Cell. Immunol.,* 65, 33, 1981.
154. Ceredig, R. and Cummings, D. E., Phenotypic and functional properties of murine thymocytes. III. Kinetic analysis of the recovery of intrathymic cytolytic T lymphocyte precursors after *in vivo* administration of hydrocortisone acetate, *J. Immunol.,* 130, 33, 1983.
155. Wylie, A. H., Glucocorticoid-induced thymocyte apoptosis is associated with endogenous endonuclease activation, *Nature (London),* 284, 555, 1980.
156. Kodama, J. and Kodama, M., Ultrastructural alterations in the liver parenchymal cells and thymus lymphocytes following the administration of hydrocortisone, *Cancer Res.,* 32, 208, 1972.
157. Miyazawa, T., Sato, C., and Kojima, K., Glucocorticoid-induced membrane alteration of thymoctyes and thymic phagocytosis, *J. Immunol.,* 127, 154, 1981.
158. Khalid, B. A. K., Pearce, P., Barr, I. G., Fraillon, D., Toh, B. H., and Funder, J. W., Dexamethasone induces different cellular protein synthetic responses in PNA⁺ and PNA⁻ mouse thymocyte subpopulations, *J. Immunol.,* 130, 115, 1983.

159. Cohen, J. J. and Duke, R. C., Glucocorticoid activation of a calcium-dependent endonuclease in thymocyte nuclei leads to cell death, *J. Immunol.*, 132, 38, 1984.

160. Weissman, I. L. and Levy, R., In vitro cortisone sensitivity of in vivo cortisone-resistant thymoctyes, *Isr. J. Med. Sci.*, 11, 884, 1975.

161. Trainin, N., Levo, Y., and Rotter, V., Resistance to hydrocortisone conferred upon thymocytes by a thymic humoral factor, *Eur. J. Immunol.*, 4, 634, 1974.

162. Astaldi, G. C. B., Astaldi, A., Groenewoud, M., Wijermans, P., Schelekenes, P. T. A., and Eijsvoogel, V. P., Effect of a human serum thymic factor on hydrocortisone-treated thymocytes, *Eur. J. Immunol.*, 7, 836, 1977.

163. Karczag, E. and Náray, A., Thymidine kinase activity in murine lymphoid organs following glucocorticoid and heparin administration, *Endokrinologie*, 74, 238, 1979.

164. Karczag, E., Kelemenics, K., Jókay, I., and Földes, I., A kinetic study of glucocorticoid-heparin interaction on the in vivo DNA-synthesis of mouse lymphatic organs, *Immunobiology*, 157, 379, 1980.

165. Draber, P., Mechanism of the inhibitory effect of hydrocortisone on concanavalin A-induced activation of thymus cells. Role of interleukins, *Int. J. Immunopharmacol.*, 4, 401, 1982.

166. Bradley, L. M. and Mishell, R. I., Selective protection of murine thymic helper T cells from glucocorticosteroid inhibition by macrophage-derived mediators, *Cell. Immunol.*, 73, 115, 1982.

167. Thurman, G. B., Rossio, J. L., and Goldstein, A. L., Thymosin-induced recovery of murine T-cell functions following treatment with hydrocortisone acetate, *Transplant. Proc.*, 9, 1201, 1977.

168. Rühl, H., Vogt, W., Rühl, U., Bochert, G., and Schmidt, S., Effects of hydrocortisone treatment and whole body irradiation of mouse lymphocyte stimulation in vitro, *Immunology*, 25, 753, 1973.

169. Cohen, P. L. and Mosier, D. E., Reactivity of steroid-resistant neonatal thymocytes, *Nature (London)*, 251, 233, 1974.

170. Thomas, N. and Bell, P. A., Glucocorticoid-induced cell-size changes and nuclear fragility in rat thymocytes, *Mol. Cell. Endocrinol.*, 22, 71, 1981.

171. Wyllie, A. H. and Morris, R. G., Hormone-induced cell death: purification and properties of thymocytes undergoing apoptosis after glucocorticoid treatment, *Am. J. Pathol.*, 109, 78, 1982.

172. Mayer, M., Galili, U., and Kaiser, N., Intracellular protease activity in glucocorticoid-mediated thymolysis, *Endocrinology*, 110, 2131, 1981.

173. Cidlowski, J. A., Glucocorticoids stimulate ribonucleic acid degradation in isolated rat thymic lymphocytes *in vitro*, *Endocrinology*, 11, 184, 1982.

174. Voris, B. P., Nicholson, M. L., and Young, D. A., Development of resistance to glucocorticoid hormones during rat thymus cell differentiation: proteins associated with emergence of the resistant state, *Cancer Res.*, 43, 1236, 1983.

175. Kaiser, N. and Mayer, M., Studies on the antiglucocorticoid action of 11-deoxysteroids in rat thymocytes: discrepancies between *in vivo* and *in vitro* effects, *J. Steroid Biochem.*, 13, 729, 1980.

176. Galili, U., Polliack, A., Okon, E., Leizerovitz, R., Gamliel, H., Korkesh, A., Schenkar, J. G., and Izak, G., Human prothymocytes. Membrane properties, differentiation patterns, glucocorticoid sensitivity and ultrastructural features, *J. Exp. Med.*, 152, 796, 1980.

177. Galili, N., Galili, U., Klein, E., Rosenthal, L., and Nordenskjöld, B., Human T lymphocytes become glucocorticoid-sensitive upon immune activation, *Cell. Immunol.*, 50, 440, 1980.

178. Galili, U., Glucocorticoid induced cytolysis of human normal and malignant lymphocytes, *J. Steroid Biochem.*, 19, 483, 1983.

179. Ranelletti, F. O., Musiani, P., Maggiano, N., Lauriola, L., and Piantelli, M., Modulation of glucocorticoid inhibitory action on human lymphocyte mitogenesis: dependence on mitogen concentration and T-cell maturity, *Cell. Immunol.*, 76, 22, 1983.

180. Kawate, T., Abo, T., Hinuma, S., and Kumagai, K., Studies on the bioperiodicity of the immune response. II. Co-variations of murine T and B cells and a role of corticosteroid, *J. Immunol.*, 126, 1364, 1981.

181. Thompson, J. and van Furth, R., The effect of glucocorticosteroids on the kinetics of mononuclear phagocytes, *J. Exp. Med.*, 131, 429, 1970.

182. Gillette, R. W. and Lance, E. M., Kinetic studies of macrophages. III. The effect of hydrocortisone upon the distribution of radiolabeled peritoneal cells, *J. Reticuloendothel. Soc.*, 12, 701, 1972.

183. Thompson, J. and van Furth, R., The effect of glucocorticosteroids on the proliferation and kinetics of promonocytes and monocytes of the bone marrow, *J. Exp. Med.*, 137, 10, 1973.

184. Oud Alblas, A. B., Linden-Schrever, B., Mattie, H., and Furth, R., The effect of glucocorticosteroids on the kinetics of pulmonary macrophages, *J. Reticuloendothel. Soc.*, 30, 1, 1981.

185. McGarry, M. P., Hydrocortisone acetate-induced eosinopenia in mice: independence from the thymus, *Cell. Immunol.*, 29, 347, 1977.

186. Slonecker, C. E. and Wan Cheng Lim, Effects of hydrocortisone on the cells in an acute inflammatory exudate, *Lab. Invest.*, 27, 123, 1972.

187. Cox, J. H. and Ford, W. L., The migration of lymphocytes across specialized vascular endothelium. IV. Prednisolone acts at several points on the recirculation pathways of lymphocytes, *Cell. Immunol.*, 66, 407, 1982.
188. Lundin, P. M. and Hedman, L. A., Influence of corticosteroids on lymphocyte recirculation, *Lymphology*, 11, 216, 1978.
189. Hedman, L. A., The effect of steroids on the circulating lymphocyte population. III. The size distribution of thoracic duct lymphocytes of the rat and guinea pig after neonatal thymectomy and prednisolone treatment, *Lymphology*, 11, 62, 1978.
190. Hedman, L. A. and Lundin, P. M., The effect of steroids on the circulating lymphocyte population. V. Effect of prednisolone treatment on cell size and life span of the thoracic duct lymphocyte population in normal and neonatally thymectomized rats — a radioisotope study, *Lymphology*, 16, 209, 1983.
191. Beer, D. J. and Center, D. M., *In vitro* corticosteroid modulation of lymphocyte migration, *Cell. Immunol.*, 55, 381, 1980.
192. Hunninghake, G. W. and Fauci, A. S., Immunologic reactivity of the lung. III. Effects of corticosteroids on alveolar macrophage cytotoxic effector cell function, *J. Immunol.*, 118, 146, 1977.
193. Fauci, A. S. and Dale, D. C., The effect of hydrocortisone on the kinetics of normal human lymphocytes, *Blood*, 46, 235, 1975.
194. Yu, D. T. Y., Clements, P. J., and Pearson, C. M., Effect of corticosteroids on exercise-induced lymphocytosis, *Clin. Exp. Immunol.*, 28, 326, 1977.
195. Abo, T., Kawate, T., Itoh, K., and Kumagai, K., Studies on the bioperiodicity of the immune response. I. Circadian rhythms of human T, B and K cell traffic in the peripheral blood, *J. Immunol.*, 126, 1360, 1981.
196. Thomson, S. P., McMahon, L. J., and Nugent, C. A., Endogenous cortisol: a regulator of the number of lymphocytes in peripheral blood, *Clin. Immunol. Immunopathol.*, 17, 506, 1980.
197. Yu, D. T. Y., Clements, P. J., Paulus, H. E., Peter, J. B., Levy, J., and Barnett, E. V., Human lymphocyte subpopulations. Effect of corticosteroids, *J. Clin. Invest.*, 53, 565, 1974.
198. Ten Berge, R. J. M., Sauerwein, H. P., Young, S. L., and Schellekens, P. T. A., Administration of prednisolone *in vivo* affects the ratio of OKT4/OKT8 and the LDH-isoenzyme pattern of human T lymphocytes, *Clin. Immunol. Immunopathol.*, 30, 91, 1984.
199. Fauci, A. S., Murakami, T., Brandon, D. D., Loriaux, D. L., and Lipsett, M. B., Mechanisms of corticosteroid action on lymphocyte subpopulations. VI. Lack of correlation between glucocorticosteroid receptor and the differential effects of glucocorticosteroids on T-cell subpopulations. *Cell. Immunol.*, 49, 43, 1980.
200. Bishop, C. R., Athens, J. W., Boggs, D. R., Warner, H. R., Cartwright, G. E., and Wintrobe, M. M., Leukokinetic studies. XIII. A non-steady-state kinetic evaluation of the mechanism of cortisone-induced granulocytosis, *J. Clin. Invest.*, 47, 249, 1968.
201. Deinard, A. S. and Page, A. R., A study of steroid-induced granulocytosis in a patient with chronic benign neutropenia of childhood, *Br. J. Haematol.*, 28, 333, 1974.
202. Rogers, P. and Matossian-Rogers, A., Differential sensitivity of lymphocyte subsets to corticosteroid treatment, *Immunology*, 46, 841, 1982.
203. Dumont, F. and Bischoff, P., Differential effect of hydrocortisone on lymphocyte populations in mouse spleen, *Biomed. Express*, 29, 28, 1978.
204. Homo, F., Dardenne, M., and Duval, D., Effect of steroids on concanavalin A-induced blast transformation of mouse lymphoid cells, *Cell. Immunol.*, 56, 381, 1980.
205. Larsson, E.-L., Cyclosporin A and dexamethasone suppress T cell response by selectively acting at distinct sites of the triggering process, *J. Immunol.*, 124, 2828, 1980.
206. Cohen, J. J. and Claman, H. N., Hydrocortisone resistance of activated initiator cells in graft versus host reaction, *Nature (London)*, 229, 274, 1971.
207. Segal, S., Cohen, I. R., and Feldman, M., Thymus-derived lymphocytes: humoral and cellular reactions distinguished by hydrocortisone, *Science*, 175, 1126, 1972.
208. Babu, U. M. and Sabbadini, E., Regulation of cell-mediated cytotoxicity. III. Synergism of corticoresistant with anti-thymocyte serum-resistant splenic T cells in the generation of cytotoxic lymphocytes in graft-vs.-host reactions, *J. Immunol.*, 119, 781, 1977.
209. Markham, R. B., Stashak, P. W., Prescott, B., Amsbaugh, D. F., and Baker, P. J., Selective sensitivity to hydrocortisone of regulatory functions that determine the magnitude of the antibody response to Type III pneumococcal polysaccharide, *J. Immunol.*, 121, 829, 1978.
210. Bradley, L. M. and Mishell, R. I., Differential effects of glucocorticoids on the functions of helper and suppressor lymphocytes-T, *Proc. Natl. Acad. Sci. U.S.A. Biol. Sci.*, 78, 3155, 1981.
211. Bradley, L. M. and Mishell, R. I., Differential effects of glucocorticoids on the functions of subpopulations of helper lymphocytes-T, *Eur. J. Immunol.*, 12, 91, 1982.
212. Schleimer, R. P., Jacques, A., Shin, H. S., Lichtenstein, L. M., and Plaut, M., Inhibition of T cell-mediated cytotoxicity by anti-inflammatory steroids, *J. Immunol.*, 132, 266, 1984.

213. Fairchild, S. S., Shannon, K., Kwan, E., and Mishell, R. I., T cell-derived glucosteroid response-modifying factor (GRMFT): a unique lymphokine made by normal T lymphocytes and a T cell hybridoma, *J. Immunol.*, 132, 821, 1984.

214. Mansour, A. and Nelson, D. S., Effect of hydrocortisone on response of rat lymphocytes to phytohaemagglutinin. III, *Aust. J. Exp. Biol. Med. Sci.*, 56, 301, 1978.

215. Noble, C. and Norbury, K. C., The differential sensitivity of rat peripheral blood T cells to immunosuppressants: cyclophosphamide and dexamethasone, *J. Immunopharmacol.*, 5, 341, 1983.

216. Yodoi, J., Hirashima, M., and Ishizaka, K., Lymphocytes bearing Fc receptors for IgE. VI. Suppressive effect of glucocorticoids on the expression of Fc receptors and glycosylation of IgE-binding factors, *J. Immunol.*, 127, 471, 1981.

217. Zeman, G. O., Cohen, G., Budrys, M., Williams, G. C., and Javor, H., The effect of plasma cortisol levels on the lymphocyte transformation test, *J. Allergy Clin. Immunol.*, 49, 10, 1972.

218. Wang, S. R. and Zweiman, B., *In vivo* and *in vitro* effects of methylprednisolone on human lymphocyte proliferation, *Immunopharmacology*, 2, 95, 1980.

219. Wang, S. R., Huang, J. H., and Wang, S., *In vitro* glucocorticoid inhibition of steroid-treated residual circulatory human lymphocytes, *Cell. Immunol.*, 65, 43, 1981.

220. Kauppila, A., Hartikainen-Sorri, A.-L., Koivisto, M., and Ryhanen, P., Cell-mediated immunocompetence of children exposed in utero to short- or long-term action of glucocorticoids, *Gynecol. Obstet. Invest.*, 15, 41, 1983.

221. Saxon, A., Stevens, R. H., Ramer, S. J., Clements, P. J., and Yu, D. T. Y., Glucocorticoids administered in vivo inhibit human suppressor T-lymphocyte function and diminish B-lymphocyte responsiveness in in vitro immunoglobulin synthesis, *J. Clin. Invest.*, 61, 922, 1978.

222. Haynes, B. F., Katz, P., and Fauci, A. S., Mechanisms of corticosteroid action on lymphocyte subpopulations. V. Effects of in vivo hydrocortisone on the circulatory kinetics and function of naturally occurring and mitogen-induced suppressor cells in man, *Cell. Immunol.*, 44, 169, 1979.

223. Duclos, H., Maillot, M. C., Kreis, H., and Galanaud, P., T-suppressor cell function impairment in peripheral blood lymphocytes from transplant recipients under azathioprine and corticosteroids, *Transplantation*, 28, 437, 1979.

224. Roberts, C., Potts, R. C., Brown, R. A., Gibbs, J. H., Browning, M. C. K., and Beck, J. W., The sensitivity of peripheral blood lymphocytes to growth inhibition by hydrocortisone is not determined by their OKT4:OKT8 ratio, *Immunol. Lett.*, 6, 227, 1983.

225. Distelhorst, C. W. and Rogers, J. C., Glucocorticoids inhibit trypsin-induced DNA release from phytohemagglutinin-stimulated blood lymphocytes, *J. Immunol.*, 123, 487, 1979.

226. Wang, S. R. and Zweiman, B., Inhibitory effects of corticosteroids and histamine on human lymphocytes, *J. Allergy Clin. Immunol.*, 67, 39, 1981.

227. Haynes, B. F., Schooley, R. T., Payling-Wright, C. R., Grouse, J. E., Dolin, R., and Fauci, A. S., Emergence of suppressor cells of immunoglobulin synthesis during acute Epstein-Barr virus-induced infectious mononucleosis, *J. Immunol.*, 123, 2095, 1979.

228. Becker, B., Shin, D. H., Palmberg, P. F., and Waltman, S. R., HLA antigens and corticosteroid response, *Science*, 194, 1427, 1976.

229. Goodwin, J. S., Changes in lymphocyte sensitivity to prostaglandin E, histamine, hydrocortisone, and X-irradiation with age: studies in a healthy elderly population, *Clin. Immunol. Immunopathol.*, 25, 243, 1982.

230. Dupont, E., Berkenboom, G., Leempoel, M., and Potvliege, P., Failure of dexamethasone to induce in vitro lysis of human mononuclear cells, *Transplantation*, 30, 387, 1980.

231. Heilman, D. H., Gambrill, M. R., and Leichner, J. P., The effect of hydrocortisone on the incorporation of tritiated thymidine by human blood lymphocytes cultured with phytohaemagglutinin and pokeweek mitogen, *Clin. Exp. Immunol.*, 15, 203, 1973.

232. Krajewski, A. S. and Wyllie, A. H., Inhibition of human lymphocyte-T colony formation by methylprednisolone, *Clin. Exp. Immunol.*, 46, 206, 1981.

233. Robertson, A. J., Gibbs, J. H., Potts, R. C., Brown, R. A., Browning, M. C. K., and Beck, J. S., Dose-related depression of PHA-induced stimulation of human lymphocytes by hydrocortisone, *Int. J. Immunopharmacol.*, 3, 21, 1981.

234. Rosner, W., Ong, K. S., and Khan, M. S., The effect of corticosteroid-binding globulin on the in vitro incorporation of thymidine into human lymphocytes, *J. Clin. Endocrinol. Metab.*, 54, 201, 1982.

235. Ogawa, K., Sueda, K., and Matsui, N., The effect of cortisol, progesterone, and transcortin on phytohemagglutinin-stimulated human blood mononuclear cells and their interplay, *J. Clin. Endocrinol. Metab.*, 56, 121, 1983.

236. Haynes, B. F. and Fauci, A. S., Mechanisms of corticosteroid action on lymphocyte subpopulations. IV. Effects of *in vitro* hydrocortisone on naturally occurring and mitogen-induced suppressor cells in man, *Cell. Immunol.*, 44, 157, 1979.

237. Tsokos, G. C., Christian, C. B., and Balow, J. E., Concanavalin-induced suppressor cells: characterization on the basis of corticosteroid and radiation sensitivity, *Immunology*, 47, 85, 1982.
238. Dwyer, J. M., Johnson, C., and Desaules, M., Behaviour of human immunoregulatory cells in culture. I. Variables requiring consideration for clinical studies, *Clin. Exp. Immunol.*, 38, 499, 1979.
239. Knapp, W. and Posch, B., Concanavalin A-induced suppressor cell activity; opposing effects of hydrocortisone, *J. Immunol.*, 124, 168, 1980.
240. Ilfeld, D. and Krakauer, R. S., Hydrocortisone reverses the suppression of immunoglobulin synthesis by concanavalin A-activated spleen cell supernatants, *Clin. Exp. Immunol.*, 48, 244, 1982.
241. Stites, D. P., Bugbee, S., and Siiteri, P. K., Differential actions of progesterone and cortisol on lymphocyte and monocyte interaction during lymphocyte activation — relevance to immunosuppression in pregnancy, *J. Reprod. Immunol.*, 5, 215, 1983.
242. Palacios, R. and Sugawara, I., Hydrocortisone abrogates proliferation of T cells in autologous mixed lymphocyte reaction by rendering the interleukin-2 producer T cells unresponsive to interleukin-1 and unable to synthesize the T-cell growth factor, *Scand. J. Immunol.*, 15, 25, 1982.
243. Kaplan, M. P., Lysz, K., Rosenberg, S. A., and Rosenberg, J. C., Suppression of interleukin-2 production by methylprednisolone. I, *Transplant. Proc.*, 15, 407, 1983.
244. Lomnitzer, R., Phillips, R., and Rabson, A. R., The effect of hydrocortisone (HC) on sodium periodate and phytohemagglutinin-induced [^{3}H]thymidine incorporation and lymphokine production by human lymphocytes, *Clin. Immunol. Immunopathol.*, 27, 378, 1983.
245. Bettens, F., Kristensen, F., Walker, C., Schwulera, U., Bonnard, G. D., and De Weck, A. L., Lymphokine regulation of activated (G_1) lymphocytes. II. Glucocorticoid and anti-Tac-induced inhibition of human T lymphocyte proliferation, *J. Immunol.*, 132, 261, 1984.
246. Bendtzen, K. and Petersen, J., Effects of cyclosporin A (CyA) and methylprednisolone (MP) on the immune response. I. T-cell activating factor abrogates CyA- but not MP-induced suppression of antigen-induced lymphokine production, *Immunol. Lett.*, 5, 79, 1982.
247. Bendtzen, K., Petersen, J., and Søeberg, B., Effects of cyclosporin A (CyA) and methylprednisolone (MP) on the immune response. II. Further studies of the monocyte — T cell interactions leading to lymphokine production, *Acta Pathol. Microbiol. Immunol. C*, 91, 159, 1983.
248. Wong, L. G., Colburn, K. K., Kacena, A., and Weisbart, R. H., Effect of methylprednisolone on the production of neutrophil migration inhibition factor by T lymphocytes (NIF-T), *Immunopharmacology*, 3, 179, 1981.
249. Guyre, P. M., Bodwell, J. E., and Munck, A., Glucocorticoid action on the immune system: inhibition of production of an Fc-receptor augmenting factor, *J. Steroid Biochem.*, 15, 35, 1981.
250. Hirschberg, H., Pfeffer, P., Hirschberg, T., and Randazzo, B., Effects of methylprednisolone on the in vitro generation of human secondary cytotoxic lymphocytes, *Transplantation*, 29, 413, 1980.
251. Hirschberg, T., Randazzo, B., and Hirschberg, H., Effects of methylprednisolone on the in vitro induction and function of suppressor cells in man, *Scand. J. Immunol.*, 12, 33, 1980.
252. Pfeffer, P. F. and Hirschberg, H., Effect of methylprednisolone on human lymphocytes primed to alloantigens, *J. Clin. Lab. Immunol.*, 10, 19, 1983.
253. Hirschberg, H., Hirschberg, T., Nousianen, H., Braathen, L. R., and Jaffe, E., The effects of corticosteroids on the antigen presenting properties of human monocytes and endothelial cells, *Clin. Immunol. Immunopathol.*, 23, 577, 1982.
254. Tillyer, C. R. and Butterworth, P. H. W., Dexamethasone enhancement of the induction of cells bearing receptors for IgM in human peripheral blood lymphocyte culture, *Clin. Exp. Immunol.*, 40, 178, 1980.
255. Maki, D. V. J., Bankhurst, A. D., Sanchez, M. E., and McLaren, L. C., Modulation of the adherence of human lymphocytes to measles-infected cells by corticosteroids, *Cell. Immunol.*, 52, 350, 1980.
256. Duncan, M. R., Sadlik, J. R., and Hadden, J. W., Glucocorticoid modulation of lymphokine-induced macrophage proliferation, *Cell. Immunol.*, 67, 23, 1982.
257. Balow, J. E. and Rosenthal, A. S., Glucocorticoid suppression of macrophage migration inhibitory factor, *J. Exp. Med.*, 137, 1031, 1973.
258. Wahl, S. M., Altman, L. C., and Rosenstreich, D. L., Inhibition of *in vitro* lymphokine synthesis by glucocorticosteroids, *J. Immunol.*, 115, 476, 1975.
259. Fast, P. E., Hatfield, C. A., Franz, C. L., Adams, E. G., Licht, N. J., and Merritt, M. V., Effects of treatment with immunomodulatory drugs on thymus and spleen lymphocyte subpopulations and serum corticosterone levels, *Immunopharmacology*, 5, 135, 1982.
260. Bona, C., Damais, C., and Chedid, L., Blastic transformation of mouse spleen lymphocytes by a water-soluble mitogen extracted from Nocardia, *Proc. Natl. Acad. Sci. U.S.A. Biol. Sci.*, 71, 1602, 1974.
261. Chedid, L., Juy, D., and Bona, C., Influence of hydrocortisone on antibody-dependent lymphoid cell mediated cytotoxicity, *Immunol. Commun.*, 3, 477, 1974.

262. Sabbele, N. R., Van Oudenaren, A., and Benner, R., The effect of corticosteroids upon the number and organ distribution of "background" immunoglobulin-secreting cells in mice, *Cell. Immunol.*, 77, 308, 1983.

263. Ulrich, R., Levy, L., Kasson, B., Harwick, H. J., and Brammer, G., Developmental changes of immunoglobulins in rats treated neonatally with hydrocortisone, *Proc. Soc. Exp. Biol. Med.*, 154, 107, 1977.

264. Ashman, R. F. and Karlan, B. R. Y., Inhibition of antigen-induced and anti-immunoglobulin-induced capping by hydrocortisone and propranolol, *Immunopharmacology*, 3, 41, 1981.

265. Cupps, T. R., Edgar, L. C., Thomas, C. A., and Fauci, A. S., Multiple mechanisms of B cell immunoregulation in man after administration of *in vivo* corticosteroids, *J. Immunol.*, 132, 170, 1984.

266. Strong, J. E. and Drewinko, B., Response to prednisolone of cultured immunoglobulin-producing human lymphoid cells, *Blood*, 44, 109, 1974.

267. Fauci, A. S., Pratt, K. R., and Whalen, G., Activation of human B lymphocytes. IV. Regulatory effects of corticosteroids on the triggering signal in the plaque-forming cell response of human peripheral blood B lymphocytes to polyclonal activation, *J. Immunol.*, 119, 598, 1977.

268. Cooper, D. A., Duckett, M., Hansen, P., Petts, V., and Penny, R., Glucocorticosteroid enhancement of immunoglobulin synthesis by pokeweed mitogen-stimulated human lymphocytes. II. Lymphocyte-T independence, *Clin. Exp. Immunol.*, 44, 129, 1981.

269. Cupps, T. R., Edgar, L. C., and Fauci, A. S., Corticosteroid-induced modulation of immunoglobulins secretion by human lymphocyte-B: potentiation of background mitogenic signals, *J. Immunopharmacol.*, 4, 255, 1982.

270. Grayson, J., Dooley, N. J., Koski, I. R., and Blaese, R. M., Immunoglobulin production induced in vitro by glucocorticoid hormones — T-cell-dependent stimulation of immunoglobulin production without B-cell proliferation in cultures of human peripheral blood lymphocytes, *J. Clin. Invest.*, 68, 1539, 1981.

271. Orson, F. M., Grayson, J., Pike, S., De Seau, V., and Blaese, R. M., T cell-replacing factor for glucocorticosteroid-induced immunoglobulin production. A unique steroid-dependent cytokine, *J. Exp. Med.*, 158, 1473, 1983.

272. Nugent, K. M. and Pesanti, E. L., Chronic glucocorticosteroid therapy impairs staphylococcal clearance from murine lungs, *Infect. Immunity*, 38, 1033, 1982.

273. Haakenstad, A. O., Case, J. B., and Mannik, M., Effect of cortisone on the disappearance kinetics and tissue localization of soluble immune complexes, *J. Immunol.*, 114, 1153, 1975.

274. Lee, K.-C., Cortisone as a probe for cell interactions in the generation of cytotoxic T cells. I. Effect on helper cells, cytotoxic T cell precursors, and accessory cells, *J. Immunol.*, 119, 1836, 1977.

275. Mantzouranis, E. and Borel, Y., Different effects of cortisone on the humoral immune response to T-dependent and T-independent antigens, *Cell. Immunol.*, 43, 202, 1979.

276. Van Dijk, H., Testerink, J., and Noordegraaf, E., Stimulation of the immune response against SRBC by reduction of corticosterone plasma levels: mediation by mononuclear phagocytes, *Cell. Immunol.*, 25, 8, 1976.

277. Norton, J. M. and Munck, A., In vitro actions of glucocorticoids on murine macrophages: effects on glucose transport and metabolism, growth in culture, and protein synthesis, *J. Immunol.*, 125, 259, 1980.

278. Reeves, W. B., Fairman, R. M., and Haurani, F. I., Influence of hormones on the release of iron by macrophages, *J. Reticuloendothel. Soc.*, 29, 173, 1981.

279. Snyder, D. S. and Unanue, E. R., Corticosteroids inhibit murine macrophage Ia expression and interleukin 1 production, *J. Immunol.*, 129, 1803, 1982.

280. Dimitriu, A., Suppression of macrophage arming by corticosteroids, *Cell. Immunol.*, 21, 79, 1976.

281. Schultz, R. M., Chirigos, M. A., Stoychkov, J. N., and Pavlidis, N. A., Factors affecting macrophage cytotoxic activity with particular emphasis on corticosteroids and acute stress, *J. Reticuloendothel. Soc.*, 26, 83, 1979.

282. van Zwet, T. L., Thompson, J., and van Furth, R., Effect of glucocorticosteroids on the phagocytosis and intracellular killing by peritoneal macrophages, *Infect. Immunity*, 12, 699, 1975.

283. Raz, A. and Goldman, R., The in vitro effect of hydrocortisone on endocytosis in cultured mouse peritoneal macrophages, *J. Reticuloendothel. Soc.*, 20, 177, 1976.

284. Nozawa, R. T., Yanaki, N., and Yokota, T., Cell growth and antimicrobial activity of mouse peritoneal macrophages in response to glucocorticoids, choleragen and lipopolysaccharide, *Microbiol. Immunol.*, 24, 1199, 1980.

285. Grasso, R. J., Klein, T. W., and Benjamin, W. R., Inhibition of yeast phagocytosis and cell spreading by glucocorticoids in cultures of resident murine peritoneal macrophages, *J. Immunopharmacol.*, 3, 171, 1981.

286. Grasso, R. J., West, L. A., Guay, R. C., and Klein, T. W., Inhibition of yeast phagocytosis by dexamethasone in macrophage cultures: reversibility of the effect and enhanced suppression in cultures of stimulated macrophages, *J. Immunopharmacol.*, 4, 265, 1982.

287. Masur, H., Murray, H. W., and Jones, T. C., Effect of hydrocortisone on macrophage response to lymphokine, *Infect. Immunity,* 35, 709, 1982.
288. Mishell, R. I., Bradley, L. M., Chen, Y.-H. U., Grabstein, K. H., Mishell, B. B., Shigi, J. M., and Shigi, S. M., Inhibition of steroid-induced immune suppression by adjuvant stimulated accessory cells, *J. Reticuloendothel. Soc.,* 24, 439, 1978.
289. Moore, R. N., Goodrum, K. J., Couch, R., Jr., and Berry, L. J., Factors affecting macrophage function: glucocorticoid antagonizing factor, *J. Reticuloendothel. Soc.,* 23, 321, 1978.
290. Stošić-Grujičić, S. and Simić, M. M., Modulation of interleukin 1 production by activated macrophages: *in vitro* action of hydrocortisone, colchicine, and *cytochalasin* B, *Cell. Immunol.,* 69, 235, 1982.
291. Belsito, D. V., Flotte, T. J., Lim, H. W., Baer, R. L., Thorbecke, G. J., and Gigli, I., Effect of glucocorticosteroids on epidermal Langerhans cells, *J. Exp. Med.,* 155, 291, 1982.
292. Pennington, J. E., Matthews, W. J., Jr., Marino, J. T., Jr., and Colten, H. R., Cyclophosphamide and cortisone acetate inhibit complement biosynthesis by guinea pig bronchoalveolar macrophages, *J. Immunol.,* 123, 1318, 1979.
293. Gaumer, H. R., Salvaggio, J. E., Weston, W. L., and Claman, H. N., Cortisol inhibition of immunologic activity in guinea pig alveolar cells, *Int. Arch. Allergy Appl. Immunol.,* 47, 797, 1974.
294. Viken, K. E., The effect of steroids on differentiation and function of cultured, mononuclear cells, *Acta Pathol. Microbiol. Scand. C,* 84, 13, 1976.
295. Rinehart, J. J., Wuest, D., and Ackerman, G. A., Corticosteroid alteration of human monocyte to macrophage differentiation, *J. Immunol.,* 129, 1436, 1982.
296. Caudle, M. R., Harbert, G. M., Jr., and Singhas, C. A., Effect of betamethasone on fetal macrophage function: depression of adherence of immunoglobulin-coated red blood cells, *Am. J. Reprod. Immunol.,* 1, 182, 1981.
297. Fries, L. F., Brickman, C. M., and Frank, M. M., Monocyte receptors for the Fc portion of IgG increase in number in autoimmune hemolytic anemia and other hemolytic states and are decreased by glucocorticoid therapy, *J. Immunol.,* 131, 1240, 1983.
298. Rinehart, J. J., Balcerzak, S. P., Sagone, A. L., and Lobuglio, A. F., Effects of corticosteroids on human monocyte function, *J. Clin. Invest.,* 54, 1337, 1974.
299. Tanner, A. R., Halliday, J. W., and Powell, L. W., Effect of long term corticosteroid therapy on monocyte chemotaxis in man, *Scand. J. Immunol.,* 11, 335, 1980.
300. Stevenson, R. D., Polymorph migration stimulator. A new factor produced by hydrocortisone-treated monocytes, *Clin. Exp. Immunol.,* 17, 603, 1974.
301. Purves, E. C. and Brown, K., Effect of cortisone acetate on effector cells for antibody-mediated cytotoxicity in mouse and rat, *Transplantation,* 25, 7, 1978.
302. Hochman, P. S. and Cudkowicz, G., Different sensitivities to hydrocortisone of natural killer cell activity and hybrid resistance to parental marrow grafts, *J. Immunol.,* 119, 2013, 1977.
303. Hochman, P. S. and Cudkowicz, G., Suppression of natural cytotoxicity by spleen cells of hydrocortisone-treated mice, *J. Immunol.,* 123, 968, 1979.
304. Cox, W. I., Holbrook, N. J., Grasso, R. J., Specter, S., and Friedman, H., Suppression of the natural killer cell activity of murine spleen cell cultures by dexamethasone, *Proc. Soc. Exp. Biol. Med.,* 171, 146, 1982.
305. Katz, P., Zaytoun, A. M., and Lee, J. H., The effects of in vivo hydrocortisone on lymphocyte-mediated cytotoxicity, *Arthritis Rheum.,* 27, 72, 1984.
306. Onsrud, M. and Thorsby, E., Influence of in vivo hydrocortisone on some human blood lymphocyte subpopulations. I. Effect on natural killer cell activity, *Scand. J. Immunol.,* 13, 573, 1981.
307. Oshimi, K., Gonda, N., Sumiya, M., and Kano, S., Effects of corticosteroids on natural killer cell activity in systemic lupus erythematosus, *Clin. Exp. Immunol.,* 40, 83, 1980.
308. Bray, R., Abrams, S., and Brahmi, Z., Studies on the mechanism of human natural killer-cell-mediated cytolysis. I. Modulation by dexamethasone and arachidonic acid, *Cell. Immunol.,* 78, 100, 1983.
309. Holbrook, N. J., Cox, W. I., and Horner, H. C., Direct suppression of natural killer activity in human peripheral blood leukocyte cultures by glucocorticoids and its modulation by interferon, *Cancer Res.,* 43, 4019, 1983.
310. Parrillo, J. E. and Fauci, A. S., Comparison of the effector cells in human spontaneous cellular cytotoxicity and antibody-dependent cellular cytoxicity: differential sensitivity of effector cells to in vivo and in vitro corticosteroids, *Scand. J. Immunol.,* 8, 99, 1978.
311. Nair, M. P. N. and Schwartz, S. A., Immunomodulatory effects of corticosteroids on natural killer and antibody-dependent cellular cytotoxic activities of human lymphocytes, *J. Immunol.,* 132, 2876, 1984.
312. Daëron, M., Sterk, A. R., Hirata, F., and Ishizaka, T., Biochemical analysis of glucocorticoid-induced inhibition of IgE-mediated histamine release from mouse mast cells, *J. Immunol.,* 129, 1212, 1982.

313. Csaba, G. and Hodinka, L., Dynamics of the cortisone-effect on mast cell formation, *Acta Morphol. Acad. Sci. Hung.*, 19, 131, 1971.

314. Marquardt, D. L. and Wasserman, S. T., Modulation of rat serosal mast cell biochemistry by in vivo dexamethasone administration, *J. Immunol.*, 131, 934, 1983.

315. Oertel, H. and Kaliner, M., The biologic activity of mast cell granules in rat skin: effects of adreno-corticosteroids on late-phase inflammatory responses induced by mast cell granules, *J. Allergy Clin. Immunol.*, 68, 238, 1981.

316. Tolone, G., Bonasera, L., and Tolone, C., Biosynthesis and release of prostaglandins by mast cells, *Br. J. Exp. Pathol.*, 59, 105, 1978.

317. Bro-Rasmussen, F., Eosinophils in the bone marrow of normal and cortisol-treated rats: quantitative and autoradiographic studies, *Acta Pathol. Microbiol. Scand. A*, 81A, 593, 1973.

318. Bro-Rasmussen, F., Effect of cortisol on the eosinophils in the rat spleen: autoradiographic studies, *Scand. J. Haematol.*, 11, 59, 1973.

319. Sabag, N., Castrillón, M. A., and Tchernitchin, A., Cortisol-induced migration of eosinophil leukocytes to lymphoid organs, *Experientia*, 34, 666, 1978.

320. Poothullil, J., Umemoto, L., Dolovich, J., Hargreave, F. E., and Day, R. P., Inhibition by prednisone of late cutaneous allergic responses induced by antiserum to human IgE, *J. Allergy Clin. Immunol.*, 57, 164, 1976.

321. Schleimer, R. P., Lichtenstein, L. M., and Gillespie, E., Inhibition of basophil histamine release by anti-inflammatory steroids, *Nature (London)*, 292, 454, 1981.

322. Schleimer, R. P., MacGlashan, D. W., Jr., Gillespie, E., and Lichtenstein, L. M., Inhibition of basophil histamine release by anti-inflammatory steroids. II. Studies on the mechanism of action, *J. Immunol.*, 129, 1632, 1982.

323. Peterson, A. P., Altman, L. C., Hill, J. S., Gosney, K., and Kadin, M. E., Glucocorticoid receptors in normal human eosinophils: comparison with neutrophils, *J. Allergy Clin. Immunol.*, 68, 212, 1981.

324. Altman, L. C., Hill, J. S., Hairfield, W. M., and Mullarkey, M. F., Effects of corticosteroids on eosinophil chemotaxis and adherence, *J. Clin. Invest.*, 67, 28, 1981.

325. MacGregor, R. R., Granulocyte adherence changes induced by hemodialysis, endotoxin, epinephrine, and glucocorticoids, *Ann. Intern. Med.*, 86, 35, 1977.

326. Perez, H. D., Kimberley, R. P., Kaplan, H. B., Edelson, H., Inman, R. D., and Goldstein, I. M., Effect of high-dose methylprednisolone infusion on polymorphonuclear leukocyte function in patients with systemic lupus erythematosus, *Arthritis Rheum.*, 24, 641, 1981.

327. Chretien, J. H. and Garagusi, V. F., Corticosteroid effect on phagocytosis and NBT reduction by human polymorphonuclear neutrophils, *J. Reticuloendothel. Soc.*, 11, 358, 1972.

328. Marone, G. and Condorelli, M., Modulation of β-adrenergic receptor by hydrocortisone in human polymorphonuclear leukocytes, *Ric. Clin. Lab.*, 12, 469, 1982.

329. Davies, A. O. and Lefkowitz, R. J., In vitro desensitization of beta-adrenergic receptors in human neutrophils — attenuation by corticosteroids, *J. Clin. Invest.*, 71, 565, 1983.

330. Klempner, M. S. and Gallin, J. I., Inhibition of neutrophil Fc receptor function by corticosteroids, *Clin. Exp. Immunol.*, 34, 137, 1978.

331. Nelson, D. H., Murray, D. K., and Brady, R. O., Dexamethasone-induced change in the sphingomyelin content of human polymorphonuclear leukocytes in vitro, *J. Clin. Endocrinol. Metab.*, 54, 292, 1982.

332. Ignarro, L. J., Glucocorticosteroid inhibition of nonphagocytic discharge of lysosomal enzymes from human neutrophils, *Arthritis Rheum.*, 20, 73, 1977.

333. Hart, D. H. L., Polymorphonuclear leukocyte elastase activity is increased by bacterial lipopolysaccharide: a response inhibited by glucocorticoids, *Blood*, 63, 421, 1984.

334. Hammerschmidt, D. E., White, J. G., Craddock, P. R., and Jacob, H. S., Corticosteroids inhibit complement-induced granulocyte aggregation: possible mechanism for their efficacy in shock states, *J. Clin. Invest.*, 63, 798, 1979.

335. Skubitz, K. M., Craddock, P. R., Hammerschmidt, D. E., and August, J. T., Corticosteroids block binding of chemotactic peptide to its receptor on granulocytes and cause disaggregation of granulocyte aggregates in vitro, *J. Clin. Invest.*, 68, 13, 1981.

336. Issekutz, A. C. and Biggar, W. D., Effect of methylprednisolone and polymyxin-B sulfate on endotoxin-induced inhibition of human neutrophil, *J. Lab. Clin. Med.*, 92, 873, 1978.

337. Forslid, J. and Hed, J., In vitro effect of hydrocortisone on the attachment and ingestion phases of immunoglobulin G- and complement component 3b-mediated phagocytosis by human neutrophils, *Infect. Immunity*, 38, 811, 1982.

338. Christie, K. E., Kjøsen, B., and Solberg, C. O., Influence of hydrocortisone on granulocyte function and glucose metabolism, *Acta Pathol. Microbiol. Scand. C*, 85, 284, 1977.

339. Capsoni, F., Meroni, P. L., Zocchi, M. R., Plebani, A. M., and Vezio, M., Effect of corticosteroids on neutrophil function: inhibition of antibody-dependent cell mediated cytotoxicity (ADCC), *J. Immunopharmacol.*, 5, 217, 1983.

340. Arie, R., Hoogervorst-Spalter, H., Kaufmann, H., Joshua, H., and Klein, A., Metabolism of cortisol by human thrombocytes, *Metabolism*, 28, 67, 1979.

341. Jorgensen, K. A. and Stoffersen, E., Hydrocortisone platelet aggregation and platelet prostaglandin metabolism, *Scand. J. Haematol.*, 25, 445, 1980.

342. JØrgensen, K. A., Freund, L., and SØrensen, P., The effect of prednisone on platelet function tests, *Scand. J. Haematol.*, 28, 118, 1982.

343. Levy, A. L. and Waldmann, J. A., The effect of hydrocortisone on immunoglobulin metabolism, *J. Clin. Invest.*, 49, 1679, 1970.

344. Elliott, E. V. and Sinclair, N. R. S. C., Effect of cortisone acetate on 19S and 7S haemolysin antibody — a time course study, *Immunology*, 15, 643, 1968.

345. Ferreira, A., Moreno, C., and Hoecker, G., Lack of correlation between the effects of cortisone on mouse spleen plaque-forming cells and circulating anti-sheep red blood cell haemolysis, *Immunology*, 24, 607, 1973.

346. Dracott, B. N. and Smith, C. E. T., Hydrocortisone and the antibody response in mice. II. Correlations between serum antibody and PFC in thymus, spleen, marrow and lymph nodes, *Immunology*, 38, 437, 1979.

347. Benner, R. and VanOudenaren, A., Corticosteroids and the humoral immune response of mice. II. Enhancement of bone marrow antibody formation to lipopolysaccharide by high doses of corticosteroids, *Cell. Immunol.*, 48, 267, 1979.

348. Ishizaka, S., Otani, S., and Morisawa, S., Identification of the corticosteroid-sensitive cells in antibody responses in mice, *J. Immunopharmacol.*, 2, 453, 1980.

349. Matuhasi, T. and Usui, M., Specific suppression of immune response to a given antigen by emulsified oil droplets containing a mixture of antigen and dexamethasone phosphate, *Nature (London) New Biol.*, 245, 213, 1973.

350. Greenberg, C. S. and Dimitrov, N. V., The effect of hydrocortisone on the immune response of mice treated with *Corynebacterium parvum*, *Clin. Immunol. Immunopathol.*, 5, 264, 1976.

351. Mantzouranis, E. C. and Borel, Y., Influence of cortisone on immunologic tolerance *in vivo*: cortisone prolongs the duration of unresponsiveness but fails to affect its induction, *Cell. Immunol.*, 74, 54, 1982.

352. Bargatze, R. F. and Katz, D. H., "Allergic breakthrough" after antigen sensitization: height of IgE synthesis is temporally related to diurnal variation in endogenous steroid production, *J. Immunol.*, 125, 2306, 1980.

353. Jókay, I., Kelemenics, K., Karczag, E., and Földes, I., Interactions of glucocorticoids and heparin on the humoral immune response of mice, *Immunobiology*, 157, 390, 1980.

354. Dracott, B. N., The effects of cortisol on the primary response of mouse spleen cell cultures to heterologous erythrocytes, *Cell. Immunol.*, 13, 356, 1974.

355. Ambrose, C. T., The requirements for hydrocortisone in antibody-forming tissue cultivated in serum-free medium, *J. Exp. Med.*, 119, 1027, 1964.

356. Mishell, R. I., Lucas, A., and Mishell, B. B., The role of activated accessory cells in preventing immunosuppression by hydrocortisone, *J. Immunol.*, 119, 118, 1977.

357. Mishell, R. I., Shiigi, J. M., Mishell, B. B., Grabstein, K. H., and Shiigi, S. M., Prevention of the immunosuppressive effects of glucocorticosteroids by cell-free factors from adjuvant activated accessory cells, *Immunopharmacology*, 2, 233, 1980.

358. Anderson, G. W. and Cerilli, J., Hormonal influences on skin graft survival in mice, *J. Surg. Res.*, 18, 321, 1975.

359. Belldegrun, A., Cohen, I. R., Frenkel, A., Servadio, C., and Zor, U., Hydrocortisone and inhibitors of prostaglandin synthesis: potentiation of allograft survival in mice, *Transplantation*, 31, 407, 1981.

360. Cohen, J. J., Fischbach, M., and Claman, H. N., Hydrocortisone resistance of graft vs. host reactivity in mouse thymus, spleen and bone marrow, *J. Immunol.*, 105, 1146, 1970.

361. Lynch, D. H., Gurish, M. F., and Daynes, R. A., Relationship between epidermal Langerhans cell density ATPase activity and the induction of contact hypersensitivity, *J. Immunol.*, 126, 1892, 1981.

362. Venetianer, A., Arányi, P., Bösze, Z., and Fachet, J., Sensitivity to glucocorticoids of lymph node cells stimulated in vivo by oxazolone, *Scand. J. Immunol.*, 8, 355, 1978.

363. Rosenau, W. and Moon, H. D., The inhibitory effects of hydrocortisone on lysis of homologous cells by lymphocytes in vitro, *J. Immunol.*, 89, 422, 1962.

364. Pavia, C., Siiteri, P. K., Perlman, J. D., and Stites, D. P., Suppression of murine allogeneic cell interactions by sex hormones, *J. Reprod. Immunol.*, 1, 33, 1979.

365. Ioachim, H. L., The cortisone-induced wasting disease of newborn rats: histopathological and autoradiographic studies, *J. Pathol.*, 104, 201, 1971.

366. Winnearls, C. G., Millard, P. R., and Morris, P. J., Effect of azathioprine and prednisolone on passive enhancement of rat renal allografts, *Transplantation*, 25, 229, 1978.

367. Cohen, I. R., Stavy, L., and Feldman, M., Glucocorticoids and cellular immunity in vitro. Facilitation of the sensitization phase and inhibition of the effector phase of a lymphocyte anti-fibroblast reaction, *J. Exp. Med.*, 132, 1055, 1970.

368. Stavy, L., Cohen, I. R., and Feldman, M., The effect of hydrocortisone on lymphocyte-mediated cytolysis, *Cell. Immunol.*, 7, 302, 1973.

369. Stavy, L., Cohen, I. R., and Feldman, M., Stimulation of rat lymphocyte proliferation by hydrocortisone during the induction of cell-mediated immunity in vitro, *Transplantation*, 17, 173, 1974.

370. Atkinson, J. P., Schreiber, A. D., and Frank, M. M., Effects of corticosteroids and splenectomy on the immune clearance and destruction of erythrocytes, *J. Clin. Invest.*, 52, 1509, 1973.

371. Balow, J. E., Hurley, D. L., and Fauci, A. S., Immunosuppressive effects of glucocorticosteroids: differential effects of acute vs. chronic administration on cell-mediated immunity, *J. Immunol.*, 114, 1072, 1975.

372. Long, D. A. and Miles, A. A., Opposite actions of thyroid and adrenal hormones in allergic hypersensitivity, *Lancet*, I, 492, 1950.

373. Weston, W. L., Claman, H. N., and Krueger, G. G., Site of action of cortisol in cellular immunity, *J. Immunol.*, 110, 880, 1973.

374. Scothorne, R. J., The effect of cortisone on the changes produced in regional lymph nodes by skin homograft, *J. Anat.*, 90, 417, 1956.

375. Friedman, E. A., Methylprednisolone therapy and allograft rejection. Comparison of daily and alternate day administration, *Transplantation*, 10, 552, 1970.

376. Rossouw, D. J., Chase, C. C., Scheepers, J. C. E., van der Walt, J. J., and Joubert, J. R., The effect of steroid therapy on the cytological and histopathological changes during experimental extrinsic allergic alveolitis, *S. Afr. Med. J.*, 60, 159, 1981.

377. Issekutz, A. C., Comparison of the effects of glucocorticoid and indomethacin treatment on the acute inflammatory reaction in rabbits, *Immunopharmacology*, 5, 183, 1983.

378. Ambrose, C. T., The essential role of corticosteroids in the induction of the immune response in vitro, in *Hormones and the Immune Response*, Wolstenholme, G. E. and Knight, J., Eds., Churchill Livingstone, London, 1970, 100.

379. Griggs, R. C., Condemi, J. J., and Vaughan, J. H., Effect of therapeutic dosages of prednisone on human immunoglobulin G metabolism, *J. Allergy Clin. Immunol.*, 49, 267, 1972.

380. Butler, W. T. and Rossen, R. D., Effects of corticosteroids on immunity in man. II. Alterations in serum protein components after methylprednisolone, *Transplant. Proc.*, 5, 1215, 1973.

381. Butler, W. T. and Rossen, R. D., Effects of corticosteroids on immunity in man. I. Decreased serum IgG concentration caused by 3 or 5 days of high doses of methylprednisolone, *J. Clin. Invest.*, 52, 2629, 1973.

382. Posey, W. C., Nelson, H. S., Branch, B., and Pearlman, D. S., Effects of acute corticosteroid therapy for asthma on serum immunoglobulin levels, *J. Allergy Clin. Immunol.*, 62, 340, 1978.

383. Settipane, G. A., Pudupakkam, R. K., and McGowan, J. H., Corticosteroid effect on immunoglobulins, *J. Allergy Clin. Immunol.*, 62, 162, 1978.

384. McMillan, R., Longmire, R., and Yelenosky, R., Effect of corticosteroids on human IgG synthesis, *J. Immunol.*, 116, 1592, 1976.

385. Tuchinda, M., Newcomb, R. W., and DeVald, B. L., Effect of prednisone treatment on the human immune response to keyhole limpet hemocyanin, *Int. Arch. Allergy Appl. Immunol.*, 42, 533, 1972.

386. Fan, P. T., Yu, D. T. Y., Clements, P. J., Fowlston, S., Eisman, J., and Bluestone, R., Effect of corticosteroids on human immune response: comparison of 1 and 3 daily 1 g intravenous pulses of methylprednisolone, *J. Lab. Clin. Med.*, 91, 625, 1978.

387. Frey, B. M., Frey, F. J., Holford, N. H. G., Lozada, F., and Benet, L. Z., Prednisolone pharmacodynamics assessed by inhibition of the mixed lymphocyte reaction, *Transplantation*, 33, 578, 1982.

388. Hahn, B. H., MacDermott, R. P., Jacobs, S. B., Pletscher, L. S., and Beale, M. G., Immunosuppressive effects of low doses of glucocorticoids: effects on autologous and allogeneic mixed leukocyte reactions, *J. Immunol.*, 124, 2812, 1980.

389. Galanaud, P., Crevon, M. C., Hillion, D., and Delfraissy, J. F., Hydrocortisone sensitivity of human in vitro antibody response: different sensitivity of the specific and the nonspecific B-cell responses induced by the same agent, *Clin. Immunol. Immunopathol.*, 18, 68, 1981.

390. Kim, Y. T., Schwartz, A., Blum, J., and Weksler, M. E., The plaque-forming cell response of human blood lymphocytes. I. PFC response of lymphocytes to formalin-treated staphylococci, *Cell. Immunol.*, 48, 308, 1979.

391. Balow, J. E., Hunninghake, G. W., and Fauci, A. S., Corticosteroids in human lymphocyte-mediated cytotoxic reactions. Effects on the kinetics of sensitization and on the cytolytic capacity of effector lymphocytes in vitro, *Transplantation*, 23, 322, 1977.

392. Ilfeld, D. N., Krakauer, R. S., and Blaese, R. M., Suppression of the human autologous mixed lymphocyte reaction by physiologic concentrations of hydrocortisone, *J. Immunol.*, 119, 428, 1977.

393. Glick, B., Cortisone, age and antibody-mediated immunity, *Int. Arch. Allergy Appl. Immunol.*, 43, 766, 1972.

394. Rollins, L. A. and McKinnell, R. G., The influence of glucocorticoids on survival and growth of allografted tumors in the anterior eye chamber of leopard frogs, *Dev. Comp. Immunol.*, 4, 283, 1980.

395. Melmon, K. L., The endocrinologic function of selected autacoids: catecholamines, acetylcholine, serotonin and histamine, in *Textbook of Endocrinology*, 6th ed., Williams, R. H., Ed., W. B. Saunders, Philadelphia, 1981, 515.

396. Mueller, R. A., Thoenen, H., and Axelrod, J., Effect of pituitary and ACTH on the maintenance of basal tyrosine hydroxylase activity in the rat adrenal gland, *Endocrinology*, 86, 751, 1970.

397. Axelrod, J. and Reisine, T. D., Stress hormones: their interaction and regulation, *Science*, 224, 452, 1984.

398. Recant, L., Hume, D. M., Forsham, P. H., and Thorn, G. W., Studies on the effect of epinephrine on the pituitary-adrenocortical system, *J. Clin. Endocrinol. Metab.*, 10, 187, 1950.

399. Labrie, F., Giguere, V., Proulx, L., and Lefevre, G., Interactions between CRF, epinephrine, vasopressin and glucocorticoids in the control of ACTH secretion, *J. Steroid Biochem.*, 20, 153, 1984.

400. Huang, X. Y. and McCann, S. M., Effect of β-adrenergic drugs on LH, FSH, and growth hormone (GH) secretion in conscious, ovariectomized rats, *Proc. Soc. Exp. Biol. Med.*, 174, 244, 1983.

401. Motulsky, H. J. and Insel, P. A., Adrenergic receptors in man: direct identification, physiologic regulation, and clinical alterations, *N. Engl. J. Med.*, 307, 18, 1982.

402. Berthelsen, S. and Pettinger, W. A., Functional basis for classification of alpha-adrenergic receptors, *Life Sci.*, 21, 595, 1977.

403. Lefkowitz, R. J., Caron, M. G., Michel, T., and Stadel, J. M., Mechanisms of hormone receptor-effector coupling: the β-adrenergic receptor and adenylate cyclase, *Fed. Proc. Fed. Am. Soc. Exp. Biol.*, 41, 2664, 1982.

404. Singh, U., Millson, D. S., Smith, P. A., and Owen, J. J. T., Identification of beta-adrenoceptors during thymocyte ontogeny in mice, *Eur. J. Immunol.*, 9, 31, 1979.

405. Johnson, D. L. and Gordon, M. A., Characteristics of adrenergic binding sites associated with murine lymphocytes isolated from spleen, *J. Immunopharmacol.*, 2, 435, 1980.

406. Loveland, B. E., Jarrott, B., and McKenzie, I. F. C., The detection of β-adrenoceptors on murine lymphocytes, *Int. J. Immunopharmacol.*, 3, 45, 1981.

407. Uzan, A., Phan, T., and Le Fur, G., Selective labeling of murine B lymphocytes by [³H]spiroperidol, *J. Pharm. Pharmacol.*, 33, 102, 1981.

408. Le Fur, G., Phan, T., Canton, T., Tur, C., and Uzan, A., Evidence for a coupling between dopaminergic receptors and phospholipid methylation in mouse B lymphocytes, *Life Sci.*, 29, 2737, 1981.

409. Marquardt, D. L. and Wasserman, S. I., Characterization of the rat mast cell: beta-adrenergic receptor in resting and stimulated cells by radioligand binding, *J. Immunol.*, 129, 2122, 1982.

410. Le Fur, G., Phan, T., and Uzan, A., Identification of stereospecific (³H)spiroperidol binding sites in mammalian lymphocytes, *Life Sci.*, 26, 1139, 1980.

411. Casale, T. B., Halonen, M., and Kaliner, M., Detection of beta-adrenergic receptors on rabbit mononuclear cells isolated free of significant contamination by other cell types, *Life Sci.*, 33, 971, 1983.

412. Watanabe, Y., Tsan Lai, R., Higuchi, H., Maeda, H., and Yoshida, H., Beta-adrenoceptors of human lymphocytes: decrease in affinity of agonist for (−)³H-dihydroalprenolol binding sites by cytoplasmic fractions, *Life Sci.*, 28, 1399, 1981.

413. Brodde, O.-E., Engel, G., Hoyer, D., Bock, K. D., and Weber, F., The β-adrenergic receptor in human lymphocytes: subclassification by the use of a new radio-ligand, (±)-¹²⁵Iodocyanopindolol, *Life Sci.*, 29, 2189, 1981.

414. Motojima, S., Fukuda, T., and Makino, S., Measurement of β-adrenergic receptors on lymphocytes in normal subjects and asthmatics in relation to β-adrenergic hyperglycaemic response and bronchial responsiveness, *Allergy*, 38, 331, 1983.

415. Pochet, R., Delespesse, G., Gausset, P. W., and Collet, H., Distribution of beta-adrenergic receptors on human lymphocyte subpopulations, *Clin. Exp. Immunol.*, 38, 578, 1979.

416. Davis, P. B., Dieckman, L., Boat, T. F., Stern, R. C., and Doershuk, C. F., Beta-adrenergic receptors in lymphocytes and granulocytes from patients with cystic fibrosis, *J. Clin. Invest.*, 71, 1787, 1983.

417. Bishopric, N. H., Cohen, H. J., and Lefkowitz, R. J., Beta-adrenergic receptors in lymphocyte subpopulations, *J. Allergy Clin. Immunol.*, 65, 29, 1980.

418. Bidart, J. M., Motte, P., Assicot, M., Bohuon, C., and Bellet, D., Catechol-o-methyltransferase activity and aminergic binding sites distribution in human peripheral blood lymphocyte subpopulations, *Clin. Immunol. Immunopathol.*, 26, 1, 1983.

419. Alexander, R. W., Cooper, B., and Handin, R. I., Characterization of human platelet alpha-adrenergic receptor: correlation of [H-3]dihydroergocryptine binding with aggregation and adenylate cyclase inhibition, *J. Clin. Invest.*, 61, 1136, 1978.

420. Grant, J. A. and Scrutton, M. C., Novel α_2-adrenoreceptors primarily responsible for inducing human platelet aggregation, *Nature (London)*, 277, 659, 1979.

421. Cooper, B., Handin, R. I., Young, L. H., and Alexander, R. W., Agonist regulation of the human platelet α-adrenergic receptor, *Nature (London)*, 274, 703, 1978.

422. Kemp, R. G., Huang, Y.-C., and Duquesnoy, R. J., Decreased epinephrine response of adenylate cyclase activity of lymphoid cells from immunodeficient pituitary dwarf mice, *J. Immunol.*, 111, 1855, 1973.

423. Gol'dshtein, M. M. and Dontsov, V. I., Reactivity of mouse splenic B lymphocytes to adrenalin during the immune response, *Bull. Exp. Biol. Med.*, 94, 1413, 1982.

424. Singh, U. and Owen, J. J. T., Studies on the maturation of thymus stem cells: the effects of catecholamines, histamine and peptide hormones on the expression of T cell alloantigens, *Eur. J. Immunol.*, 6, 59, 1976.

425. Ito, M., Sless, F., and Parrott, D. M. V., Evidence for control of complement receptor rosette-forming cells by α- and β-adrenergic agents, *Nature (London)*, 266, 633, 1977.

426. Johnson, D. L., Ashmore, R. C., and Gordon, M. A., Effects of beta-adrenergic agents on the murine lymphocyte response to mitogen stimulation, *J. Immunopharmacol.*, 3, 205, 1981.

427. Melmon, K. L., Bourne, H. R., Weinstein, Y., Shearer, G. M., Kram, J., and Bauminger, S., Hemolytic plaque formation by leukocytes *in vitro:* control by vasoactive hormones, *J. Clin. Invest.*, 53, 13, 1974.

428. Depelchin, A. and Letesson, J. J., Adrenaline influence on the immune response. I. Accelerating or suppressor effects according to the time of application, *Immunol. Lett.*, 3, 199, 1981.

429. Braun, W. and Rega, M. J., Adenyl cyclase-stimulating catecholamines as modifiers of antibody formation, *Immunol. Commun.*, 1, 523, 1972.

430. Besedovsky, H. O., del Rey, A., Sorkin, E., Da Prada, M., and Keller, H. H., Immunoregulation mediated by the sympathetic nervous system, *Cell. Immunol.*, 48, 346, 1979.

431. Pierpaoli, W. and Maestroni, G. J. M., Pharmacologic control of the hormonally modulated immune response. III. Prolongation of allogeneic skin graft rejection and prevention of runt disease by a combination of drugs acting on neuroendocrine functions, *J. Immunol.*, 120, 1600, 1978.

432. Guirgis, H. M. and Townley, R. G., Effect of pertussis and beta-adrenergic-blocking agents on mast cells, *J. Allergy Clin. Immunol.*, 58, 241, 1976.

433. Joasoo, A. and McKenzie, J. M., Stress and the immune response in rats, *Int. Arch. Allergy Appl. Immunol.*, 50, 659, 1976.

434. Thevathassan, O. J. and Gordon, A. S., Adrenocortical-medullary interactions on the blood eosinophils, *Acta Haematol.*, 19, 162, 1958.

435. Podolec, Z., Vetulani, J., Bednarczyk, B., and Szczeklik, A., Central dopamine receptors regulate blood eosinophilia in the rat, *Allergy*, 34, 103, 1979.

436. Alm, P. E. and Bloom, G. D., Effects of norepinephrine on transmembrane calcium transport in rat mast cells, *Int. Arch. Allergy Appl. Immunol.*, 66, 427, 1981.

437. Alm, P. E. and Bloom, G. D., Catecholamine inhibition of rat mast cell histamine secretion: a process independent of cyclic AMP levels and counteracted by glucose, *Life Sci.*, 32, 307, 1983.

438. Ernstrom, U. and Sandberg, G., Effects of adrenergic alpha- and beta-receptor stimulation on the release of lymphocytes and granulocytes from the spleen, *Scand. J. Haematol.*, 11, 275, 1973.

439. Ernstrom, U. and Sandberg, G., Adrenaline-induced release of lymphocytes and granulocytes from the spleen, *Biomedicine*, 21, 293, 1974.

440. Verghese, M. W. and Snyderman, R., Hormonal activation of adenylate cyclase in macrophage membranes is regulated by guanine nucleotides, *J. Immunol.*, 130, 869, 1983.

441. Crary, B., Hauser, S. L., Borysenko, M., Kutz, I., Hoban, C., Ault, K. A., Weiner, H. L., and Benson, H., Epinephrine-induced changes in the distribution of lymphocyte subsets in a peripheral blood of humans, *J. Immunol.*, 131, 1178, 1983.

442. Tonnesen, E., Tonnesen, J., and Christensen, N. J., Augmentation of cytotoxicity by natural killer (NK) cells after adrenaline administration in man, *Acta Pathol. Microbiol. Immunol. B*, 92, 81, 1984.

443. Steel, C. M., French, E. B., and Aitchison, W. R. C., Studies on adrenaline-induced leucocytosis in normal man. I. The role of the spleen and of the thoracic duct, *Br. J. Haematol.*, 21, 413, 1971.

444. French, E. B., Steel, C. M., and Aitchison, W. R. C., Studies on adrenaline-induced leucocytosis in normal man. II. The effects of α- and β-adrenergic blocking agents, *Br. J. Haematol.*, 21, 423, 1971.

445. Saran, R., Effect of adrenaline and isoprenaline on circulating eosinophils in tropical pulmonary eosinophilia, *Indian J. Med. Res.*, 67, 439, 1978.

446. Aarons, R. D., Nies, A. S., Gal, J., Hegstrand, L. R., and Molinoff, P. B., Elevation of beta-adrenergic receptor density in human lymphocytes after propranolol administration, *J. Clin. Invest.*, 65, 949, 1980.

447. Colucci, W. S., Alexander, R. W., Williams, G. H., Rude, R. E., Holman, B. L., Konstam, M. A., Wynne, J., Mudge, G. H., Jr., and Braunwald, E., Decreased lymphocyte beta-adrenergic-receptor density in patients with heart failure and tolerance to the beta-adrenergic agonist pirbuterol, *N. Engl. J. Med.*, 305, 185, 1981.

448. Lee, T.-P., Regulation of beta-adrenergic response in human lymphocytes: agonists induced subsensitivity, *Res. Comm. Chem. Pathol. Pharmacol.*, 22, 233, 1978.

449. Parker, C. W., Huber, M. G., and Baumann, M. L., Alterations in cyclic AMP metabolism in human bronchial asthma. III. Leukocyte and lymphocyte responses to steroids, *J. Clin. Invest.*, 52, 1342, 1973.

450. Lee, T. P., Busse, W. W., and Reed, C. E., Effect of beta adrenergic agonist, prostaglandins, and cortisol on lymphocyte levels on cyclic adenosine monophosphate and glycogen: abnormal lymphocytic metabolism in asthma, *J. Allergy Clin. Immunol.*, 59, 408, 1977.

451. Sherman, N. A., Smith, R. S., and Middleton, E., Jr., Effect of adrenergic compounds, aminophylline and hydrocortisone, on in vitro immunoglobulin synthesis by normal human peripheral lymphocytes, *J. Allergy Clin. Immunol.*, 52, 13, 1973.

452. Galant, S. P., Underwood, S. B., Lundak, T. C., Groncy, C. C., and Mouratides, D. I., Heterogeneity of human lymphocyte subpopulations to pharmacologic stimulation. I. Lymphocyte responsiveness to beta-adrenergic agents, *J. Allergy Clin. Immunol.*, 62, 349, 1978.

453. Crary, B., Borysenko, M., Sutherland, D. C., Kutz, I., Borysenko, J. Z., and Benson, H., Decrease in mitogen responsiveness of mononuclear cells from peripheral blood after epinephrine administration in humans, *J. Immunol.*, 130, 694, 1983.

454. Lad, P. M., Glovsky, M. M., Smiley, P. A., Klempner, M., Reisinger, D. M., and Richards, J. H., The β-adrenergic receptor in the human neutrophil plasma membrane: receptor-cyclase uncoupling is associated with amplified GTP activation, *J. Immunol.*, 132, 1466, 1984.

455. Anderson, R. and Van Rensburg, A. J., The in vitro effects of propranolol and atenolol on neutrophil motility and post-phagocytic metabolic activity, *Immunology*, 37, 15, 1979.

456. Schopf, R. E. and Lemmel, E.-M., Control of the production of oxygen intermediates of human polymorphonuclear leukocytes and monocytes by β-adrenergic receptors, *J. Immunopharmacol.*, 5, 203, 1983.

457. Szentivanyi, A., The beta adrenergic theory of the atopic abnormality in bronchial asthma, *J. Allergy*, 42, 208, 1968.

458. Szentivanyi, A., Radioligand binding approach in the study of lymphocytic adrenoreceptors and the constitutional basis of atopy, *J. Allergy Clin. Immunol.*, 65, 5, 1980.

459. Kaliner, M., Orange, R. P., and Austen, K. F., Immunological release of histamine and slow reacting substance of anaphylaxis from human lung. IV. Enhancement by cholinergic and alpha adrenergic stimulation, *J. Exp. Med.*, 136, 556, 1972.

460. Assem, E. S. K. and Schild, H. O., β-adrenergic receptors concerned with the anaphylactic mechanism, *Int. Arch. Allergy Appl. Immunol.*, 45, 62, 1973.

461. Mansfield, L. E. and Nelson, H. S., Effect of beta-adrenergic agents on immunoglobulin-G levels in asthmatic subjects, *Int. Arch. Allergy Appl. Immunol.*, 68, 13, 1982.

462. Shereff, R. H., Harwell, W., Lieberman, P., Rosenberg, E. W., and Robinson, H., Effect of beta adrenergic stimulation and blockade on immediate hypersensitivity skin test reactions, *J. Allergy Clin. Immunol.*, 52, 328, 1973.

463. Kram, J. A., Bourne, H. R., Maibach, H. I., and Melmon, K. L., Cutaneous immediate hypersensitivity in man: effects of systemically administered adrenergic drugs, *J. Allergy Clin. Immunol.*, 56, 387, 1975.

464. Brooks, S. M., Mcgowan, K., Bernstein, I. L., Altenau, P., and Peagler, J., Relationship between numbers of beta-adrenergic receptors in lymphocytes and disease severity in asthma, *J. Allergy Clin. Immunol.*, 63, 401, 1979.

465. Scarpace, P. J., Littner, M. R., Tashkin, D. P., and Abrass, I. B., Lymphocyte beta-adrenergic refractoriness induced by theophylline or metaproterenol in healthy and asthmatic subjects, *Life Sci.*, 31, 1567, 1982.

466. Fraser, C. M., Venter, J. C., and Kaliner, M., Autonomic abnormalities and autoantibodies to beta-adrenergic receptors, *N. Engl. J. Med.*, 305, 1165, 1981.

467. Venter, J. C., Fraser, C. M., and Harrison, L. C., Autoantibodies to β_2-adrenergic receptors: a possible cause of adrenergic hyporesponsiveness in allergic rhinitis and asthma, *Science*, 207, 1361, 1980.

468. Kafka, M. S., Tallman, J. F., Smith, C. C., and Costa, J. L., Alpha-adrenergic receptors on human platelets, *Life Sci.*, 21, 1429, 1977.

469. Campbell, W. B., Johnson, A. R., Callahan, K. S., and Graham, R. M., Anti-platelet activity of beta-adrenergic antagonists: inhibition of thromboxane synthesis and platelet aggregation in patients receiving long-term propranolol treatment, *Lancet*, II, 1382, 1981.

470. Homer, J. T. and Cain, W. A., Enhancement of IgE antibody formation in the rabbit by adrenergic antagonists, *Int. Arch. Allergy Appl. Immunol.*, 59, 121, 1979.
471. Schmidt-Gayk, H. E., Jakobs, K. H., and Hackenthal, E., Cyclic AMP and phagocytosis in alveolar macrophages: influence of hormones and dibutyryl cyclic AMP, *J. Reticuloendothel. Soc.*, 17, 251, 1975.
472. Hodgson, R. M., Clothier, R. H., Ruben, L. N., and Balls, M., Effects of alpha-adrenergic and beta-adrenergic agents on spleen cell antigen in 4 amphibian species, *Eur. J. Immunol.*, 8, 348, 1978.
473. Gordon, M. A., Cohen, J. J., and Wilson, I. B., Muscarinic cholinergic receptors in murine lympho-cytes: demonstration by direct binding, *Proc. Natl. Acad. Sci. U.S.A. Biol. Sci.*, 75, 2902, 1978.
474. Ueno, S., Wada, K., Takahashi, M., and Tarui, S., Acetylcholine receptor in rabbit thymus: anti-genic similarity between acetylcholine receptors of muscle and thymus, *Clin. Exp. Immunol.*, 42, 463, 1980.
475. Fuchs, S., Schmidt-Hopfeld, I., Tridente, G., and Tarrab-Hazdai, R., Thymic lymphocytes bear a surface antigen which crossreacts with acetylcholine receptor, *Nature (London)*, 287, 162, 1980.
476. Galant, S. P., Lundak, R. L., and Eaton, L., Enhancement of early human E rosette formation by cholinergic stimuli, *J. Immunol.*, 117, 48, 1976.
477. Strom, T. B., Sytkowski, A. J., Carpenter, C. B., and Merrill, J. P., Cholinergic augmentation of lymphocyte-mediated cytotoxicity: a study of the cholinergic receptor of cytotoxic T lymphocytes, *Proc. Natl. Acad. Sci. U.S.A. Biol. Sci.*, 71, 1330, 1974.
478. Whaley, K., Lappin, D., and Barkas, T., C2 synthesis by human monocytes is modulated by a nico-tinic cholinergic receptor, *Nature (London)*, 293, 580, 1981.
479. Fantozzi, R., Masini, E., Blandina, P., Mannaioni, P. F., and Bani-Sacchi, T., Release of histamine from rat mast cells by acetylcholine, *Nature (London)*, 273, 473, 1978.
480. Kaliner, M., Cholinergic nervous system and immediate hypersensitivity. I. Eccrine sweat responses in allergic patients, *J. Allergy Clin. Immunol.*, 58, 308, 1976.
481. Kaplan, A. P., Natbony, S. F., Tawil, A. P., Fruchter, L., and Foster, M., Exercise-induced ana-phylaxis as a manifestation of cholinergic urticaria, *J. Allergy Clin. Immunol.*, 68, 319, 1981.
482. Abe, J., Ichikawa, Y., Yamasaki, K., Homme, M., and Nomura, M., Plasma corticosterone level in runt disease, *J. Natl. Cancer Inst.*, 48, 119, 1972.
483. Hoot, G. P., Head, J. R., and Griffin, W. S. T., Increased free plasma corticosterone and adrenal hyperactivity associated with graft-versus-host disease, *Transplantation*, 35, 478, 1983.
484. Levine, S., Sowinski, R., and Steinetz, B., Effects of experimental allergic encephalomyelitis on thymus and adrenal: relation to remission and relapse, *Proc. Soc. Exp. Biol. Med.*, 165, 218, 1980.
485. Belliveau, J. F., Tschaen, D. M., Ferrante, K. J., and O'Leary, G. P., Jr., The plasma corticosteroid profile in the adjuvant induced arthritic rat model, *FEBS Lett.*, 139, 136, 1982.
486. Besedovsky, H., Sorkin, E., Keller, M., and Muller, J., Changes in blood hormone levels during the immune response, *Proc. Soc. Exp. Biol. Med.*, 150, 466, 1975.
487. Shek, P. N. and Sabiston, B. H., Neuroendocrine regulation of immune processes: change in circu-lating corticosterone levels induced by the primary antibody response in mice, *Int. J. Immunophar-macol.*, 5, 23, 1983.
488. Simensen, E., Olson, L. D., Ryan, M. P., Vanjonack, W. J., and Johnson, H. D., Plasma corticos-terone concentrations in turkeys inoculated with *Pasteurella multocida* and maintained in high and low environmental temperatures, *Avian Dis.*, 24, 833, 1980.
489. Moberg, G. P., Site of action of endotoxins on hypothalamic-pituitary-adrenal axis, *Am. J. Physiol.*, 220, 397, 1971.
490. Seltzer, A. and Donoso, A. O., Involvement of specific receptors in the histamine stimulation of the pituitary-corticoadrenal system in the rat, *Neuroendocrinol. Lett.*, 4, 299, 1982.
491. Badger, A. M., Griswold, D. E., Dimartino, M. J., and Poste, G., Inhibition of antibody synthesis by histamine in concanavalin A-treated mice: the possible role of glucocorticosteroids, *J. Immunol.*, 129, 1017, 1982.
492. Besedovsky, H. O., del Rey, A., and Sorkin, E., Lymphokine-containing supernatants from Con A-stimulated cells increase corticosterone blood levels, *J. Immunol.*, 126, 385, 1981.
493. Duff, G. W. and Durum, S. K., Fever and immunoregulation: hyperthermia, interleukins 1 and 2, and T-cell proliferation, *Yale J. Biol. Med.*, 55, 437, 1982.
494. Jampel, H. D., Duff, G. D., Gershon, R. K., Atkins, E., and Durum, S. K., Fever and immunore-gulation. III. Hyperthermia augments the primary in vitro humoral immune response, *J. Exp. Med.*, 157, 1229, 1983.
495. Liddle, G. W., The adrenals, in *Textbook of Endocrinology*, 6th ed., Williams, R. H., Ed., W. B. Saunders, Philadelphia, 1981, 249.
496. Sivas, A., Uysal, M., and Oz, H., The hyperglycemic effect of thymosin-F5, a thymic hormone, *Hormone Metab. Res.*, 14, 330, 1982.

497. Healy, D. L., Hodgen, G. D., Schulte, H. M., Chrousos, G. P., Loriaux, D. L., Hall, N. R., and Goldstein, A. L., The thymus-adrenal connection: thymosin has corticotropin-releasing activity in primates, *Science,* 222, 1353, 1983.

498. Vahouny, G. V., Kyeyune-Nyombi, E., McGillis, J. P., Tare, N. S., Huang, K.-Y., Tombes, R., Goldstein, A. L., and Hall, N. R., Thymosin peptides and lymphokines do not directly stimulate adrenal corticosteroid production in vitro, *J. Immunol.,* 130, 791, 1983.

499. Pedernera, E. A., Romano, M., Besedovsky, H. O., and Del Carmen Aguilar, M., The bursa of Fabricius is required for normal endocrine development in chicken, *Gen. Comp. Endocrinol.,* 42, 413, 1980.

500. Pouplard, A., Bottazzo, G.-F., Doniach, D., and Roitt, I. M., Binding of human immunoglobulins to pituitary ACTH cells, *Nature (London),* 261, 142, 1976.

501. Boyd, W. H., Peters, A., and Morris, G., Binding bovine immunoglobulins to anterior lobe cells of hypophysis, *Experientia,* 34, 1090, 1978.

502. Boyd, W. H., Peters, A., and Morris, G., Binding of bovine immunoglobulins to pituitary intermediate lobe cells, *Endocrinol. Exp.,* 13, 3, 1979.

503. Boyd, W. H. and Peters, A., Low molecular weight protein in bovine anterior pituitary similar to immunoglobulin M, *Endocrinol. Exp.,* 14, 83, 1980.

504. Smith, E. M., Meyer, W. J., and Blalock, J. E., Virus-induced corticosterone in hypophysectomized mice: a possible lymphoid adrenal axis, *Science,* 218, 1311, 1982.

505. Blalock, J. E., Opinion. The immune system as a sensory organ, *J. Immunol.,* 132, 1067, 1984.

506. Smith, E. M. and Blalock, J. E., Human lymphocyte production of corticotropin and endorphin-like substances: association with leukocyte interferon, *Proc. Natl. Acad. Sci. U.S.A. Biol. Sci.,* 78, 7530, 1981.

507. Johnson, H. M., Smith, E. M., Torres, B. A., and Blalock, J. E., Regulation of the in vitro antibody response by neuroendocrine hormones, *Proc. Natl. Acad. Sci. U.S.A. Biol. Sci.,* 79, 4171, 1982.

508. Johnson, H. M., Torres, B. A., Smith, E. M., Dion, L. D., and Blalock, J. E., Regulation of lymphokine (γ-interferon) production by corticotropin, *J. Immunol.,* 132, 246, 1984.

509. Keri, G., Parameswaren, V., Trunkey, D. D., and Ramachandran, J., Effects of septic shock plasma on adrenocortical cell function, *Life Sci.,* 28, 1917, 1981.

510. Mathison, J. C., Schreiber, R. D., La Forest, A. C., and Ulevitch, R. J., Suppression of ACTH-induced steroidogenesis by supernatants from LPS-treated peritoneal exudate macrophages, *J. Immunol.,* 130, 2757, 1983.

Chapter 5

THE EFFECTS OF GROWTH HORMONE AND RELATED HORMONES ON THE IMMUNE SYSTEM

I. Berczi

TABLE OF CONTENTS

I. INTRODUCTION

Growth hormone, somatomedins, somatostatin, and insulin will be discussed in this chapter. Recent evidence indicates that somatomedins, or in other words insulin-like growth factors, which mediate the action of growth hormone on a variety of target tissues, are very similar, both in structure and in function, to insulin.[1,2] Moreover, there is a long standing observation in medicine which is supported by recent data, that insulin and growth hormone act as antagonists on glucose metabolism and that there is a regulatory interaction between these two hormones.[3-8] Indeed, there is evidence for altered pituitary function in diabetics.[9-10] Therefore, these hormones may be regarded as a functionally related unit governing growth and glucose metabolism.

II. GROWTH HORMONE (GH)

A. Early Observations

Early investigators noted that GH increased the size of thymus in both intact and hypophysectomized (Hypox) animals. A specific thymotropic function was suggested for GH, since Hypox animals treated with GH had larger thymuses than operated control animals. Prolonged GH treatment of Hypox rats also stimulated lymph node and spleen growth in addition to that of thymus. However, other investigators observed extensive increase of thymic and lymph node weight in Hypox animals, as compared to controls, which seemed to contradict the above results. Furthermore, GH was found to be ineffective in starved animals and in intact rats.[11]

Around the turn of this century some pathologists regarded acromegaly to be associated with lymphatic hyperplasia, suggesting a stimulatory influence of the pituitary gland on the thymus.[12] However, it was recognized that in addition to hormonal changes a great number of diverse conditions influence the size of the thymus and of lymphatic organs, which cast serious doubts on the validity of these observations.

B. Growth Hormone Receptors in Lymphoid Tissue

Lesniak and co-workers[13,14] demonstrated the specific binding of ^{125}I-human growth hormone (HGH) to the human lymphocyte cell line IM-9. ^{125}I-HGH bound to IM-9 cells could only be displaced by HGH and not by bovine, ovine, or rat GH, which are biologically inactive in man, or by bovine TSH. Sheep prolactin showed slight displacement of ^{125}I-HGH at a concentration of 50 μg/mℓ. The ability of a variety of HGH preparations to inhibit binding of ^{125}I-HGH to IM-9 was proportional to the biological potency of the material. Tryptic digestion destroyed the capacity of cells to bind HGH. Approximately 4000 binding sites per cell were estimated with an affinity constant of 1.3×10^9 M^{-1}. The same group of investigators were unable to show binding of labeled HGH to circulating blood cells.

Arrenbrecht[15] described the specific binding of bovine ^{125}I-HGH to calf and mouse thymocytes, and 10 to 20,000 binding sites per cell were proposed. These results were questioned by Herington and Faragher[16] who were unable to find GH receptors on rat thymocytes and suggested that the results of Arrenbrecht were due to the absorption of tracer onto the incubation tube, rather than to the thymocytes.

Stewart et al.[17] extracted peripheral lymphocytes of pituitary dwarf children with Triton® X100 and demonstrated binding of GH by the solubilized material, which was increased after GH treatment of these patients. The receptor detected was extremely elusive, and it was proposed by the investigators that GH receptors released by the liver were taken up by lymphocytes and rapidly released again.

In our laboratory two myeloid cell lines, one monocyte line, three B cell lines, and three T cell lines, all of human origin, were examined for the presence of lactogenic or

GH receptors, using ^{125}I-HGH as a tracer in radioreceptor assay. Rat lymph node, spleen, thymus, and bone marrow cells were examined similarly, both as fresh preparations or after stimulation with PHA or LPS. No clearly detectable receptors were found.[18] Therefore, while certain lymphoid cell lines express specific and high avidity receptors for GH, this does not seem to be a general rule for other cultured cells of lymphoid origin, and it is uncertain at the present time, whether or not normal lymphocytes express GH receptors.

C. The Effect of Growth Hormone on the Thymus and Bone Marrow

There is a marked reduction of DNA synthesis in the thymus and other lymphoid organs of rats 15 weeks after hypophysectomy. Administration of bovine growth hormone (BGH) leads to the enhancement of DNA synthesis, whereas the injection of rabbit anti-BGH globulin over 5 days caused a drop in the weight of the thymus and in the rate of the DNA synthesis in these organs. After a single injection of BGH to Hypox animals, the stimulation of DNA synthesis was observed earlier in the thymus than in the spleen or lymph nodes. Furthermore, BGH stimulated DNA and RNA synthesis by thymocytes in vitro.[19]

Lymphoid cell suspensions were transferred into normal or thymectomized suckling mice, which were also treated with GH. After immunization, the number of antibody forming cells were determined in the spleen. GH enhanced the helper function of normal thymocytes, but not of lymph node and spleen cells or of hydrocortisone resistant thymocytes.[20] A high frequency of wasting disease occurred in the offspring of inbred Weimaraner dogs, which was associated with a small thymus, lack of antibody response, and impaired response of lymphocytes to PHA. Such deficient pups lacked a normal increase in plasma GH concentration after stimulation with clonidine, which indicates that these animals had concurrent abnormalities of thymus dependent immune function and GH metabolism.[21]

Prepubertal hypopituitary dwarf children are anemic and have reduced levels of erythropoietin stimulating factor (ESF) in the urine. Treatment with HGH in doses sufficient to produce a linear growth induces bone marrow lymphocytosis and increased erythropoiesis, which is associated with increased concentrations of ESF in the urine, increased transferrin levels, and expansion of the plasma volume.[22]

D. The Effect of Growth Hormone on Immunity
1. Mouse

Baroni and co-workers[23] were the first to call attention to the immunodeficiency of hereditary pituitary recessive dwarf mice of Snell-Bagg strain. These animals are characterized by early involution of the thymus, hypocellularity in peripheral lymphoid tissues and bone marrow, and impaired immune responses. Treatment of such animals with GH and thyroxin prevented the thymus involution and the cellular depletion in lymphoid organs and also normalized the immune response. Similar results were obtained on the same mouse strain by Fabris and co-workers.[24,25] These authors proposed that the immunodeficiency of Snell-Bagg dwarf mouse was due to the arrested ontogenic development of the thymus due to the failure of the pituitary to produce certain hormones, especially GH. They confirmed that dwarf mice can be normalized immunologically by GH and thyroxin treatment, which restores completely the structure of the thymus and of peripheral lymphoid tissues. The action of hormones was not exerted, if dwarf mice were thymectomized in adult age. Dumont et al.[26] also studied Snell-Bagg dwarf mice and found essentially normal thymocyte population but slightly decreased frequency of T cells and lowered frequency of B lymphocytes in the spleen, but with normal response to T and B cell mitogens. High mobility splenic cells had a smaller modal volume in dwarf mice than in control animals, but this difference was not corrected by treatment with GH and thyroxin. When expressed as a function of body weight, the numbers of splenic T and B lymphocytes in untreated mice were about half the corresponding values in hormone reconstituted or normal littermates. Hormone treatment exerted little direct effect on the thymus in adult life but rather influenced the size of the pool of both peripheral T and B lymphocytes.

Spleen cells from Hypox mice showed a persistent depression of the immune reactivity to antigen in vitro. Treatment of Hypox animals with GH prior to cell culture resulted in an almost normal immune reactivity. Furthermore, in Hypox animals exogenous GH could interfere with the effect of increased endogenous corticosterone.[27] Spleen natural killer (NK) cell activity was reduced in mice hypophysectomized 4 to 8 weeks earlier. The percentage of null cells and of target binding cells in spleens from hypophysectomized and sham-operated animals were not significantly different. Administration of ovine GH (100 μg/day i.p. for 10 days) resulted in a marked recovery of NK activity in Hypox animals. The NK activity was mediated by non-T, non-B lymphocytes.[28]

In mixed culture of mouse lymphocytes the presence of insulin, but not of GH, was necessary for the generation of blastogenic response. However, the presence of GH during a 5-day culture allowed for the generation of cytotoxic T lymphocytes. Further studies revealed that GH was needed to be present during the first 2 days of culture before the entry of the cytotoxic cell precursors into cell division.[29]

2. Rat

Lymph node and thymus, but not spleen cells, of Hypox rats incorporated less ³H-thymidine than did cells from intact rats. Furthermore, cortisol-induced leukopenia did not return to normal within 6 hr in Hypox animals, but did so in their normal counterparts. An increased concentration of an unidentified factor that promotes leukocytic proliferation was found in the plasma of intact cortisol treated rats, which also stimulated ³H-thymidine uptake by thymus and lymph node tissue in vitro. Treatment of Hypox animals with GH opposed cortisol-induced leukopenia. It was suggested that GH release is a normal leukocytopoietic stimulus following cortisol-induced lymphopenia and that GH mediates a normal response to stress.[30]

The turnover of DNA showed a sharp reduction in the spleen, a significant but smaller decrease in the thymus, and it remained largely unchanged in the lymph nodes of rats after hypophysectomy. Formalin injection into normal animals gave rise to lymph follicle proliferation in the spleen and the appearance of high concentrations of pyroninophil cells in the lymphoid organs. Similar changes were absent in Hypox animals but could be elicited by the administration of GH and/or thyroxin.[31]

Hayashida and Li[32] were the first to observe that ACTH and GH have an antagonistic effect on the humoral immune response of rats. Young adult rats were immunized with an extract of *Pasteurella pestis*. ACTH treatment alone, in daily doses just sufficient to prevent body weight increase, suppressed the antibody response significantly. The administration of GH alone resulted in a marked increase in body weight and a slight increase in antibody levels. When GH and ACTH were given simultaneously, body weight was maintained at a level slightly above that of controls, and GH counteracted effectively the depression of antibody production.

The production of precipitating antibodies was impaired and skin allograft rejection was delayed in rats following hypophysectomy. Daily injections of GH restored normal responses, if the thymus was present. In Hypox and thymectomized animals it was necessary to give thymic hormone in addition to GH for immune restoration.[33,34] A marked reduction in plaque-forming cells and hemagglutination titers was observed in rats 15 weeks after hypophysectomy. The administration of BGH to Hypox animals led to the recovery of the immune response.[19] Immunization of weanling rats with

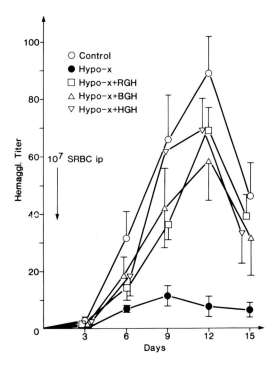

FIGURE 1. Reconstitution of the antibody response in hypophysectomized rats by various growth hormone preparations. The combined results of two identical experiments performed on female Fischer rats are presented in this Figure. Groups of four animals were used in the first and groups of five in the second experiment. Sheep red blood cells (SRBC; 10⁷ i.p.) were injected 3 weeks after hypophysectomy (Hypo-X), along with a group of normal controls. Treatment of the appropriate groups with 40 μg daily s.c. doses of rat growth hormone (RGH), bovine growth hormone (BGH), and human growth hormone (HGH) was started at the time of antigen injection and maintained for 10 days. Animals included in the final evaluation: O — 9, ●— 8, □ — 8, △ — 7, ▽ — 7. Mean haemagglutination titers ± SE are indicated in the Figure. *Statistical analysis* (*t*-test): control compared with Hypo-X — P<0.001 throughout the experiment. No significant difference occurred between the reactivity of controls and the hormone treated groups.[18]

sheep red blood cells (SRBC) led, within 24 hr, to an increase in DNA synthesis in the spleen, which was further increased significantly when the antigen was given together with GH, insulin, and estradiol. When the hormones were administered singularly, only GH and insulin increased DNA synthesis in the spleen; but not in the lymph nodes.[35]

Scott et al.[36] observed that long-term hypophysectomized rats responded better to immunization with SRBC than did their aging unoperated littermates. The Hypox animals were maintained on corticosterone, deoxycorticosterone, and thyroxin, with salt supplements in the drinking water. One week prior to immunization additional daily doses of 100 μg/kg of BGH were given for the duration of the experiments.

During our initial studies on the hormonal reconstitution of humoral immunity in Hypox rats, BGH was less effective than bovine prolactin. However, in subsequent experiments rat-, bovine-, and human GH were compared for the reconstitution of the anti-SRBC antibody response in Hypox animals and were found to be equally effective. GH was able to reconstitute humoral immunity in Hypox rats to the level of controls and no other pituitary hormone was necessary (Figure 1).[18,37] Essentially, identical results were obtained with delayed-type hypersensitivity reactions induced by di-

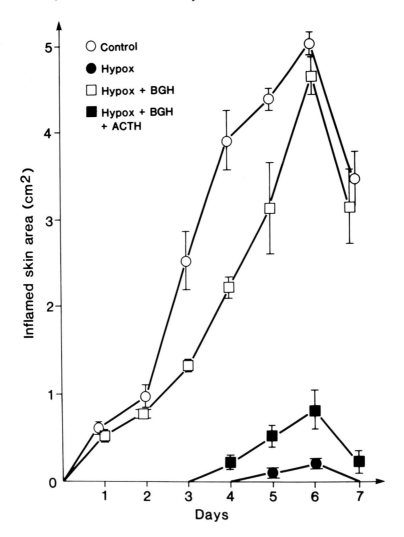

FIGURE 2.   The antagonistic effect of growth hormone and ACTH on DNCB contact sensitivity. Groups of five female Wistar Furth rats were used. (Please see legend to Figure 1 for more details.) BGH and ACTH were given s.c. at 40 μg daily doses for 5 days, commencing on the day of sensitization with dinitrochlorobenzene (DNCB; 2 mg dissolved in 10 μℓ of acetone was painted on the shaved dorsal skin), and maintained for 5 days. *Statistics:* Control group was significantly different ($P < 0.1$) from Hypo-X, Hypo-X + BGH + ACTH on days 1 to 7; and from Hypo-X + BGH on days 3 to 5. Hypo-X compared to Hypo-X + BGH: $P < 0.01$ on days 1 to 7; Hypo-X compared to Hypo-X + BGH + ACTH: $P < 0.01$ on days 4 to 6; Hypo-X + BGH compared to Hypo-X + BGH + ACTH: $P < 0.01$ on days 1 to 7.[38]

nitrochlorobenzene (DNCB). Hypox rats did not develop contact sensitivity to this agent, but they did so readily if BGH was given, commencing on the day of skin painting with DNCB and maintained for 5 days. Maximum reaction occurred 5 to 6 days after skin painting. Histologically the lesions of GH treated animals were indistinguishable from those of controls. If ACTH was given in addition to GH to Hypox animals, the reaction was inhibited, indicating that these two hormones act antagonistically on contact sensitivity reactions (Figures 2 and 3).[38]

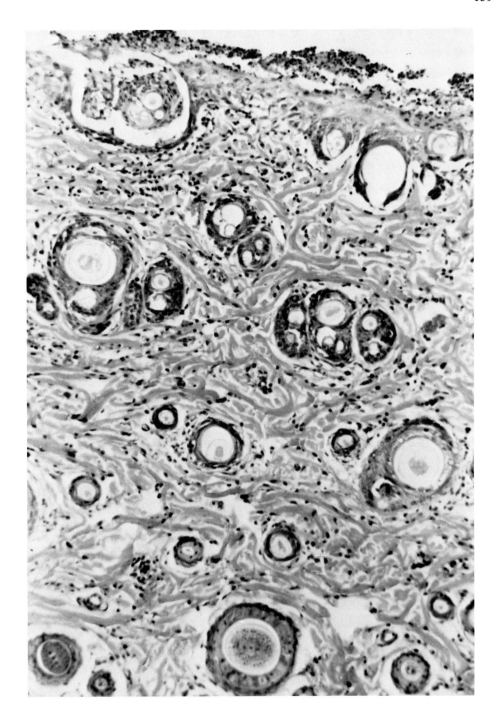

FIGURE 3.   Skin reaction to DNCB in Hypo-X rat given GH therapy. Histology of DNCB skin reaction in hypophysectomized rat given GH therapy reveals an inflammatory infiltrate composed of polymorphonuclear and mononuclear leukocytes involving the dermis, primarily in a perivascular and periappendageal distribution. The surface is covered by fibrin and inflammatory cells; however, there is no ulceration in this case. (Hematoxylin-eosin stain; original magnification × 32.) (Courtesy of Drs. S. L. Asa and K. Kovacs, Department of Pathology, University of Toronto.)

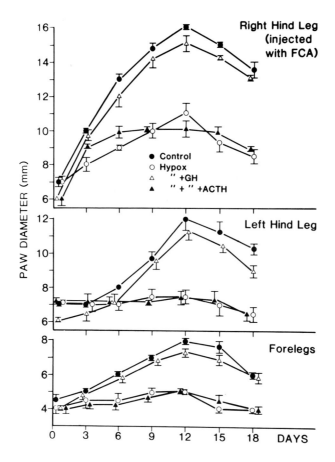

FIGURE 4.   The antagonistic effect of GH and ACTH on the development of adjuvant arthritis. Groups of ten female Fischer animals were used; hypophysectomy was performed 3 weeks prior to the induction of arthritis by 0.1 mℓ of Freund's complete adjuvant (containing 5 mg/mℓ of *Mycobacterium tuberculosis)* injected into the right hind paw. Hormone treatment was initiated on the day of arthritis induction: bovine growth hormone (BGH) was given at 40 μg daily doses s.c. and porcine ACTH at 0.02 IU s.c., and maintained for 18 days. The final evaluation included eight to ten animals from each group. Mean paw diameters are shown in the figure. *Statistics:* For the forelegs and right hind legs, controls and Hypox + GH differed significantly ($P < 0.01$) from Hypox and from Hypox + GH + ACTH on days 6 to 18 and for the left hind legs, on days 9 to 18. No consistently significant differences occurred between control and Hypox + GH or between Hypox and Hypox + GH + ACTH. See Figure 1 for abbreviations.[39]

Adjuvant arthritis in the rat is a popular model for rheumatoid arthritis. This autoimmune reaction is also inhibited by hypophysectomy, and GH treatment of Hypox animals restores their sensitivity to the arthritis reaction. Furthermore, the restoring effect of GH is inhibited again by ACTH (Figures 4 and 5).[39]

Treatment of rats with the dopaminergic ergot alkyloid, bromocriptine (BRC), inhibited immune reactions as much as did hypophysectomy. Additional treatment of BRC-suppressed animals with BGH restored their immune reactivity, which could again be inhibited by ACTH treatment (Figure 6).[40] This was an unexpected finding for two reasons. First, BRC is known to inhibit prolactin (PRL) secretion only, and second, little or no effect can be demonstrated on GH secretion.[41,42] If indeed this is the case at the doses applied in our experiments (5 mg/kg daily), the observed immunodeficiency must be due to the lack of PRL secretion. In this case the restoring effect

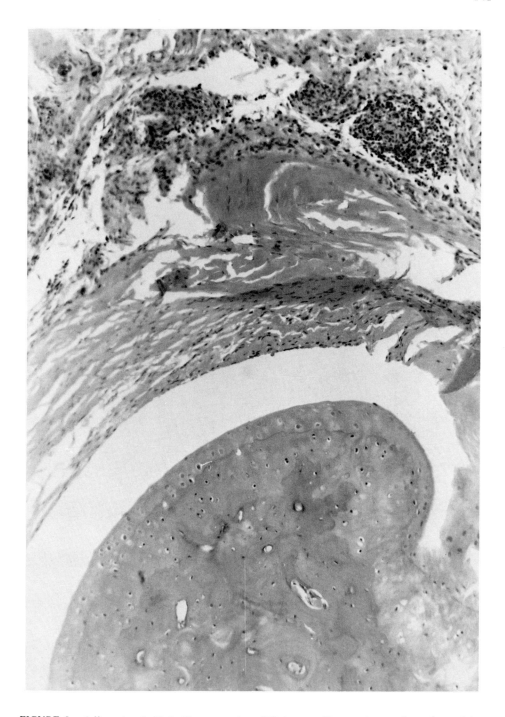

FIGURE 5. Adjuvant arthritis in Hypox rat given GH therapy. The s.c. tissue and muscle overlying bone is infiltrated by polymorphonuclear and mononuclear inflammatory cells. (Hematoxylin-eosin stain; original magnification × 32.) (Courtesy of Drs. S. L. Asa and K. Kovacs, Department of Pathology, University of Toronto.)

of GH can only be explained by its modest PRL content (3%). This is unlikely, however, because in all of our experiments comparable doses of GH and PRL were necessary for restoring a variety of immune reactions in Hypox animals. In such doses (200

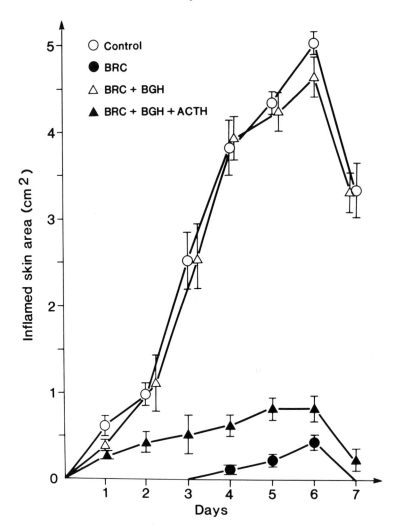

FIGURE 6.   Restoration of the contact sensitivity reaction in bromocriptine-suppressed rats by GH is antagonized by ACTH. Groups of five female Wistar Furth rats were treated with 5 mg/kg bromocriptine s.c., commencing 1 week before the induction of DNCB contact sensitivity and treatment was maintained until the end of the experiment. Injections of ovine prolactin (40 μg/day/animal s.c.) and of porcine ACTH (40 μg/day/animal s.c.) were initiated on the day of DNCB application and maintained for 5 days. All animals survived and were included in the final evaluation of this experiment. *Statistics:* Control was significantly different $P <$ 0.01) from the BRC-treated group on days 4 to 6, and from the BRC + BGH + ACTH group on days 2 to 7, but did not differ significantly at any time from the group treated with BRC + BGH: the BRC-treated group was significantly different from BRC + BGH and from BRC + BGH + ACTH on days 4 to 6.[40]

μg/kg) the PRL contamination of GH was far less than the minimum dose of PRL capable of restoring immunocompetence (100 μg/kg). Therefore, one must consider the possibility, that GH was also affected by BRC treatment. Indeed, some observations in man would support this assumption.[43,44] This explanation is more compatible with our results, obtained in Hypox animals, where GH was as effective in restoring immune activity as PRL, and only one of these hormones was needed for complete restoration. Nevertheless, further studies are required to clarify these points.[18]

3. Man

Fleisher and co-workers[45] studied a family with X-linked hypogammaglobulinemia and isolated GH deficiency. Two brothers and their two maternal uncles had this disorder. All patients had short stature and related bone age during childhood, and the adults had delayed onset of puberty. Two patients had recurrent sinopulmonary infections. The immunodeficiency was characterized by the absence of antibody formation in vivo and impaired immunglobulin secretion in vitro. Three of the four patients lacked circulating B lymphocytes, although tonsils were present. All patients had deficient GH reponses to insulin, arginine, or levodopa. The immunodeficiency of these patients differed from the usual X-linked immune disorders and the World Health Organization classification in that it was associated with GH deficiency without other endocrine abnormality. Gupta et al.[46] found that patients with isolated GH deficiency had increased proportions of suppressor/cytotoxic T lymphocytes and surface immunoglobulin bearing B lymphocytes. Proliferative response to phytohemagglutinin (PHA) was normal, but in mixed lymphocyte reactions, T cells from three of four patients responded poorly and three out of four patients' non T cells showed poor stimulation in the system. Con A activated suppressor cell activity was also normal.

Thrombin induces an abrupt increase of oxygen consumption by platelets, which was significantly reduced in pituitary dwarfs. During GH treatment the response of platelets from dwarfs to thrombin was similar to that of controls.[47]

Granulocytes isolated from the peripheral blood of pituitary dwarfs had a low level of tetrazolium reductase activity under resting conditions and also after stimulation of phagocytosis by starch. Two hours after the i.m. administration of HGH, the resting and stimulated tetrazolium reductase activity was significantly increased. An increase of both activities was found also in patients with acromegaly. A modest increase of tetrazolium reductase activity was observed after adding GH to isolated granulocytes in vitro.[48]

Allergic patients reacted with a significantly lower rise of serum GH levels after stimulation with L-dopa; compared with controls. L-Dopa treatment induced a significant elevation of eosinophil counts in healthy subjects 30 to 60 min after administration, but not in allergic patients. Another GH releasing agent, apomorphine (0.75 mg), elicited increase in GH in 9 of 10 control individuals, but only in 6 of the 11 ectopic patients studied. These results indicate that central dopaminergic stimulation of GH release is often impaired in allergic patients; this may be among the causes of failure to respond to L-dopa.[49]

Vanderschueren-Lodeweyckx and co-workers[50] reported that HGH did not stimulate lymphocytes in vitro from normal donors or from patients with hypopituitarism. The PHA response of lymphocytes from the same donors was not potentiated either by GH. Schimpff and co-workers[51] observed that GH dependent factors are present in human serum that potentiate the response of lymphocytes to PHA. However, subsequent investigations revealed that this effect was probably due to L-glutamine, which is increased in acromegalics and reduced in hypopituitary patients.[52] Mercola et al.[53] observed that nanogram concentrations of HGH potentiated colony formation by normal human T cells, which was species specific. A T cell leukemia-derived lymphoblast line also showed augmented colony growth in the presence of HGH. Ovine prolactin was stimulatory in two of the four individuals tested. Human placental lactogen also showed some activity. Kiess et al.[54] demonstrated that HGH itself induced lymphoproliferation with maximal responses at 50 ng/mℓ concentration and after 7 days of exposure. In contrast, HGH reduced the proliferative response of peripheral blood lymphocytes to PHA. Both of these effects were neutralized by HGH specific antisera.

4. Other Species

An autosomal dwarf and a sex-linked dwarf line of white Leghorn strain of chicken were examined for immunocompetence, in comparison with normally growing white Leghorn chickens. Autosomal dwarf animals responded normally to SRBC during primary immunization and following a secondary antigen challenge. On the other hand, the males of the sex-linked dwarf strain produced less antibody to low antigen dosages, in both the primary and secondary response, but as antigen dose was increased, the humoral response was no longer depressed. Antibody titers were normal in females, but PFC formation was impaired significantly both in males and females.[55] One-day-old male chicks were treated either with thyroxin feed supplements, or by daily injections of GH, or by a combination of these treatments. In sex-linked dwarf animals GH enhanced significantly the humoral immune responsiveness and bursal growth, whereas thyroxin stimulated thymic growth as well as overall growth. GH and/or thyroxin treatments had no specific effects on primary lymphoid organ growth in the autosomal dwarf strain, but either treatments separately resulted in significant increase in overall body size. None of the treatments affected any of the above parameters in control animals. No differences were found between the dwarf and control strains in endogenous GH levels, although mammalian GH treatments did produce significant changes in serum T3 and T4 levels within the control strain.[56]

III. SOMATOMEDIN AND SOMATOSTATIN

A. Somatomedin

Specific receptor sites for somatomedin, distinct from insulin receptor sites, have been described on circulating human mononuclear cells, on cord blood lymphocytes, and on the IM-9 human leukemia cell line.[57-59] Fetal lymphocytes bound more ^{125}I-somatomedin C than did adult lymphocytes. Somatomedins are similar structurally and functionally to insulin, and for this reason they are also called insulin-like growth factors (IGF-I, IGF-II). Insulin competed for the IGF-I receptor on IM-9 insulin receptor with displacement of ^{125}I-insulin, which was concentration dependent. Insulin and somatomedin peptides not only bind to each other's receptors, but regulate each receptor, which is proportional to their ability to occupy that receptor.[58,59]

There are no firm data for the possible biological effect of somatomedins on lymphoid cells. Lymphocytes from constitutionally tall children responded to lectins in a similar manner to children with normal growth.[60] A GH dependent serum factor capable of enhancing the thymidine uptake by lectin activated human lymphocytes has been described by Thierito-Prévost and Schimpff.[61] Subsequent studies revealed that the enhancing factor is likely to be identical with L-glutamine.[52]

B. Somatostatin

Somatostatin is a cyclic tetradecapeptide, first isolated from hypothalamic tissue, but subsequently found to be widely distributed in various tissues. Its designation stems from its inhibitory action on GH release. Somatostatin also inhibits the secretion of a number of hormones and neurotransmitters.

Somatostatin stimulated macrophage endocytic function in perfused livers of rats, as revealed by the uptake of carbon particles. Glucagon had a similar effect, whereas insulin reduced phagocytosis.[62] Somatostatin strongly stimulated the secretion of histamine from rat peritoneal mast cells. Stimulation was energy, temperature, and calcium dependent.[63] Vasoactive intestinal polypeptide was found to be a potent stimulator of adenylate cyclase activity in rat lymphocytes, which was antagonized by somatostatin.[64]

IV. INSULIN

A. Insulin Receptors in Lymphoid Cells

Resting T and B lymphocytes have very few, if any, insulin receptors on their surface. If, however, the cells are activated by specific antigen, or mitogens, high affinity $(K_d = 1.1$ n $M)$ insulin receptors will appear on both cell types. Thus, the appearance of insulin receptors can be regarded as a marker of cellular activation. Inhibition of DNA synthesis with mitomycin C, the disruption of micro- and spindle-tubules by colchicine, and the disruption of microfilaments by cytochalasin B, do not affect the expression of insulin receptors by T cells. The expression of receptors during the generation of killer T cells in culture preceded the appearance of effector function by 24 hr. When the insulin receptor was removed from killer T cells by trypsin digestion, effector function ceased.[65-68]

Established B cell lines of mouse and human origin have more insulin receptors on their surfaces than their normal, unstimulated counterparts. A mouse B cell line (1605L) was estimated to have 16,600 insulin receptor sites per cell with an affinity of 1.9 nM^{-1}. The Epstein Barr virus (EBV)-negative human lymphoma cell line, Ramos, has a low concentration of insulin receptors. Sublines derived from this cultured cell line through EBV infection expressed variable, but usually high, insulin binding capacity.[69-73] The exposure of human cultured lymphoid cells to insulin in vitro is followed by internalization, or shedding and degradation, of both receptor and insulin molecules.[74-77]

The insulin receptor of cultured human B lymphocytes contained two different chains of glycoproteins, with molecular weights of 126,000 and 90,000 daltons, respectively. The expression of both chains was decreased (down regulated) after exposure of the cells to insulin.[78]

Investigations with mouse lymphocytes revealed that B cells express insulin receptors under the influence of activated T cells of the helper phenotype. This cell interaction is genetically restricted and governed by the immune response region of the major histocompatibility complex.[79]

Hyperinsulinemia was created in patients with type I diabetes mellitus by means of continuous subcutaneous insulin infusion. A progressive fall in the number of insulin receptors, expressed by T lymphocytes after lectin treatment, was observed 14 days after the initiation of hyperinsulinemia. However, the level of lectin stimulation and the time course of the PHA response was not altered.[80]

Peripheral blood monocytes bind approximately 20 times more insulin than do circulating lymphocytes. The ratio between insulin binding to lymphocytes and monocytes is constant from person to person. High and low affinity receptors were detected on human monocytes, the total number being 70,000 sites per cell, of which 2000 are high affinity sites with an affinity constant of 2.5 nM. Apparently, the insulin receptor on monocytes is remarkably similar to receptors present in other tissues, such as fat, liver, muscle cells, etc. For this reason monocytes were used frequently for insulin receptor studies in man. There is a diurnal variation in insulin binding to human monocytes, which can be eliminated by total fasting. Insulin sensitivity in normal subjects is greatest in the morning, decreasing to a minimum in the late afternoon. Changes of receptor affinity due to the sucrose and fat content of the diet is responsible for the most part for changes in insulin binding, although alterations of the number of receptors per cell, as well as in the number of circulating monocytes, also have an influence. Experimental hyperinsulinemia, or the hyperinsulinemia present in obese subjects, cause a decrease (down regulation) of insulin receptors by an enhanced degradation of receptor protein. Acute exercise causes an increase in insulin binding, parallel to the increase in insulin sensitivity.[81,82]

Hormonal factors also influence the level of monocyte insulin receptors. Thus, in acromegalic patients, the total receptor concentration per cell was inversely related to the basal level of insulin. In acromegalics with normal glycemia, an increase in receptor affinity could also be demonstrated, which was not found in their hyperglycemic counterparts.[83,84] Monocyte insulin binding was increased in patients with chronic glucocorticoid excess, or after chronic treatment with prednisone. Prednisone treatment caused an increase in receptor concentration, whereas in patients with adrenocortical hyperfunction, an increase in receptor affinity could be demonstrated.[84] In young women, a higher monocyte insulin binding was found during the follicular menstrual phase as compared to the luteal phase,[85] which suggests that female sex hormones may have an influence on insulin receptors.

Normal human mononuclear cells were activated with PHA, or T cell growth factor and established as B and T lymphoblastoid cell lines. Glucagon and insulin receptors increased 15- and 36-fold, respectively, and peaked after 5 days of PHA activation, parallel with the rise in thymidine incorporation. Cells cultured with TCGF showed a modest rise in insulin binding and a striking and progressive rise, up to 50-fold in glucagon binding, due to both increased receptor number and affinity. This finding suggests that TCGF selects out a T lymphoblast subset with very high glucagon receptors. Glucagon binding was sevenfold higher, whereas insulin binding was sevenfold lower, in T lymphoblasts compared to B lymphoblastoid cells. T cell lines had twice the number of glucagon receptors, whereas B lines had fourfold higher number of insulin receptors with much greater affinity for insulin than those T line receptors.[86]

B. The Effect of Insulin on the Immune System
1. Mouse
Insulin enhanced the Con A reactivity of mouse lymphocytes and once the cells were activated, insulin was capable of replacing Con A for the continued stimulation of the cells, which led to the generation of nonspecific cytotoxic T lymphocytes. However, insulin did not influence the PHA responsiveness of lymphocytes.[87,88] Others found that insulin inhibited the initial proliferation induced by either Con A or lipopolysaccharide (LPS). However, a 50% increase in antibody forming cells was found in LPS plus insulin treated cultures. Thus, insulin appears to favor the differentiation of activated cells.[89]

Insulin, in doses which did not influence the blood sugar level, potentiated the anaphylactic shock in mice and moderately inhibited the carrageenan-induced paw edema.[90]

2. Man
In human mixed lymphocyte reactions, performed in serum free medium, physiologic concentrations of insulin and transferrin synergistically potentiated DNA synthesis.[91] Insulin inhibited the lysis of erythrocyte target cells by antibody dependent cytotoxicity, whereas the lysis of tumor target cells was not influenced.[92] Physiological concentrations of insulin enhanced significantly the fibrinolytic activity of monocytes and stimulated the phagocytosis of inert particles. Lysozyme secretion was unaffected.[93]

Lymphocytes from lymph nodes of rats, rabbits, pigs, cows, and from human tonsils elaborated a proinflammatory factor termed as anaphylactoid inflammation promoting factor (AIPF), after exposure to insulin. Thymus cells showed no such activity. The molecular weight of AIPF was estimated to be 67,000 daltons and its activity was abolished by heat treatment or incubation by DNase, or chymotrypsin, but not by RNase. AIPF, by itself, did not induce increased vascular permeability and proved to be distinct from the permeability factors present in the lysate of lymph node cells.[94]

3. Other Species

Physiologic concentrations of insulin enhanced the cytotoxic effect of rat lymphocytes.[95] Rat lymph node cells, incubated in the presence of insulin, released a factor(s) that was capable of increasing dextran induced anaphylactoid reaction in vivo.[96] On guinea pig macrophages, the existing Fc receptors were not blocked by insulin, but the increase in receptor expression during culture was inhibited in a dose related manner.[97]

Chronic treatment of rats with insulin depressed significantly (by 48%) the intravascular phagocytosis of colloidal carbon, whereas glucagon an somatostatin stimulated macrophage endocytic function (by 32 and 26%, respectively) compared to the control value. Acute treatment with the three pancreatic hormones, 30 min before the administration of carbon, yielded similar results; insulin depressed glucagon and somatostatin stimulated phagocytosis. When isolated rat livers were perfused with near physiologic concentrations of these hormones (20 ng/mℓ of insulin, 10 ng/mℓ of glucagon and 5 ng/mℓ of somatostatin), and with colloidal carbon, reduction of phagocytosis occurred after insulin and enhancement after glucagon and somatostatin administration.[62]

C. Insulin Dependent Diabetes

In man, juvenile diabetes is an autoimmune disease of complex etiology, in which genetic factors and environmental insults (viral infections) seem to play important roles. The association of diabetes mellitus with certain HLA phenotypes led to the common belief that inherited immune abnormalities are fundamental to this endocrine disorder.[98] However, it was also pointed out by Mirakian et al.[99] that juvenile onset diabetes is frequently associated with pituitary abnormalities that are possibly caused by autoantibodies. Similar genetic deficiencies seem to be involved in most, if not all, the animal models of diabetes. Although there are numerous papers on diabetes related alterations of immune reactivity, both in man and in animals, the relevance of these investigations to the physiological role of insulin in immunoregulation is limited, because of the difficulties of assessing the impact of genetic abnormalities associated with diabetes. For this reason, the effect of diabetes on immune reactions will be discussed only briefly here, on the basis of some selected papers. For more detailed information the reader is referred to recent reviews on this topic.[100-103]

1. Mouse

Alloxan treated diabetic mice had a reduced number of leukocytes and exhibited impaired humoral and cell mediated immune responses, whereas the nonspecific inflammatory response was normal.[104-106]

Diabetic mice cannot develop contact sensitivity, or efficient graft rejection. Administration of insulin partially restores these responses. After the sensitization of diabetic mice with picryl chloride, there is a preferential recruitment of suppressor T cells. Such suppressor cells are capable of canceling the transmission of contact sensitivity by immunized T cells after mixing and transferring the cell mixture into normal recipients.[107-109] Diabetic mice do not easily develop anaphylactic shock and form very little, if any, IgE antibodies. Mice sensitized as normoglycemic and then made diabetic are protected from anaphylaxis to a great extent, although they form minute amounts of IgE antibodies. Immune cells transferred into diabetic mice lose their ability to form IgE, whereas cells of primed diabetic animals acquire IgE forming capacity after transfer into normal recipients. Massive doses of glucose given to normoglycemic mice, which increase their glucose levels to that seen in diabetic animals, prevent local anaphylactic reactions elicited with monoclonal IgE antibodies.[110] Macrophages of alloxan-diabetic mice have more Fc receptors and phagocytose heavily opsonized SRBC better than do normal macrophages. However, the reverse is true when suboptimally opsonized SRBC is used. No differences are found between normal and diabetic macrophages in the rate of digestion of engulfed antigen.[111] Alloxan treated diabetic mice and genetically diabetic C57BL/KsJ mice both show an increased susceptibility to *Candida albicans* infection. In the genetically diabetic animals, the numbers of lymphocytes and peritoneal macrophages are decreased, lymphocytes respond poorly to Con A, and the phagocytosis of yeast cells by macrophages is depressed. The in vivo production of lymphokines and delayed-type hypersensitivity reactions are also depressed. All these parameters are within the normal range in alloxan-diabetic animals.[112]

2. Rat

Macrophages from diabetic rats exhibited a decreased sensitivity to murine migration inhibition factor and a decreased phagocytic activity. Insulin treatment for 10 to 15 days significantly improved these parameters toward normal.[113] In rats, rendered hyperglycemic with alloxan, an increased proliferation of mast cells was noted in the pancreas, thyroid, skin, and mesentery. Insulin treatment reduced the number of mast cells in these organs.[114] Rats with streptozotocin induced diabetes of 4 weeks duration showed an increased mitogenesis in normal connective tissue, which was mediated by mast cells.[115]

IgG began to accumulate in glomeruli of rats, beginning 1 month after diabetes induction by alloxan. IgG was associated with complement in the glomerulus and its amount was directly proportional to the severity of diabetes.[116]

Allogeneic skin graft rejection and PHA or mixed lymphocyte culture (MLC) responses were strongly depressed in pancreatectomized rats. The cellularity of the thymus and of the thymus dependent areas in lymph nodes and spleen, as well as the number of peripheral blood lymphocytes, were significantly reduced after pancreatectomy. Immunological recovery from high doses of cortisone was also greatly impaired. Daily treatment with insulin prevented these immunological alterations. By contrast the number of antibody producing cells in the spleen, or antibody titers, were normal in diabetic rats.[117]

A diabetic syndrome has been discovered in the BB strain of rats, which is considered to be the best available animal model for human insulin-dependent diabetes. This strain is characterized by an extreme susceptibility to opportunistic infections and to the development of autoimmune reactions. BB rats exhibit a severe T cell deficiency with depression of both the helper and cytotoxic/suppressor T lymphocyte subsets and an inversion of the helper T cell to cytotoxic/suppressor T lymphocyte ratio, in all animals with increasing maturity. T cell mediated immune responses are severely impaired, as demonstrated by the poor rejection of allografts, the poor response of splenic, or peripheral blood lymphocytes, to mitogens and to allogeneic cells in cultures. A variety of autoantibodies that include antibodies to islet cell surface, to lymphocytes, and to thymocytes, were also demonstrated in BB animals. Autoantibodies were present in the majority of rats at an age when neither morphological nor metabolic evidence of the diabetic syndrome was yet detected. Genetic studies indicated that the immune defects and insulin dependent diabetic syndrome of these rats are linked to the major histocompatibility complex, although the involvement of at least two non-MHC linked genes was also suggested.[118-122]

3. Man

As already pointed out, insulin-dependent diabetes, which is also known as type I or juvenile-onset diabetes, has an autoimmune etiology with humoral and cell mediated immunity against the insulin secreting cells. Genetic factors, especially the genes involved in immunoregulation, as well as environmental insults (virus infections or toxins) are implicated in the pathogenesis of type I diabetes. On the other hand, noninsulin-dependent diabetes, which is also known as type II or maturity-onset diabetes, has a different, as yet unclarified etiology, without the apparent role of immune mechanisms. Type I diabetes may be associated with other immune and endocrine abnormalities, malabsorption, and coeliac disease.[123-132]

Insulin-dependent diabetic patients frequently have antibodies in pancreatic islets that secrete insulin[133-137] to the insulin receptor,[138-144] to insulin itself. This may occur without exogenous insulin administration,[145-149] thyroglobulin and microsomal autoantibodies,[150-153] and autoantibodies to somatostatin and glucagon producing cells as well as in a variety of endocrine organs.[154,155]

Peripheral blood lymphocytes were shown to home to the pancreas specifically in patients with acute onset insulin-dependent diabetes mellitus[156] and to respond specifically in the leukocyte migration test to fetal calf pancreatic extract.[157] B lymphocytes from diabetics, with associated autoimmune disease, were shown to inhibit pancreatic B cell function in vitro.[158] Finally, in diabetic patients with neuropathy, cell mediated immunity to the nervous system has been demonstrated by specific lymphocyte transformation in vitro.[159] Cellular hypersensitivity to liver mitochondria was also demonstrated in diabetics with high frequency.[160] Black diabetic patients had an increased T cell population compared to white control patients. No difference was demonstrated in the percentage of B lymphocytes in any of the above groups.[161] The percentage of T cells (E-rosette forming) and B cells (erythrocyte-antibody-complement-rosette forming) was significantly decreased in poorly controlled juvenile diabetics, whereas cells with Fc receptors for IgG were decreased in both well controlled and poorly controlled patients. Mitogen stimulation was not different from controls, but it was significantly lower in poorly controlled, than in well controlled, diabetics and high concentrations of glucose had an inhibitory effect on mitogen stimulation.[162]

Insulin-dependent controlled diabetic patients had a significantly decreased response to PHA stimulation and a lower ratio of thymus derived to bone marrow derived lymphocytes, when compared to similar but nondiabetic patients, who were awaiting elective operations. Serum IgA, IgG, and IgM levels were comparable.[163]

The comparison of IgA, IgG, and IgM and complement (C3) levels in 46 diabetic patients with 19 matched controls revealed that IgG and complement levels were significantly depressed in insulin-dependent diabetics, whereas IgA and complement were elevated in noninsulin-dependent diabetics.[164] The prevalence of IgA deficiency in children with juvenile onset insulin-dependent diabetes is significantly increased, but not in patients with adult insulin-dependent diabetes. Juvenile diabetics with IgA deficiency frequently have other immune associated diseases, such as thyroiditis, hepatitis, and infections. Autoantibodies to endocrine organs can also be detected with high frequency.[155] Antibacterial antibody formation was severely impaired in insulin-dependent diabetic patients, but was almost normal in blood relatives of insulin-dependent diabetics. Therefore, the humoral antibacterial immunodeficiency observed in diabetics is likely to be a disease associated process, which is probably independent of major histocompatibility complex linked genes.[165]

The release of migration inhibitory factor (MIF) triggered by PPD from cells of well controlled insulin-dependent diabetic, nonketotic diabetic, and nonhyperglycemic obese subjects was 100 ± 8, 48 ± 17, and $36 \pm 17\%$ of control values, respectively.[166]

A number of investigators demonstrated that patients newly diagnosed with insulin-dependent diabetes are deficient in nonspecific (Con A inducible) and antigen specific (islet cell inducible) suppressor cell function. Studies with monoclonal antibodies also indicated that a significant proportion (40%) of diabetic patients are deficient in suppressor T cells, which leads to an increase of the helper/suppressor cell ratio. There is no evidence for polyclonal activation of B lymphocytes in normal diabetics, but a significant increase in the number of spontaneous plaque forming cells (PFC) in patients suffering from both diabetes and Hashimoto's thyroiditis was observed. Apparently, suppressor cell function was normal during remission periods of diabetes and in long-term diabetics.[167-176] Interestingly enough, the mitogenic response of lymphocytes from prematurely born infants of diabetic mothers was found significantly higher than in age-matched premature controls and in full term newborns and remained so at 1 month of age.[177] In contrast to the above observations, one group of investigators found that diabetics have a moderate, but significant, reduction of the proportions of total T lymphocytes at the expense of the helper T cell subset, whereas the proportions of suppressor/cytotoxic cells were normal. This abnormality was not related to the duration of diabetes, the control of the disease, nor to the presence of autoimmune phenomena.[178] Others observed an increase in circulating Ia antigen bearing T cells in patients with type I diabetes.[179] Diabetic lymphocytes exhibited a decreased blast transformation in response to PHA, Con A, and pokeweed mitogen (PWM) when compared to normal human lymphocytes. Added insulin increased the diabetic lymphocyte response to each of the mitogens, but blast transformation never reached the level of that of controls.[180,181]

Diabetes influences insulin receptors on monocytes: there may be either an increased or a decreased insulin binding by monocytes in newly diagnosed diabetics, whereas insulin treated outpatients have normal insulin binding.[182] Monocyte insulin receptors increase twofold during pregnancy. A further increase can be observed in pregnant women with abnormal glucose tolerance, but with normal fasting plasma glucose levels. On the other hand, untreated diabetic pregnant patients have markedly reduced receptor sites, which can be restored by insulin treatment to normal pregnant levels.[183] Normal infants, and infants born to gestational diabetic mothers, have about four and ten times, respectively, as many insulin receptor sites per monocyte than found in monocytes from normal adults. Receptor affinity is also increased.[184]

The total number of circulating monocytes was lower in diabetic patients than in healthy individuals. The phagocytosis of *C. albicans* by patients' monocytes was depressed, whereas latex particles and SRBC were phagocytosed normally. The chemotactic response was found to be enhanced by some and to be depressed by other investigators.[185,186] The clearance of microaggregated iodinated serum albumin was significantly reduced in diabetics with severe microangiopathy, in comparison with patients without angiopathy, or with normal subjects. Positive correlations were found between reduced colloid clearance and increased levels of circulating immune complexes, as determined by the Clq solid phase method.[187,188]

Some investigators found that antibody-dependent cellular cytotoxicity was significantly decreased in diabetic children and was more severe in poorly balanced than in well controlled patients.[189] However, others found a significant increase in K cell and antibody dependent cellular cytotoxicity (ADCC) reactions, both in newly diagnosed and in unaffected siblings.[190]

Diabetic granulocytes phagocytose *Staphylococcus aureus* less efficiently and are impaired with regards to the intracellular killing of these bacteria in comparison with controls. The chemotactic reaction is also reduced. Bacterial killing capacity improves significantly with better control of diabetes.[191,192]

Granulocytes of diabetic patients exhibited a markedly reduced mobilization reaction, as revealed in vivo by the skin latex particles, and killing of *Escherichia coli* bacteria were impaired only in decompensated patients, whereas it was normal in patients in compensated metabolism.[193] Neutrophil granulocyte chemotaxis was found to be normal in diabetics.[194] The conversion of lysolecithin to lecithin was deficient[194] by neutrophils from diabetic patients, and extracts of polymorphonuclear leukocytes of diabetics exhibited less collagenolytic activity than extracts from normoglycemic control subjects.[196] Platelets from diabetics are more prone to aggregation than those of normal individuals.[197,198]

The levels of the complement components C3 activator, C3 and C4, were increased both in diabetics and in individuals with glucose intolerance. In glucose intolerant subjects, elevation occurred without fasting hyperglycemia, but it was positively correlated with fasting plasma glucose. An age-related increase of complement components was also observed, but the diabetic complement increase was still detectable when compared to age-matched nondiabetics.[199] The occurrence of a rare properdin factor (BfSl) was significantly increased in insulin-dependent diabetic patients in north India (21 vs. 3.5%).[200]

4. Guinea Pig

The response of lymphocytes from spontaneously diabetic guinea pigs to PHA and Con A was significantly depressed, compared to normal controls. On remission of diabetes the proliferative response of lymphocytes returned to normal, or to above control levels.[201]

V. THE INFLUENCE OF THE IMMUNE SYSTEM ON GROWTH HORMONE AND INSULIN SECRETION

Children with juvenile rheumatoid arthritis, rheumatic fever, inflammatory bowel disease, and asthma frequently exhibit growth failure due to deficient GH secretion.[3,202-205]

Colloidal carbon blockage of the reticuloendothelial system in rats resulted in acute hyperinsulinemia and functional hyperinsulinism. The removal of ^{125}I-insulin was not altered by colloidal carbon blockage, but pancreata from treated rats manifested enhanced insulin secretion. Furthermore, culture media conditioned by macrophages enhanced glucose mediated insulin secretion in vivo and in the isolated perfused rat pancreas. It was suggested that the hyperinsulinemia of reticuloendothelium system (RES) blockage is due to a macrophage-derived monokine.[206]

REFERENCES

1. Phillips, L. S. and Vassilopoulou-Sellin, R., Somatomedins, *N. Engl. J. Med.,* 302, 371, 1980.
2. Blundell, T. I. and Humbel, R. F., Hormone families: pancreatic hormones and homologous growth factors, *Nature (London),* 287, 5785, 1980.
3. Daughaday, W. H., The adrenohypophysis, in *Textbook of Endocrinology,* 6th ed., Williams, R. D., Ed., W. B. Saunders, Philadelphia, 1981, 73.
4. Maes, M. and Ketelslegers, J. -M., Effects of diabetes on somatogenic and lactogenic receptors in rat liver, *Ann. Endocrinol.,* 42, 295, 1981.
5. Horner, J. M., Kemp, S. F., and Hintz, R. L., Growth hormone and somatomedin in insulin-dependent diabetes mellitus, *J. Clin. Endocrinol. Metab.,* 53, 1148, 1981.
6. Ceda, G. P., Speroni, G., Dall'Aglio, E., Valenti, G., and Butturini, U., Nonspecific growth hormone responses to thyrotropin-releasing hormone in insulin-dependent diabetes: sex-related and age-related pituitary responsiveness, *J. Clin. Endocrinol. Metab.,* 55, 170, 1982.
7. LeBlanc, J., Nadeau, A., Richard, D., and Tremblay, A., Variations in plasma glucose, insulin, growth hormone and catecholamines in response to insulin in trained and non-trained subjects, *Metabolism,* 31, 453, 1982.
8. Grecu, E. O., Spencer, E. M., White, V. A., and Sheikholislam, B. M., Exaggerated somatomedin-C response to human growth hormone infusion in patients with type-II diabetes mellitus, *Am. J. Med. Sci.,* 287, 7, 1984.
9. Cerasola, G. A., Donatelli, M., Sinagra, D., Russo, V., Amico, L. M., and Lodato, G., Study of pituitary secretion in relation to retinopathy in patients with juvenile diabetes mellitus, *Acta Diabetol. Lat.,* 18, 319, 1981.

10. Dasmahapatra, A., Urdanivia, E., and Cohen, M. P., Growth hormone response to thyrotropin-releasing hormone in diabetes, *J. Clin. Endocrinol. Metab.*, 52, 859, 1981.
11. Dougherty, T. F., Effect of hormones on lymphatic tissue, *Physiol. Rev.*, 32, 379, 1952.
12. Hammar, J. A., The new views as to the morphology of the thymus gland and their bearing on the problem of the function of the thymus, *Endocrinology*, 5, 543, 731, 1921.
13. Lesniak, M. A., Roth, J., Gorden, P., and Gavin, J. R., III, Human growth hormone radioreceptor assay using cultured human lymphocytes, *Nature (London)*, 241, 20, 1973.
14. Lesniak, M. A., Gorden, P., Roth, J., and Gavin, J. R., III, Binding of ^{125}I-human growth hormone to specific receptors in human cultured lymphocytes, *J. Biol. Chem.*, 249, 1661, 1974.
15. Arrenbrecht, S., Specific binding of growth hormone to thymocytes, *Nature (London)*, 252, 255, 1974.
16. Herington, A. C. and Faragher, I. G., Binding of growth hormone to isolated rat thymocytes: a reassessment, *IRCS Med. Sci. Biochem.*, 9, 1147, 1981.
17. Stewart, C., Clejan, S., Fugler, L., Cheruvanky, T., and Collipp, P. J., Growth hormone receptors in lymphocytes of growth hormone-deficient children, *Arch. Biochem. Biophys.*, 220, 309, 1983.
18. Nagy, E., Berczi, I., and Friesen, H. G., Regulation of immunity in rats by lactogenic and growth hormones, *Acta Endocrinol.*, 102, 351, 1983.
19. Pandian, M. R. and Talwar, G. P., Effect of growth hormone on the metabolism of thymus and on the immune response against sheep erythrocytes, *J. Exp. Med.*, 134, 1095, 1971.
20. Arrenbrecht, S. and Sorkin, E., Growth hormone-induced T cell differentiation, *Eur. J. Immunol.*, 3, 601, 1973.
21. Roth, J. A., Lomax, L. G., Altszuler, N., Hampshire, J., Kaeberle, M. L., Shelton, M., Draper, D. D., and Ledet, A. E., Thymic abnormalities and growth hormone deficiency in dogs, *Am. J. Vet. Res.*, 41, 1256, 1980.
22. Jepson, J. H. and McGarry, E. E., Hemopoiesis in pituitary dwarfs treated with human growth hormone and testosterone, *Blood*, 39, 238, 1972.
23. Baroni, C. D., Fabris, N., and Bertoli, G., Effects of hormones on development and function of lymphoid tissues. Synergistic action of thyroxin and somatotropic hormone in pituitary dwarf mice, *Immunology*, 17, 303, 1969.
24. Fabris, N., Pierpaoli, W., and Sorkin, E., Hormones and the immunological capacity. III. The immunodeficiency disease of the hypopituitary Snell-Bagg dwarf mouse, *Clin. Exp. Immunol.*, 9, 209, 1971.
25. Fabris, N., Pierpaoli, W., and Sorkin, E., Hormones and the immunological capacity. IV. Restorative effects of developmental hormones or of lymphocytes on the immunodeficiency syndrome of the dwarf mouse, *Clin. Exp. Immunol.*, 9, 227, 1971.
26. Dumont, F., Robert, F., and Bischoff, P., T and B lymphocytes in pituitary dwarf Snell-Bagg mice, *Immunology*, 38, 23, 1979.
27. Gisler, R. H. and Schenkel-Hulliger, L., Hormonal regulation of the immune response. II. Influence of pituitary and adrenal activity on immune responsiveness *in vitro*, *Cell. Immunol.*, 2, 646, 1971.
28. Saxena, Q. B., Saxena, R. K., and Adler, W. H., Regulation of natural killer activity in vivo. III. Effect of hypophysectomy and growth hormone treatment on the natural killer activity of the mouse spleen cell population, *Int. Arch. Allergy Appl. Immunol.*, 67, 169, 1982.
29. Snow, C. E., Feldbush, T. L., and Oaks, J. A., The effect of growth hormone and insulin upon MLC responses and the generation of cytotoxic lymphocytes, *J. Immunol.*, 126, 161, 1981.
30. Chatterton, R. T., Jr., Murray, C. L., and Hellman, L., Endocrine effects on leukocytopoiesis in the rat. I. Evidence for growth hormone secretion as the leukocytopoietic stimulus following acute cortisol-induced lymphopenia, *Endocrinology*, 92, 775, 1973.
31. Enerback, L., Lundin, P. M., and Mellgren, J., Pituitary hormones elaborated during stress: action on lymphoid tissues, serum proteins and antibody titres, *Acta Pathol. Microbiol. Scand.*, Suppl. 144, 141, 1961.
32. Hayashida, T. and Li, C. -H., Influence of adrenocorticotropic and growth hormone on antibody formation, *J. Exp. Med.*, 105, 93, 1957.
33. Comsa, J., Schwarz, J. A., and Neu, H., Interaction between thymic hormone and hypophyseal growth hormone on production of precipitating antibodies in the rat, *Immunol. Commun.*, 3, 11, 1974.
34. Comsa, J., Leonhardt, H., and Schwarz, J. A., Influence of the thymus-corticotropin-growth hormone interaction on the rejection of skin allografts in the rat, *Ann. N.Y. Acad. Sci.*, 249, 387, 1975.
35. Maor, D., Englander, T., Eylan, E., and Alexander, P., Participation of hormone in the early stages of the immune response, *Acta Endocrinol.*, 75, 205, 1974.
36. Scott, M., Bolla, R., and Denckla, W. D., Age-related changes in immune function of rats and the effect of long-term hypophysectomy, *Mech. Age. Dev.*, 11, 127, 1979.
37. Berczi, I., Nagy, E., Kovacs, K., and Horvath, E., Regulation of humoral immunity in rats by pituitary hormones, *Acta Endocrinol.*, 98, 506, 1981.

38. Berczi, I., Nagy, E., Asa, S. L., and Kovacs, K., Pituitary hormones and contact sensitivity in rats, *Allergy,* 38, 325, 1983.

39. Berczi, I., Nagy, E., Asa, S. L., and Kovacs, K., The influence of pituitary hormones and adjuvant arthritis, *Arthritis Rheum.,* 27, 682, 1984.

40. Nagy, E., Berczi, I., Wren, G. E., Asa, S. L., and Kovacs, K., Immunomodulation by bromocriptine, *Immunopharmacology,* 6, 231, 1983.

41. Meites, J. and Clemens, J. A., Hypothalamic control of prolactin secretion, *Vitam. Horm.,* 30, 165, 1972.

42. Parkes, D., Drug therapy: bromocriptine, *N. Engl. J. Med.,* 301, 873, 1979.

43. Bansal, S. A., Lee, L. A., and Woolf, P. D., Dopaminergic stimulation and inhibition of growth hormone secretion in normal man: studies of the pharmacologic specificity, *J. Clin. Endocrinol. Metab.,* 53, 1273, 1981.

44. Bazan, M. C., Barontini, M., Domene, H., Stafano, F. J., and Bergada, C., Effects of α-bromoergocriptine on pituitary hormone secretion in children, *J. Clin. Endocrinol. Metab.,* 53, 314, 1981.

45. Fleisher, T. A., White, R. M., Broder, S., Nissley, S. P., Blaese, R. M., Mulvihill, J. J., Olive, G., and Waldmann, T. A., X-linked hypogammaglobulinemia and isolated growth hormone deficiency, *N. Engl. J. Med.,* 302, 1429, 1980.

46. Gupta, S., Fikrig, S. M., and Noval, M. S., Immunological studies in patients with isolated growth hormone deficiency, *Clin. Exp. Immunol.,* 54, 87, 1983.

47. DelPrincipe, D., Boscherini, B., Menichelli, A., Giardini, O., Mastracchio, F., Malvaso, M., Gabriotti, M., and Spadoni, G. L., Blood platelet oxygen consumption pituitary in dwarfs, *Nouv. Presse Med.,* 10, 2015, 1981.

48. Rovenský, J., Vigaš, M., Lokaj, J., Čunčik, P., Lukáč, P., and Takáč, A., Effect of growth hormone on the metabolic activity of phagocytes of peripheral blood in pituitary dwarfs and acromegaly, *Endocrinol. Exp.,* 16, 129, 1982.

49. Szezklik, A., Sieradzki, J., Serwonska, M., and Podolek, Z., Impaired responses of growth hormone and blood eosinophils to L-dopa in atopy, *Acta Allergol.,* 32, 382, 1977.

50. Vanderschueren-Lodeweyckx, M., Stet, B., Van den Berghe, H., Eggermont, E., and Eeckels, R., Growth hormone and lymphocyte transplantation, *Lancet,* I, 441, 1973.

51. Schimpff, R. M., Thieriot-Prévost, G., and Job, J. C., Thymidine uptake in activated human lymphocytes: effects of GH-dependent serum factors (somatomedin), *Pathol. Biol.,* 29, 347, 1981.

52. Salvatoni, A., Schimpff, R. -M., Delvigne, and Job, J. C., Growth hormone dependency of the effect of human serum on thymidine uptake by lectin-activated human lymphocytes: the role of dialyzable factors (L-glutamine), *Horm. Res.,* 19, 5, 1984.

53. Mercola, K. E., Cline, M. J., and Golde, D. W., Growth hormone stimulation of normal and leukemic human T-lymphocyte proliferation in vitro, *Blood,* 58, 337, 1981.

54. Kiess, W., Holtmann, H., Butenandt, O., and Eife, R., Modulation of lymphoproliferation by human growth hormone, *Eur. J. Pediatr.,* 140, 47, 1983.

55. Marsh, J. A., Assessment of antibody production in sex-liked and autosomal dwarf chickens, *Dev. Comp. Immunol.,* 7, 535, 1983.

56. Marsh, J. A., Gause, W. C., Sandhu, S., and Scanes, C. G., Enhanced growth and immune development in dwarf chickens treated with mammalian growth hormone and thyroxine, *Proc. Soc. Exp. Biol. Med.,* 175, 351, 1984.

57. Thorsson, A. V. and Hintz, R. L., Specific ^{125}I-somatomedin receptor on circulating human mononuclear cells, *Biochem. Biophys. Res. Commun.,* 74, 1566, 1977.

58. Rosenfeld, R., Thorsson, A. V., and Hintz, R. L., Increased somatomedin receptor sites in newborn circulating mononuclear cells, *J. Clin. Endocrinol. Metab.,* 48, 456, 1979.

59. Rosenfeld, R. G., Hintz, R. L., and Dollar, L. A., Insulin-induced loss of insulin-like growth factor-I receptors on IM-9 lymphocytes. I, *Diabetes,* 31, 375, 1982.

60. Bozzola, M., Schimpff, R. M., Thieriot-Prévost, G., Leduc, B., and Job, J. C., Plasma somatomedin activity measured as thymidine factor in normal children with average and constitutionally tall stature, *Horm. Metab. Res.,* 14, 372, 1982.

61. Thieriot-Prévost, G. and Schimpff, R. M., A hormonally controlled serum factor stimulating the thymidine uptake into lectin-activated lymphocytes, *Acta Endocrinol.,* 98, 358, 1981.

62. Cornell, R. P. and McClellan, C. C., Modulation of hepatic reticuloendothelial system phagocytosis by pancreatic hormones, *J. Reticuloendothel. Soc.,* 32, 397, 1982.

63. Theoharides, T. C. and Douglas, W. W., Somatostatin induces histamine secretion from rat peritoneal mast cells, *Endocrinology,* 102, 1637, 1978.

64. O'Dorisio, M. S., Hermina, N. S., O'Dorisio, T. M., Balcerzak, S. P., Vasoactive intestinal polypeptide modulation of lymphocyte adenylate cyclase, *J. Immunol.,* 127, 2551, 1981.

65. Helderman, J. H. and Strom, T. B., Specific insulin binding site on T and B lymphocytes as a marker of cell activation, *Nature (London),* 274, 62, 1978.

66. Helderman, J. H. and Strom, T. B., Absence of a role for the cellular exoskeleton in the emergence of the T lymphocyte insulin receptor, *Exp. Cell. Res.,* 123, 119, 1979.

67. Helderman, J. H., Reynolds, T. C., and Strom, T. B., Insulin receptor as a universal marker of activated lymphocytes, *Eur. J. Immunol.,* 8, 589, 1978.

68. Helderman, J. H., Strom, T. B., and Dupuy-D'Angeac, A., A close relationship between cyctotoxic T lymphocytes generated in the mixed lymphocyte culture and insulin receptor-bearing lymphocytes: enrichment by density gradient centrifugation, *Cell. Immunol.,* 46, 247, 1979.

69. Åman, P., Lundin, G., Hall, K., and Klein, G., Insulin receptors on human lymphoid lines of B-cell origin, *Cell. Immunol.,* 65, 307, 1981.

70. Galbraith, R. A., Buse, M. G., and Marchalonis, J. J., Insulin binding to cultured B- and T-lymphocytes, *Immunol. Lett.,* 4, 141, 1982.

71. Gavin, J. R., III, Roth, J., Jen, P., and Freychet, P., Insulin receptors in human circulating cells and fibroblasts, *Proc. Natl. Acad. Sci. U.S.A.,* 69, 747, 1972.

72. Lang, U., Kahn, C. R., and Chrambach, A., Characterization of the insulin receptor and insulin-degrading activity from human lymphocytes by quantitative polyacrylamide gel electrophoresis, *Endocrinology,* 106, 40, 1980.

73. Spira, G., Åman, P., Koide, N., Lundin, G., Klein, G., and Hall, K., Cell-surface immunoglobulin and insulin receptor expression in an EBV-negative lymphoma cell line and its EBV-converted sublines, *J. Immunol.,* 126, 122, 1981.

74. Goldfine, I. D., Jones, A. L., Hradek, G. T., Wong, K. Y., and Mooney, J. S., Entry of insulin into human cultured lymphocytes: electron microscope autoradiographic analysis, *Science,* 202, 760, 1978.

75. Kasuga, M., Kahn, C. R., Hedo, J. A., Van Obberghen, E., and Yamada, K. M., Insulin-induced receptor loss in cultured human lymphocytes is due to accelerated receptor degradation, *Proc. Natl. Acad. Sci. U.S.A. Biol Sci.,* 78, 6917, 1981.

76. Berhanu, P. and Olefsky, J. M., Photoaffinity labeling of insulin receptors in viable cultured human lymphocytes: demonstration of receptor shedding and degradation. I. *Diabetes,* 31, 410, 1982.

77. Maegawa, H., Kobayashi, M., Ohgaku, S., Yasuda, H., Iwasaki, M., Watanabe, N., and Shigeta, Y., Evidence of the lack of receptor-mediated insulin degradation in human cultured lymphocytes (RPMI-1788 line), *Endocrinol. Jpn.,* 30, 679, 1983.

78. Harrison, L. C., Itin, A., Kasuga, M., and Van Obberghen, E., The insulin receptor on the human lymphocyte: insulin-induced down-regulation of 126,000 and 90,000 glycosylated subunits, *Diabetologia,* 22, 233, 1982.

79. Helderman, J. H., T cell cooperation for the genesis of B cell insulin receptors, *J. Immunol.,* 131, 644, 1983.

80. Helderman, J. H., Pietri, A. O., and Raskin, P., In vitro control of T-lymphocyte insulin receptors by in vivo modulation of insulin, *Diabetes,* 32, 712, 1983.

81. Schwartz, R. H., Raffale Bianco, A., Handwerger, B. S., and Kahn, C. R., A demonstration that monocytes rather than lymphocytes are the insulin-binding cells in preparations of human peripheral blood mononuclear leukocytes: implications for studies of insulin-resistant states in man, *Proc. Natl. Acad. Sci. U.S.A.,* 72, 474, 1975.

82. Beck-Nielsen, H., Insulin receptors in man. The monocyte as model for insulin receptor studies, *Dan. Med. Bull.,* 27, 173, 1980.

83. Muggeo, M., Saviolakis, G. A., Businaro, V., Valerio, A., Moghetti, P., and Crepaldi, G., Insulin receptor on monocytes from patients with acromegaly and fasting hyperglycemia, *J. Clin. Endocrinol. Metab.,* 56, 733, 1983.

84. Muggeo, M., Saviolakis, G. A., Wachslicht-Rodbard, H., and Roth, J., Effects of chronic glucocorticoid excess in man on insulin binding to circulating cells: differences between endogenous and exogenous hypercorticism, *J. Clin. Endocrinol. Metab.,* 56, 1169, 1983.

85. DePirro, R., Fusco, A., Bertoli, A., Greco, A. V., and Lauro, R., Insulin receptors during menstrual cycle in normal woman, *J. Clin. Endocrinol. Metab.,* 47, 1387, 1978.

86. Bhathena, S. J., Gazdar, A. F., Schechter, G. P., Russell, E. K., Soehnlen, F. E., Gritsman, A., and Recant, L., Expression of glucagon receptors on T- and B-lymphoblasts: comparison with insulin receptors, *Endocrinology,* 111, 684, 1982.

87. Snow, E. C., Feldbush, T. L., and Oaks, J. A., The role of insulin in the response of murine T lymphocytes to mitogenic stimulation in vitro, *J. Immunol.,* 124, 739, 1980.

88. Kumagai, J. I., Akiyama, H., Iwashita, S., Iida, H., and Yahara, I., In vitro regeneration of resting lymphocytes from stimulated lymphocytes and its inhibition by insulin, *J. Immunol.,* 126, 1249, 1981.

89. Diaz-Espada, F. and Lopez-Alarcon, L., Mitogen-induced changes in glycolytic enzymes of mouse lymphocytes: influence of insulin on cell activation in vitro, *Immunology,* 46, 705, 1982.

90. Ottlecz, A., Koltai, M., Blazsó, G., and Minker, E., Contributions to the regulatory role of insulin in inflammation and anaphylaxis, *Int. Arch. Allergy Appl. Immunol.,* 56, 284, 1978.

91. Strom, T. B. and Bangs, J. D., Human serum-free mixed lymphocyte response: the stereo-specific effect of insulin and its potentiation by transferrin, *J. Immunol.,* 128, 1555, 1982.

92. Gelfand, E. W., Ipp, M. M., and Riordan, J. R., Insulin modulation of antibody-dependent cytotoxicity and the detection of antireceptor antibodies, *J. Lab. Clin. Med.,* 99, 39, 1982.

93. Ghezzo, F., Garbarino, G., and Ioverno, L., Insulin modulates human mononuclear adherent cell fibrinolytic and phagocytic activities *Scand. J. Haematol.,* 30, 379, 1983.

94. Koltai, M., Blazsó, G., Minker, E., Lonovics, J., and Ottlecz, A., Anaphylactoid-inflammation-promoting factor: an insulin-induced factor derived from non-sensitized lymphocytes increases anaphylactoid inflammation in rats, *Int. Arch. Allergy Appl. Immunol.,* 49, 358, 1975.

95. Strom, T. B., Bear, R. A., and Carpenter, C. B., Insulin-induced augmentation of lymphocyte-mediated cytotoxicity, *Science,* 187, 1206, 1975.

96. Koltai, M., Ottlecz, A., Minker, E., and Blazsó, G., Sensitization by insulin of the anaphylactoid inflammation in rats, *Int. Arch. Allergy Appl. Immunol.,* 46, 261, 1974.

97. Rhodes, J., Modulation of macrophage Fc receptor expression in vitro by insulin and cyclic nucleotides, *Nature (London),* 257, 597, 1975.

98. Nerup, J. and Christie, M., HLA and diabetes mellitus, in *HLA in Endocrine and Metabolic Disorders,* Farid, N. R., Ed., Academic Press, New York, 1981, 69.

99. Mirakian, R., Bottazzo, G. F., Gudworth, A. G., Richardson, C. A., and Doniach, D., Autoimmunity to anterior pituitary cells and the pathogenesis of insulin-dependent diabetes mellitus, *Lancet,* I, 755, 1982.

100. Cahill, G. F., Jr., Diabetes mellitus: a brief overview, *Johns Hopkins Med. J.,* 143, 155, 1978.

101. Vialettes, B., Beaume, D., and Vague, P., Auto-immunity and insulin dependent diabetes, *Diabete. Metab.,* 8, 349, 1982.

102. Kromann, H., Aspects of the aetiology and pathogenesis of insulin dependent diabetes mellitus: a brief overview, *Dan. Med. Bull.,* 29, 257, 1982.

103. Marliss, E. B., Nakhooda, A. F., Poussier, P., and Sima, A. A. F., The diabetic syndrome of the BB Wistar rat: possible relevance to Type-1 (insulin-dependent) diabetes in man, *Diabetologia,* 22, 225, 1982.

104. Pavelić, K., Slijepčević, M., and Pavelić, J., Recovery of immune system in diabetic mice after treatment with insulin, *Horm. Metab. Res.,* 10, 381, 1978.

105. Ptak, W., Czarnik, Z., and Hanczakowska, M., Contact sensitivity in alloxan-diabetic mice, *Clin. Exp. Immunol.,* 19, 319, 1975.

106. Ptak, W., Hanczakowska, M., Różycka, R., and Różycka, D., Impaired antibody responses in alloxan diabetic mice, *Clin. Exp. Immunol.,* 29, 140, 1977.

107. Ptak, W., Rewicka, M., and Kollat, M., Development of specific suppressor cells in hypoinsulinaemic mice, *Nature (London),* 283, 199, 1980.

108. Ptak, W., Rewicka, M., Kollat, M., and Walicki, W., Ease of induction of cells producing TNP-specific suppressor factor in hypoinsulinemic mice, *Clin. Immunol. Immunopathol.,* 19, 447, 1981.

109. Mahmoud, A. A. F., Rodman, H. M., Mandel, M. A., and Warren, K. S., Induced and spontaneous diabetes mellitus and suppression of cell mediated immunologic responses, *J. Clin. Invest.,* 57, 362, 1976.

110. Ptak, W., Rewicka, M., Strzyzewska, J., and Kollat, M., Alleviation of IgE-mediated immune reactions in hypoinsulinaemic and hyperglycaemic mice, *Clin. Exp. Immunol.,* 52, 54, 1983.

111. Ptak, W., Rewicka, M., and Bielecka, J., Macrophage function in alloxan-diabetic mice: expression and activity of Fc receptors, *J. Clin. Lab. Immunol.,* 5, 121, 1981.

112. Pasko, K. L., Salvin, S. B., and Winkelstein, A., Mechanisms in the *in vivo* release of lymphokines. V. Responses in alloxan-treated and genetically diabetic mice, *Cell. Immunol.,* 62, 205, 1981.

113. Jones, C. A., Seifert, M. F., Dixit, P. K., Macrophage migration inhibition in experimental diabetes, *Proc. Soc. Exp. Biol. Med.,* 170, 298, 1982.

114. Maiti, A. K. and Dasgupta, S. R., Mast cells in different tissues of alloxan diabetic rat, *Indian J. Exp. Biol.,* 18, 1152, 1980.

115. Norrby, K., Delayed mast cell mediated mitogenic reactivity in diabetic rats, *Virchows Arch. B Cell Pathol.,* 41, 39, 1982.

116. Hägg, E., Occurrence of immunoglobulin and complement in the glomeruli of rats with long-term alloxan diabetes — an immunofluorescence study, *Acta Pathol. Microbiol. Scand. A,* 82, 220, 1974.

117. Fabris, N. and Piantanelli, L., Differential effect of pancreatectomy on humoral and cell-mediated immune responses, *Clin. Exp. Immunol.,* 28, 315, 1977.

118. Like, A. A., Rossini, A. A., Guberski, D. L., and Appel, M. C., Spontaneous diabetes mellitus; reversal and prevention in the BB/W rat with antiserum to rat lymphocytes, *Science,* 206, 1421, 1979.

119. Elder, M. E. and MacLaren, N. K., Identification of profound peripheral T lymphocyte immunodeficiencies in the spontaneously diabetic BB rat, *J. Immunol.,* 130, 1723, 1983.

120. Jackson, R., Rassi, N., Crump, T., Haynes, B., and Eisenbarth, G. S., The BB diabetic rat: profound T-cell lymphocytopenia, *Diabetes,* 30, 887, 1981.

121. Dyrberg, T., Poussier, P., Nakhooda, F., Marliss, E. B., and Lernmark, A., Islet cell surface and lymphocyte antibodies often precede the spontaneous diabetes in the BB rat, *Diabetologia*, 26, 159, 1984.

122. Guttmann, R. D., Colle, E., Michel, F., and Seemayer, T., Spontaneous diabetes mellitus syndrome in the rat. II. T lymphopenia and its association with clinical disease and pancreatic lymphocytic infiltration, *J. Immunol.*, 130, 1732, 1983.

123. Arky, R. A., Antibodies and disorders of glucose metabolism: a courting couple, *N. Engl. J. Med.*, 307, 1445, 1982.

124. Bottazzo, G. F., Florin-Christensen, A., and Doniach, D., Islet-cell antibodies in diabetes mellitus with autoimmune polyendocrine deficiencies, *Lancet*, II, 1279, 1974.

125. Van Thiel, D. H., Smith, W. I., Rabin, B. S., Fisher, S. E., and Lester, R., A syndrome of immunoglobulin A deficiency, diabetes mellitus, malabsorption, and a common HLA haplotype, *Ann. Intern. Med.*, 86, 10, 1977.

126. Champsaur, H. F., Botazzo, G. F., Bertrams, J., Assan, R., and Bach, C., Virologic, immunologic, and genetic factors in insulin-dependent diabetes mellitus, *J. Pediatr.*, 100, 15, 1982.

127. Craighead, J. E., Current views on the etiology of insulin-dependent diabetes mellitus, *N. Engl. J. Med.*, 299, 1439, 1978.

128. Rayfield, E. J. and Seto, Y., Viruses and pathogenesis of diabetes mellitus, *Diabetes*, 27, 1126, 1978.

129. Handwerger, B. S., Fernandes, G., and Brown, D. M., Immune and autoimmune aspects of diabetes mellitus, *Hum. Pathol.*, 11, 338, 1980.

130. Kahn, R., Autoimmunity and the aetiology of insulin dependent diabetes mellitus, *Nature (London)*, 299, 15, 1982.

131. Huang, S.-W. and MaClaren, N. K., Insulin-dependent diabetes: a disease of autoaggression, *Science*, 192, 64, 1976.

132. Shanahan, F., McKenna, R., McCarthy, C. F., and Drury, M. I., Coeliac disease and diabetes mellitus — a study of 24 patients with HLA typing, *Q. J. Med.*, 51, 329, 1982.

133. Bottazzo, G. F., Mann, J. I., Thorogood, M., Baum, J. D., and Doniach, D., Autoimmunity in juvenile diabetics and their families, *Br. Med. J.*, 2, 165, 1978.

134. Rittenhouse, H. G., Oxender, D. L., Pek, S., and Ar, D., Complement-mediated cytotoxic effects on pancreatic islets with sera from diabetic patients, *Diabetes*, 29, 317, 1980.

135. Sai, P., Boitard, C., Debray-Sachs, M., Pouplard, A., Assan, R., and Hamburger, J., Complement-fixing islet cell antibodies from some diabetic patients alter insulin release in vitro, *Diabetes*, 30, 1051, 1981.

136. Kobayashi, T., Sawano, S., Itoh, T., Sugimoto, T., Tanaka, T., and Suwa, S., The prevalence of islet-cell antibodies and complement-fixing islet-cell antibodies in Japanese diabetics, *Endocrinol. Jpn.*, 28, 429, 1981.

137. Mustonen, A., Knip, M., and Akerblom, H. K., An association between complement-fixing cytoplasmic islet cell antibodies and endogenous insulin secretion in children with insulin-dependent diabetes mellitus, *Diabetes*, 32, 743, 1983.

138. Flier, J. S., Kahn, C. R., Roth, J., and Bar, R. S., Antibodies that impair insulin receptor binding in an unusual diabetic syndrome with severe insulin resistance, *Science*, 190, 63, 1975.

139. Flier, J. S., Kahn, C. R., and Roth, J., Receptors, antireceptor antibodies and mechanisms of insulin resistance, *N. Engl. J. Med.*, 300, 413, 1979.

140. Taylor, S. I., Grundberger, G., Marcus-Samuels, B., Underhill, L. H., Dons, R. F., Ryan, J., Roddam, R. F., Rupe, C. E., and Gorden, P., Hypoglycemia associated with antibodies to the insulin receptor, *N. Engl. J. Med.*, 307, 1422, 1982.

141. Van Obberghen, E. and Kahn, C. R., Autoantibodies to insulin receptors, *Mol. Cell. Endocrinol.*, 22, 277, 1981.

142. Van Obberghen, E., Grunfeld, C., Harrison, L. C., Karlsson, A., Muggeo, M., and Kahn, C. R., Autoantibodies to the insulin receptor and insulin-resistant diabetes, *Horm. Res.*, 16, 280, 1982.

143. Jennette, J. C., Wilkman, A. S., and Bagnell, C. R., Insulin receptor autoantibody-induced pancreatic islet-Beta (B)-cell hyperplasia, *Arch. Pathol. Lab. Med.*, 106, 218, 1982.

144. Maron, R., Elias, D., de Jongh, B. M., Bruining, G. J., van Rood, J. J., Shechter, Y., and Cohen, I. R., Autoantibodies to the insulin receptor in juvenile onset insulin-dependent diabetes, *Nature (London)*, 303, 817, 1983.

145. Rovira, A., Valverde, I., Escorihuela, R., and Lopez-Linares, M., Autoimmunity to insulin in a child with hypoglycemia, *Acta Paediatr. Scand.*, 71, 343, 1982.

146. Falholt, K., Determination of insulin specific IgE in serum of diabetic patients by solid-phase radioimmunoassay, *Diabetologia*, 22, 254, 1982.

147. Keilacker, H., Rjasanowski, I., Ziegler, M., Michaelis, D., Woltanski, K. P., and Besch, W., Insulin antibodies in juvenile diabetes mellitus: correlations to diabetic stability, insulin requirement and duration of insulin treatment, *Horm. Metab. Res.*, 14, 227, 1982.

157

148. Zeidler, A., Frasier, S. D., Kumar, D., and Loon, J., Histocompatibility antigens and immunoglobulin-G insulin antibodies in Mexican-American insulin-dependent diabetic patients, *J. Clin. Endocrinol. Metab.*, 54, 569, 1982.
149. Wilkin, T. J. and Nicholson, S., Autoantibodies against human insulin, *Br. Med. J.*, 288, 349, 1984.
150. Nagaoka, K., Sakurami, T., Nabeya, N., Imura, H., and Kuno, S., Thyroglobulin and microsomal antibodies in patients with insulin dependent diabetes mellitus and their relatives, *Endocrinol. Jpn.*, 26, 213, 1979.
151. Kokkonen, J., Kiuttu, J., Mustonen, A., and Rasanen, O., Organ-specific antibodies in healthy and diabetic children and young adults, *Acta Paediatr. Scand.*, 71, 223, 1982.
152. De Mario, U., Ventriglia, L., Iavicoli, M., Guy, K., and Andreani, D., The correlation between insulin antibodies and circulating immune complexes in diabetics with and without microangiopathy, *Clin. Exp. Immunol.*, 52, 575, 1983.
153. Di Mario, U., Irvine, W. J., Borsey, D. G., Kyner, J. L., Weston, J., and Galfo, C., Immune abnormalities in diabetic patients not requiring insulin at diagnosis, *Diabetologia*, 25, 392, 1983.
154. Kaldany, A., Autoantibodies to islet cells in diabetes mellitus, *Diabetes*, 28, 102, 1979.
155. Smith, W. I., Rabin, B. S., Huellmantel, A., Van Thiel, D. H., and Drash, A., Immunopathology of juvenile-onset diabetes mellitus. I. IgA deficiency and juvenile diabetes, *Diabetes*, 27, 1092, 1978.
156. Kaldany, A., Hill, T., Wentworth, S., Brink, S. J., D'Elia, J. A., Clouse, M., and Soeldner, J. S., Trapping of peripheral blood lymphocytes in the pancreas of patients with acute-onset insulin-dependent diabetes mellitus. I, *Diabetes*, 31, 463, 1982.
157. Nerup, J., Andersen, O. O., Bendixen, G., Egeberg, J., and Poulsen, J. E., Anti-pancreatic, cellular hypersensitivity in diabetes mellitus: antigenic activity of fetal calf pancreas and correlation with clinical type of diabetes, *Acta Allergol.*, 28, 223, 1973.
158. Boitard, C., Chatenoud, L. -M., and Debray-Sachs, M., In vitro inhibition of pancreatic B cell function by lymphocytes from diabetics with associated autoimmune diseases: a T cell phenomenon, *J. Immunol.*, 129, 2529, 1982.
159. Segal, P., Teitelbaum, D., and Ohry, A., Cell-mediated immunity to nervous system antigens in diabetic patients with neuropathy, *Isr. J. Med. Sci.*, 19, 7, 1983.
160. Richens, E. R., Ancil, R. J., Gough, K. R., and Hartog, M., Cellular hypersensitivity to mitochondrial antigens in diabetes mellitus, *Clin. Exp. Immunol.*, 13, 1, 1973.
161. Glassman, A. B., Lindsay, J. H., Jr., Levine, J. H., and Bennett, C. L., T and B lymphocyte subpopulations in black patients with diabetes mellitus, *Ann. Clin. Lab. Sci.*, 8, 467, 1978.
162. Selam, J. L., Clot, J., Andary, M., and Mirouze, J., Circulating lymphocyte subpopulations in juvenile insulin-dependent diabetes: correction of abnormalities by adequate blood glucose control, *Diabetologia*, 16, 35, 1979.
163. Eliashiv, A., Olumide, F., Norton, L., and Eiseman, B., Depression of cell-mediated immunity in diabetes, *Arch. Surg.*, 113, 1180, 1978.
164. Farid, N. R. and Anderson, J., Immunoglobulins and complement in diabetes mellitus, *Lancet*, 2, 92, 1973.
165. Schernthaner, G., Ludwig, H., Mayr, W. R., and Eibl, M., Humoral antibacterial immunity in first degree relatives of insulin-dependent diabetics, *Diabete. Metab.*, 4, 163, 1978.
166. Kolterman, O. G., Olefsky, J. M., Kurahara, C., and Taylor, K., A defect in cell-mediated immune function in insulin-resistant diabetic and obese subjects, *J. Lab. Clin. Med.*, 96, 535, 1980.
167. Slater, L.M., Murray, S. L., Kershnar, A., and Mosier, M. A., Immunological suppressor cell activity in insulin dependent diabetes, *J. Clin. Lab. Immunol.*, 3, 105, 1980.
168. Lederman, M. M., Ellner, J. J., and Rodman, H. M., Defective suppressor cell generation in juvenile onset diabetes, *J. Immunol.*, 127, 2051, 1981.
169. Fairchild, R. S., Kyner, J. L., and Abdou, N. I., Specific immunoregulation abnormality in insulin-dependent diabetes mellitus, *J. Lab. Clin. Med.*, 99, 175, 1982.
170. Gupta, S., Fikrig, S. M., Khanna, S., and Orti, E., Deficiency of suppressor T-cells in insulin-dependent diabetes mellitus: an analysis with monoclonal antibodies, *Immunol. Lett.*, 4, 289, 1982.
171. Horita, M., Suzuki, H., Onodera, T., Ginsberg-Fellner, F., Fauci, A. S., and Notkins, A. L., Abnormalities of immunoregulatory T cell subsets in patients with insulin-dependent diabetes mellitus, *J. Immunol.*, 129, 1426, 1982.
172. Buschard, K., Madsbad, S., and Rygaard, J., Depressed suppressor cell activity in patients with newly diagnosed insulin-dependent diabetes mellitus, *Clin. Exp. Immunol.*, 41, 25, 1980.
173. Buschard, K., Madsbad, S., Krarup, T., and Rygaard, J., Glycaemic control and suppressor cell activity in patients with insulin-dependent diabetes mellitus, *Clin. Exp. Immunol.*, 48, 189, 1982.
174. Buschard, K., Madsbad, S., and Rygaard, J., Suppressor cell activity in patients with newly diagnosed insulin-dependent diabetes mellitus — a prospective study, *J. Clin. Lab. Immunol.*, 8, 19, 1982.
175. Buschard, K., Madsbad, S., and Rygaard, J., Suppressor cell activity and beta-cell function in insulin-dependent diabetics, *Acta Pathol. Microbiol. Immunol. C*, 90, 53, 1982.

176. Buschard, K., Röpke, C., Madsbad, S., Mehlsen, J., Sørensen, T. B., and Rygaard, J., Alterations of peripheral lymphocyte-T subpopulations in patients with insulin-dependent (Type-1) diabetes mellitus, *J. Clin. Lab. Immunol.,* 10, 127, 1983.

177. El Mohandes, A., Touraine, J. L., Touraine, F., Shukry, A. S., and Salle, B., Lymphocyte populations and responses to mitogens in infants of diabetic mothers, *J. Clin. Lab. Immunol.,* 8, 25, 1982.

178. Mascart-Lemone, F., Delepesse, G., Dorchy, H., Lemiere, B., and Servais, G., Characterization of immunoregulatory lymphocytes-T in insulin-dependent diabetic children by means of monoclonal antibodies, *Clin. Exp. Immunol.,* 47, 296, 1982.

179. Jackson, R. A., Morris, M. A., Haynes, B. F., and Eisenbarth, G. S., Increased circulating Ia-antigen-bearing T cells in type I diabetes mellitus, *N. Engl. J. Med.,* 306, 785, 1982.

180. Glassman, A. B., Lindsay, J. H., Jr., Bennett, C. E., and Hodges, E. R., Jr., Effects of insulin on phytohemagglutinin-P, concanavalin-A, and pokeweed mitogen in diabetic and nondiabetic lymphocytes, *Ann. Clin. Lab. Sci.,* 11, 9, 1981.

181. Delespesse, G., Duchateau, J., Bastenie, P. A., Lauvaux, J. P., Collet, H., and Govaerts, A., Cell-mediated immunity in diabetes mellitus, *Clin. Exp. Immunol.,* 18, 461, 1974.

182. Pedersen, O., Beck-Nielsen, H., and Heding, L., Insulin receptors on monocytes from patients with ketosis-prone diabetes mellitus, *Diabetes,* 27, 1098, 1978.

183. Gratacos, J. A., Neufeld, N., Kumar, D., Artal, R., Paul, R. H., and Mestman, J., Monocyte insulin binding studies in normal and diabetic pregnancies, *Am. J. Obstet. Gynecol.,* 141, 611, 1981.

184. Neufeld, N. D., Kaplan, S. A., Lippe, B. M., and Scott, M., Increased monocyte receptor binding of (I-125) insulin in infants of gestational diabetic mothers, *J. Clin. Endocrinol. Metab.,* 47, 590, 1978.

185. Geisler, C., Almdal, T., Bennedsen, J., Rhodes, J. M., and Kolendorf, K., Monocyte functions in diabetes mellitus, *Acta Pathol. Microbiol. Immun. C,* 90, 33, 1982.

186. Hill, H. R., Augustine, N. H., Rallison, M. L., and Santos, J. I., Defective monocyte chemotactic responses in diabetes mellitus, *J. Clin. Immunol.,* 3, 70, 1983.

187. Iavicoli, M., Di Mario, U., Pozzilli, P., Canalese, J., Vetriglia, L., Galfo, C., and Andreani, D., Impaired phagocytic function and increased immune complexes in diabetics with severe microangiopathy, *Diabetes,* 31, 7, 1982.

188. Andreani, D., Di Mario, U., Galfo, C., Ventriglia, L., and Iavicoli, M., Circulating immune complexes in diabetics with severe microangiopathy — evaluation by 2 different methods, *Acta Endocrinol.,* 99, 239, 1982.

189. Sabioncello, A., Rabatic, S., Kadrnka-Lovrencic, M., Oberiter, V., and Dekaris, D., Decreased phagocytosis and antibody-dependent cellular cytotoxicity (ADCC) in type-1 diabetes, *Biomed. Express,* 35, 227, 1981.

190. Sensi, M., Pozzilli, P., Gorsuch, A. N., Bottazzo, G. F., and Cudworth, A. G., Increased killer cell activity in insulin dependent (Type-1) diabetes mellitus, *Diabetologia,* 20, 106, 1981.

191. Niethammer, D., Heinze, E., Teller, W., Kleihauer, E., Wildfeuer, A., and Haferkamp, O., Impairment of granulocyte function in juvenile diabetes, *Klin. Wochenschr.,* 53, 1057, 1975.

192. Nolan, C. M., Beaty, H. N., and Bagdade, J. D., Further characterization of impaired bactericidal function of granulocytes in patients with poorly controlled diabetes, *Diabetes,* 27, 889, 1978.

193. Viollier, A. -F. and Senn, H. J., Granulocytic defence machanisms in diabetes mellitus with special reference to bacterial killing, *Schweiz. Med. Wochenschr.,* 109, 1896, 1979.

194. Valerius, N. H., Eff, C., Hansen, N. E., Karle, H., Nerup, J., Soeberg, B., and Sorensen, S. F., Neutrophil and lymphocyte function in patients with diabetes mellitus, *Acta Med. Scand.,* 211, 463, 1982.

195. Subbaiah, P. V. and Bagdade, J. D., Host defense in diabetes mellitus — defective membrane synthesis during phagocytosis, *Horm. Metab. Res.,* 14, 445, 1982.

196. Nicoll, G. A., Gollapudi, G. M., Ramamurthy, N. S., and Golub, L. M., Suppressed collagenolytic activity in polymorphonuclear leucocytes from diabetic humans, *Experientia,* 37, 315, 1981.

197. Lagarde, M., Berciaud, P., Burtin, M., and Dechavanne, M., Refractoriness of diabetic platelets to inhibitory prostaglandins, *Prostagland. Med.,* 7, 341, 1981.

198. Davis, J. W., Hartman, C. R., Davis, R. F., Kyner, J. L., Lewis, H. D., and Phillips, P. E., Platelet aggregate ratio in diabetes mellitus, *Acta Haematol.,* 67, 222, 1982.

199. McMillan, D. E., Elevation of complement components in diabetes mellitus, *Diabete. Metab.,* 6, 265, 1980.

200. Kirk, R. L., Ranford, P. R., Theophilus, J., Ahuja, H. M. S., Mehra, N. K., and Vaidya, M. C., The rare factor BfSl of the properdin system strongly associated with insulin-dependent diabetes in north India, *Tissue Antigen,* 20, 303, 1982.

201. Singh, S. B., Lang, C. M., and Rapp, F., Defective cell-mediated immune response in spontaneous diabetes mellitus in the guinea pig, *J. Clin. Lab. Immunol.,* 10, 113, 1983.

202. Falliers, C. J., Tan, L. S., Szentivanyi, J., Jorgensen, J. R., and Bukantz, S. C., Childhood asthma and steroid therapy as influences on growth, *Am. J. Dis. Child.,* 105, 127, 1963.

203. Snyder, R. J., Collipp, P. J., and Greene, J. S., Growth and ultimate height of children with asthma, *Clin. Pediatr.*, 6, 389, 1967.
204. Green, J. R. B., O'Donoghue, D. P., Edwards, C. R. W., and Dawson, A. M., A case of apparent hypopituitarism complicating chronic inflammatory bowel disease, *Acta Paediatr. Scand.*, 66, 643, 1977.
205. Ferguson, A. C. and Murray, A. B., Short stature and delayed skeletal maturation in children with allergic disease, *J. Allergy Clin. Immunol.*, 69, 461, 1982.
206. Filkins, J. P. and Yelich, M. R., Mechanism of hyperinsulinemia after reticuloendothelial system phagocytosis, *Am. J. Physiol.*, 242, E115, 1982.

Chapter 6

PROLACTIN AND OTHER LACTOGENIC HORMONES

I. Berczi and Eva Nagy

TABLE OF CONTENTS

I. INTRODUCTION

Prolactin (PRL) is present in all vertebrates, but its function in lower animals has not been established with certainty. Osmoregulatory, integumentary, growth, developmental, and metabolic functions have been proposed for cold-blooded animals, but none of these seem to be predominant, major actions. On the other hand, in mammals and birds, the physiological role of PRL is clearly related to reproductive functions. The crop milk production in pigeons and doves and the incubation or brood patch development in many species is regulated by PRL. In mammals, PRL is involved in the stimulation of mammary gland growth and lactation; it has a luteotropic and luteolytic effect and also stimulates the growth and secretion of male accessory sex organs. In addition, the osmoregulatory functions of PRL are important to the mammalian fetus.[1]

PRL is related structurally to growth hormone (GH) and placental lactogen (PL). GH is generally considered the principal hormone that promotes body growth and regulates a variety of associated anabolic processes. On the other hand, PRL is viewed as a hormone of reproductive significance. However, if one compares all the known functions of these hormones on an evolutionary scale, it is clear that there is a considerable overlap. For instance, primate GH has a lactogenic effect, which can be readily demonstrated in a variety of species. The functional differences of GH and PRL seem to be greatest in ungulates, yet ungulate PRL is capable of supporting limb regeneration in the newt, tail growth in the tadpole, and body growth in the lizard. Although lactogenic and GH receptors are different, some cross-reactivity of GH and PRL with each other's receptor has been demonstrated, which emphasizes further the similarities of these two hormones. It has been estimated that PRL and GH diverged by gene duplication from a common ancestral gene at least 380 million years ago. Placental lactogen also belongs to this hormonal family. Recent studies showed that several forms of PRL and GH exist, which may have different biological functions. It remains to be seen whether or not these isohormones will have a family of corresponding isoreceptors on various target tissues.[2] There seems to be a complete functional overlap between PRL, GH, and PL with regard to their capacity of restoring the immunocompetence of hormonally altered animals.

II. PROLACTIN RECEPTORS ON LYMPHOID CELLS

Studies of crude membrane preparations of various tissues of monkey, rat, guinea pig, rabbit, sheep, pigeon, and frog, for the presence of PRL receptors, using ^{125}I-labeled human GH and ovine PRL, showed clear indications for the presence of receptors in the liver and mammary gland, but yielded negative results in spleen.[3] Similarly, search for PRL receptors in different rat tissues (by immunohistochemistry, radioautography, and radioreceptor assay) revealed specific binding sites on cells of the convoluted tubules of the kidney, hepatocytes of the liver, glandular cells of the zona reticularis, zona fasciculata, zona glomerulosa of the adrenal cortex, interstitial cells of the testes, and epithelial cells of the choroid plexus. Again, no indication of PRL receptors in lymphoid tissue was found.[4] In this laboratory, two myeloid cell lines, a monocyte line, three B cell lines, and three T cell lines, all of human origin, were examined by radioreceptor assay for the presence of lactogenic or GH receptors, using ^{125}I-human GH as tracer. Furthermore, rat lymph node, spleen, thymus, and bone marrow cells were examined as fresh preparations, or after stimulation with phytohemagglutinin (PHA) or lipopolysaccharide (LPS), using identical methodology. None of these experiments provided clear evidence for the presence of lactogenic receptors on any of the lymphoid cells tested.[5] However, the estrogen induced rat lymphoma, Nb2, was found to require lactogenic hormones for proliferation in vitro.[6,7] This tumor cell line was subsequently shown to have approximately 12,000 high affinity ($K_d = 75$ p M) receptor sites per cell. The affinity of the Nb_2 PRL receptor is approximately 20-fold higher than that of the receptors in other cell types.[8] The Nb2 lymphoma has T cell surface markers and is frozen at an intermediate state of differentiation.[9] Recently, Russel and co-workers[10] reported the presence of PRL receptors on peripheral blood T- and B-lymphocytes, as well as on monocytes. The calculated receptor number was 360 per cell with approximate K_d of 1.66 nM. Certain concentrations of cyclosporin enhanced the specific binding of ^{125}I-PRL to human lymphoid cells, whereas other concentrations were inhibitory. PRL treatment of lymphocytes induced ornithine decarboxylase, which is a growth regulatory enzyme.

III. PROLACTIN AND IMMUNITY

A. Regulation of Mammary Immune Function

Birds and mammals provide their young with antibodies as protection against environmental pathogens.[11] In birds, immunoglobulins are transferred to the egg, whereas in mammals, the transfer of antibodies to the offspring is achieved through the placenta and/or the colostrum and milk.[12,13] Hooved animals (horses, pigs, sheep, goats, cattle, etc.) protect theirs exclusively by antibodies secreted into the colostrum, since the placental transmission cannot take place in these animals because of anatomical barriers. It is a long-standing observation in veterinary medicine that newborn calves and piglets succumb to infection due to ubiquitous germs if deprived of colostrum. Alternatively, they can be protected by orally administered antibodies, especially if given within the first 36 hr after birth when the intestinal mucosa is capable of absorbing antibodies, which will then appear in the circulation.[14] Some carnivorous animals, (e.g., cat, dog, ferret) provide their young with antibodies through the placenta. However, the immunoglobulins secreted by the mammary gland remain a significant factor in protection of the young, since intestinal absorption is possible for some 10 days. The situation is similar in the rat and mouse, except that antibodies will absorb unaltered from the gastrointestinal tract up to 20 days. In rats and mice the transmission of immunoglobulins across the neonatal intestine is selective, and it is mediated by specific Fc receptors.[15,16] Rabbits, guinea pigs, and primates transmit immunoglobulins into the blood stream of the offspring prenatally through the placenta. The intestinal mucosa of the young of these animals and of human babies is unable to absorb biologically active immunoglobulins.

Even though there is no gastrointestinal absorption of immunoglobulins in the human infant, it is clear that the colostrum provides significant protection against various gastrointestinal infections, enterotoxins, and viruses. Furthermore, colostral immune factors may be instrumental in the prevention of other pathological abnormalities, such as food allergy, protein losing enthropathy, and inflammatory bowel disease.[17-20] The major immunoglobulin in human colostrum and milk is secretory IgA, although all the other immunoglobulin classes are present. Highest levels were found immediately after delivery, with a significant decrease within the next few days, which is followed by more or less constant levels.[19-21] Local production, or selective excretion, was proposed for all immunoglobulin classes on the basis of concentration differences between milk and serum. Human colostrum was found to contain numerous cells producing IgA antibodies against the O antigen of commonly encountered *Escherichia coli* bacteria. Furthermore, oral administration of nonpathogenic strain of *E. coli* led to the rapid appearance of colostral cells producing anti-*O*-antibodies.[22] High levels of colostrum IgA agglutinins to *Salmonella typhimurium* have been found in three patients after clinical gastrointestinal infections during pregnancy.[23] These and similar observations in man and in animals led to the concept that the mammary gland is integrated into the "common mucosal immune system".[24] According to this concept, IgA-forming lymphocytes that are stimulated by antigen in the gastrointestinal tract or in the bronchial mucosa migrate to the lactating mammary gland and produce secretory IgA. Cell mediated immunity, (e.g., tuberculin sensitivity) is also transferred by breast feeding to the child.[25,26] Experiments in rats and mice showed that both immunostimulation and immunosuppression can be transmitted from mother to offspring through the placenta and/or the milk. IgG antibodies, antigen, and nonimmunoglobulin factors crossing the placenta or excreted into the milk were indicated in the transfer of immunosuppression to the offspring.[27-31]

The development and function of the mammary gland is regulated by PRL and steroid hormones.[32-36] The immune function of the mammary gland is also hormonally regulated, as revealed by the studies of Weisz-Carrington and co-workers.[37-39] They studied the localization of immunoglobulin forming plasma cells and epithelial immunoglobulins in the mammary gland of mice. In male or female virgin animals, only occasional plasma cells and very low amounts of intraepithelial immunoglobulins were present. During pregnancy, the mammary gland increased 6-fold in weight and the number of IgA plasma cells increased 150-fold per unit area. This amounted to a 900-fold estimated increase of plasma cells in the mammary gland. This increment paralleled the development and proliferation of the glandular epithelium, which was associated with the plasma cells. The intraepithelial content of IgA was also maximal, when the glandular epithelium was most developed. Weaning, or deliberate interruption of suckling for more than 10 days, resulted in a sharp decrease of IgA plasma cells and involution of the epithelium with declining immunoglobulin content. When mice were immunized orally to produce IgA antibodies against ferritin, antibody forming plasma cells were detected in the intestinal mucosa, in the lactating mammary gland, salivary gland, and respiratory tract. Lymphocytes were transferred from mesenteric lymph nodes and peripheral lymph nodes of orally immunized donors into nonimmunized recipients. Cells forming IgA antibodies to ferritin homed to exocrine targets, whereas IgM and IgG antibody-forming cells homed to the peripheral nodes. These findings were compatible with the concept of generalized and interrelated secretory immune system.[39]

The secretory immune system of the mammary gland could be activated in female or in castrated male mice by combined treatment with progesterone, estrogen, and PRL. Development of the glandular epithelium occurred with concomitant increase in the number of IgA secreting plasma cells and of intraepithelial IgA. Treatment with any one of the hormones alone, or with progesterone and estrogen combined, caused minimal to moderate increases in the number of IgA plasma cells. The greatest induction of development was observed by PRL treatment, as a single hormone. Combined hormone treatment of female virgin recipients induced a preferential localization of lymphocytes from mesenteric, but not peripheral, lymph nodes in the mammary gland. Testosterone treatment of lactating mothers inhibited the localization of mesenteric lymphocytes in the mammary gland.[38] Mammary tissue was taken from lactating mice and cultured in the presence of insulin, progesterone, estrogen, and PRL. Such cultured mammary epithelial cells bound specifically and internalized dimeric serum IgA, as assessed by immunofluorescence and enzyme immunoassay. Only a minimal amount of IgA was bound in the absence of PRL, but IgA binding increased 25 times, if PRL was added to the culture medium.[40]

Klareskog and co-workers[41] treated virgin guinea pigs with estradiol, progesterone, and ovine PRL, which induced the expression of Ia antigens on the mammary gland epithelium. The expression of Ia molecules could be reversed by the administration of testosterone. Therefore, the expression of Ia molecules by the mammary gland epithelium is under hormonal control. Since Ia antigens are known to have immunoregulatory function, the authors suggested that this hormone induced expression of Ia antigen may play a fundamental role in the activation of mammary immune system.

The effect of menstrual cycle on the immunoglobulin content of the mammary gland was studied in 53 women. Immunoglobulin localization in sections of mammary glands was determined by direct immunofluorescence, with antibodies specific for IgG, IgA, IgM, and IgA secretory component. Immunoglobulin A, its secretory component, and IgM concentrations increased significantly in the preovulatory phase of the cycle. No significant IgG localization was noted, and there was no correlation between IgA and IgM localization and plasma cell infiltration. Plasma cell infiltration was not influenced by menstrual cycle phase.[42]

The number of leukocytes in rat mammary epithelium during pregnancy was constant (3.5%). However, with the onset of lactation, the percentage of leukocytes was significantly increased (8.7%). Although the total percentage of intraepithelial leukocytes was increased, the number of labeled cells 4 days after the injection of 1 μCi of ^{3}H-thymidine was unchanged between 20 days of gestation and 2 days post partum, and actually showed a significant decrease between 2 to 6 days post partum. This decrease in the incidence of labeled cells, during the period of increased alveolar infiltration of leukocytes, indicate that many of these cells had been formed elsewhere, prior to the thymidine injection, and are redistributed to the mammary gland in response to the onset of lactation.[43]

Lactation has a systemic effect on the immune system, which manifests both in morphological signs and in functional alterations. Thus, in rats a sudden decrease of corticosteriod binding globulin (CBG) activity was observed on the 3rd day of lactation, which resulted in an increase of free corticosterone and thus, caused a marked decrease in thymus weight. CBG levels were inversely related to the number of pups per litter during lactation. CBG activity returned to virgin level four days after weaning, but thymus weight and resting corticosterone concentrations reached virgin levels much later.[44] A decrease in the number of bone marrow lymphocytes was observed in mice during pregnancy, which gradually increased to normal levels 20 days after delivery. Lymphocyte frequency was restored to normal levels earlier in nonlactating than in lactating animals. During pregnancy the spleen weight increases in mice to reach a peak at 15 days of gestation. Spleen weight returns to normal 20 days after delivery. Both the red and white pulp increase in volume during pregnancy, the white pulp rapidly returning to normal after parturition. However, the red pulp remains greater in lactating females when compared to nonlactating animals, where the red pulp decreases even more rapidly in volume after parturition. Splenic plasma cells increase in number during pregnancy and are accumulated in large number in the marginal zone and periarterial area. Plasma cells decrease rapidly in number after delivery. The weight of mesenteric lymph nodes also increases significantly during pregnancy and decreases both in lactating and nonlactating animals after parturition. During pregnancy, numerous plasma cells are present in the medullary cord of lymph nodes, which decrease rapidly after parturition. Plasma cells are also markedly increased during pregnancy in the iliac lymph nodes, but not in the axillary and popliteal lymph nodes.[45,46]

Experimental glomerulonephritis was suppressed in rats by lactation. Five out of six lactating animals did not develop proteinuria after the injection of nephrotoxic serum, whereas four of five nonlactating, nonpregnant rats showed the proteinuric response. The amount of heterologous IgG deposit was similar in both groups, but lactating rats had less autologous IgG localized in the glomerular basal membrane.[47] The half-life of immune complexes (consisting of dinitrophenyl-(DNP)ovalbumin and mouse anti-DNP antibody) was 4 min in lactating mice compared with 8 min in normal female animals. Tissue distribution studies showed that by 2 hr the mammary gland had sequestered three- to fourfold more immune complexes than the liver. Lactating mice transferred immune complexes to their milk, and small quantities of the complexes could be demonstrated in the circulation of nursing neonates.[48]

The response of spleen cells of lactating mice to mitogens was not altered, but their graft-vs.-host (GVH) reactivity in vivo was decreased. However, significant changes occurred in thymus cell populations, in the mitogen and mixed leukocyte responsiveness of thymocytes, and in their capacity to induce GVH reactions. Thymocytes of 12-day pregnant animals responded more to PHA and in mixed lymphocyte reactions than did thymocytes of virgin animals. There was a further, and remarkable, increase in both responses 1 to 3 days post partum, and at 21 days they were still higher than either the virgin or the 12-day pregnant responses. Similarly post partum thymocytes were more efficient in inducing GVH reactions than were virgin thymocytes, increasing the spleen index ratio to 150% of controls.[49]

The self cure of breeding female rats was inhibited, if primary infection with *Nippostrongylus brasiliensis* coincided with lactation. The majority of worms persisted to day 34 when lactation was prolonged. A normal self cure occurred during pregnancy, or when litters were removed at birth, or when the suckling litter was limited to three.[50] Lactating rats, infected with *N. brasiliensis,* showed significant increases in worm fecundity and total worm burdens in comparison with infected controls. Immune mesenteric lymph node cells were obtained from nulliparous female donors on day 15 of primary infection. When such cells were transferred to lactating recipients, they suppressed invariably worm fecundity and induced a rejection of a substantial proportion of worms by day 10. This indicates that immune cells were functional in lactating animals. Mesenteric lymph node cells, obtained from infected lactating donors, also caused suppression of worm fecundity and reduced the number of parasites in nulliparous recipients, but such cells were substantially less effective in lactating recipients, causing the expulsion of 51% of worms by day 10 compared to 99% in the nulliparous group. Therefore, potentially immune lymphoid cells were present in the mesenteric nodes of lactating females, but the rejection mechanism was severely impaired.[51] Castrated male rats were treated twice daily with 1 mg of ovine PRL during a primary infection with *N. brasiliensis.* Survival of the worms in the small intestine was prolonged, which suggested that PRL inhibited rejection of the parasite. Syngeneic lymphocyte transfer experiments showed that PRL treatment caused a deficient immune response to the parasite. The most impressive difference in mean worm counts occurred when normal recipients of immune cells were compared with PRL-treated recipients (mean worm counts 39 vs. 329 in nine and seven animals, respectively). Mesenteric lymph node cells from PRL-treated, infected donors were less efficient in the same recipient combination (worm counts 307 in normal and 439 in PRL-treated recipients).[52] Spleen cells from mice immunized with *Trichinella spiralis* were not functional in syngeneic lactating recipients, but were functional in syngeneic nonlactating recipients. Furthermore, spleen cells from lactating donors that had been previously sensitized to *T. spiralis* were not functional when transferred into syngeneic nulliparous recipient mice.[53]

The serum of lactating rats not infected with the protozoan parasite, *Trypanosoma lewisi,* contained a rheumatoid-factor-like IgM, which amplified the specific IgG response to the parasite after exposure. This IgM was responsible for the unusual resistance of previously uninfected, lactating rats to *T. lewisi.* Lactating rats, infected with *T. lewisi,* resolved parasitemia in 9 days, compared with 21 days of nonlactating females. This heightened resistance was transferred to the rat pups infected with *T. lewisi* and *Hemobartonella muris.* Suckling pups were protected to a large extent (82.5%), whereas only 6.6% survived when solid food was provided to supplement milk. Supplementary food did not reduce survival in pups infected with only *T. lewisi.* Lactating rat serum agglutinated the "adult form" of *T. lewisi,* and parasite immunity could be passively transferred with lactating rat serum to animals already weaned.[54,55]

Rat pups were infected with *T. lewisi* from the age of 2 to 40 days and some of the animals were allowed to suckle their mother, while others were weaned. Nursing pups infected on days 2, 10, 20, or 30 resisted the parasites very well, whereas 85 and 76% of weaned animals, infected at the age of 20 and 30 days respectively, died. Weaned animals 40-days-old, resisted infection. The resistance of young rats could be increased artificially by implanting the pituitary glands of adult nonimmune rats i.m., or by injecting oestrin subcutaneously. Rats twenty-days-old, given pituitary grafts were protected completely, whereas 89% of the untreated sibling controls died during the first 3 weeks of infection. Animals, twenty-days-old, receiving oestrin were also able to withstand infection much better than did their untreated siblings. Only 1 of 20 treated animals died, whereas 14 of the 17 controls (82.3%) died during the first 3 weeks of infection.[56]

An autoimmune disease of the pituitary gland, lymphocytic hypophysitis, occurs most frequently in young women in association with pregnancy and lactation. It may mimic prolactin-producing pituitary adenomas clinically and may be accompanied by mild hyperprolactinemia. Hypersecretion of other pituitary hormones has not been reported. Histologically the disease is characterized by a massive lymphocytic infiltration and a widespread adenohypophysial cell damage. Most of the infiltrating cells are lymphocytes, although plasma cells and macrophages are also present. Occasionally multinucleated giant cells and epithelioid cells can be detected, which may form noncauseating granulomas. Sometimes lymphoid follicles with germinal centers can be recognized. Electron microscopically the interdigitation of activated lymphocytes with adenohypophysial cells has been observed. No immune complex deposits could be found, and vascular impairment or thrombus formation was not noticed. In patients with lymphocytic hypophysitis, hypopituitarism occurs, which is not restricted to the secretion of PRL.[57]

B. The Immunoregulatory Role of Prolactin

During our initial attempts to reconstitute the immunocompetence of hypophysectomized animals, we transplanted syngeneic pituitary glands under the kidney capsule, induced humoral, cell mediated, or autoimmune reactions in such animals. It became apparent very quickly that syngeneic pituitary grafts are capable of reconstituting the antibody response of Hypox animals to sheep red blood cells (SRBC), contact sensitivity reactions to dinitrochlorobenzene (DNCB), or the ability to develop adjuvant arthritis. It has been established earlier by other investigators that ectopic pituitary glands secrete significant amounts of PRL, whereas the production of other known pituitary hormones is grossly impaired.[58] Indeed, the transplanted glands in our experiments could readily be stained by the immunoperoxidase technique for PRL, whereas the number of GH containing cells was conspicuously decreased. Subsequent experiments revealed that bovine PRL is capable of restoring the immune reactivity of Hypox animals with an efficiency similar to that of syngeneic pituitary grafts (SPG).[59-61] In some experiments, we compared rat PRL with bovine PRL and human placental lactogen (PL) for their ability to restore the antibody response and contact sensitivity reactions in Hypox animals. Each hormone was able to restore immunocompetence without the necessity of additional hormone supplementation (Figures 1 and 2).[5] The restoration of DNCB reactions in Hypox rats by bovine PRL (Figure 3) was dose-dependent and the minimum effective dose was found to be 100 μg/kg/day. This was estimated to be approximately ten times lower than the dose required for the induction of lactation. The restoration of the contact sensitivity reaction in Hypox animals by

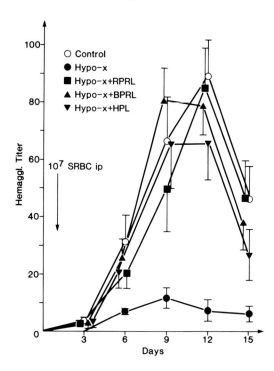

FIGURE 1.   Reconstitution of the antibody response in hypophysectomized rats by lactogenic hormones. The combined results of two identical experiments performed on female Fischer rats are presented in this Figure. Groups of four animals were used in the first and groups of five in the second experiment. Sheep red blood cells (SRBC; 10⁷ i.p.) were injected 3 weeks after hypophysectomy (Hypo-X), along with a group of normal controls. Treatment of the appropriate groups with 40 µg daily s.c. doses of rat prolactin (RPRL), bovine prolactin (BPRL), and human placental lactogen (HPL) was started at the time of antigen injection and maintained for 10 days. Animals included in the final evaluation: O — 9, ● — 8, ■ — 8, ▲ — 8, ▼ — 7. Mean haemagglutination titers ± SE are indicated in the Figure. *Statistical analysis (t-test):* control compared with Hypo-X — $P<0.001$ throughout the experiment. No significant difference occurred when the reactivity of controls was compared with the hormone treated groups.[5]

PRL was antagonized by simultaneously administered ACTH (Figure 4).[62] This was also true for the restoration of the adjuvant arthritis reaction (Figure 5).[63]

PRL secretion can be inhibited selectively, both in man and laboratory rats, by the dopamine agonist drug, bromocriptine (BRC).[64,65] Treatment of intact rats with BRC inhibited the development of contact sensitivity reaction to DNCB in a dose-dependent fashion. Additional treatment with bovine PRL restored the immune reactivity of BRC suppressed animals to normal levels and ACTH antagonized the restoring effect of PRL. Virtually identical results were obtained in similar experiments on antibody formation against SRBC and the development of adjuvant arthritis. All these reactions could be inhibited by BRC treatment, restored by additional PRL injections, and antagonized by the simultaneous administration of ACTH (Figures 3, 6, and 7).[66,63]

Spangelo and co-workers[67] immunized male mice with SRBC. A direct effect of PRL on the primary immune response was determined by injections (200 µg/day for 3 days) during the time of immunization. PRL treatment induced a significant increase in antibody production. Furthermore, serum PRL levels were decreased significantly during the course of immune response. As antibody titers fell on days 5 through 7, the concentration of PRL returned to control values.

PRL was measured in 13 untreated and 42 treated patients suffering from coeliac disease, a condition of food allergy. Raised PRL values were found in four of the five untreated male patients, whereas the eight untreated female patients had normal levels.

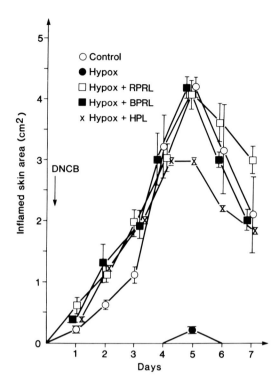

FIGURE 2. Reconstitution of hypophysectomized rats for contact sensitivity by lactogenic hormones. Three weeks after hypophysectomy (Hypo-X), groups of five Fischer rats were sensitized with dinitrochlorobenzene (DNCB) dissolved in acetone (200 mg/mℓ), by applying 2 mg DNCB onto approximately 1 cm^2 of the shaved dorsal skin, along with five normal controls. Hormone treatment was started on the day of sensitization, at 40 μg/rat/day s.c., and maintained for 7 days. Animals included in the final evaluation after combining the results of two identical experiments: O — 9, ● — 8, □ — 8, ■ — 8, X — 7. *Statistical analysis:* control vs. Hypo-X — $p < 0.001$ throughout the experiment; hormone treated groups responded somewhat better than controls on days 1 to 3 ($P < 0.02$) but not on days 4 to 7, except the RPRL group on day 7 ($P < 0.02$). HPL treated animals did not peak as high as did controls ($P < 0.02$).[5]

Levels of PRL were elevated in all 35 patients responding favorably to a gluten-free diet. In contrast, significantly lower PRL levels were found in seven patients not responding to the diet. No other known cause of hyperprolactinemia could be defined.[68] Circulating thyroglobulin, microsomal antibodies, and thyroid function have been evaluated in 92 hyperprolactinemic patients, 4 of which had acromegaly. High titers of thyroglobulin and microsomal antibodies were found in one acromegalic, and in 12 women with either adenomatose or idiopathic hyperprolactinemia. Low titers of one or both antibodies were found in nine other euthyroid women. In a control population of 185 subjects studied with the same methods, the prevalence of thyroglobulin and microsomal antibodies was 3.3% in females and 2.5% in males. Thus, autoimmune thyroid disorders, especially asymptomatic autoimmune thyroiditis, occur in hyperprolactinemic women with a prevalence far exceeding that in the general population.[69] A 54-year-old man with hyperprolactinemia was found to have a large chromophobe pituitary adenoma that concurred with a granulomatose hypophysitis.[70]

Karmali and Horrobin[71] described that PRL inhibited the PHA induced transformation of normal human peripheral blood lymphocytes. However, in our laboratory, the response of rat lymph node and spleen cells (to several mitogens that included PHA and in the mixed lymphocyte reaction) was not influenced by either bovine or rat PRL. Physiological concentrations and up to 20 times higher levels of hormone were included in the culture medium.[72]

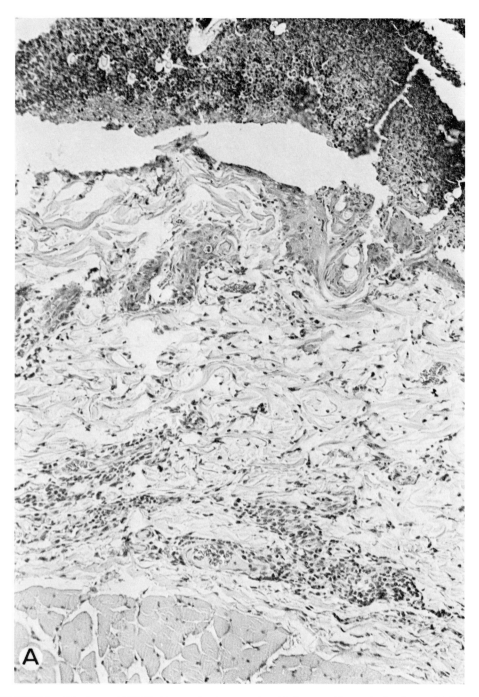

FIGURE 3.   Histology of DNCB skin reaction in normal and in hormonally manipulated rats. (A) Photomicrograph showing intense reactions to DNCB in skin of a nonhypophysectomized control rat; an ulcer is
covered by necrotic debris, fibrin, polymorphonuclear and mononuclear leukocytes. The dermis is edema-
tous and there is perivascular infiltration by lymphocytes and macrophages (Hematoxylin-eosin stain; original magnification × 100.)

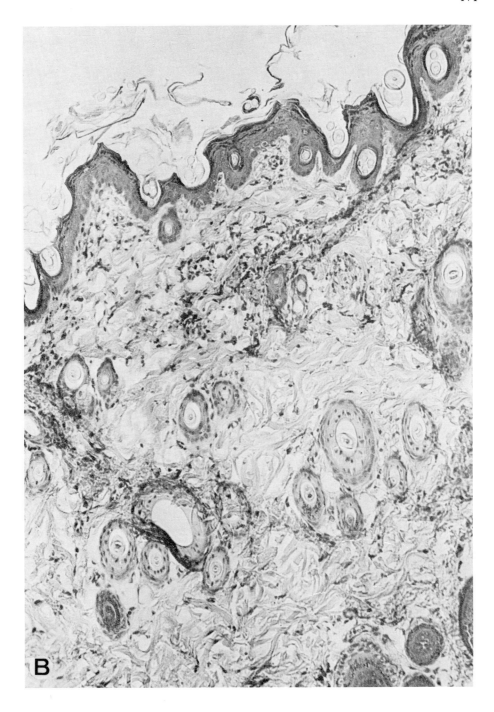

FIGURE 3(B).   Photomicrograph showing skin of Hypo-X rat with slight dermal edema, minimal inflammation and no ulceration. (Hematoxylin-eosin stain; original magnification × 100.)

Altered chemotaxis of leukocytes was observed in two of three patients with hyperprolactinemia. When normal leukocytes from 12 donors were exposed to high concentrations (1 to 2000 ng/mℓ) of PRL, statistically significant suppression of chemotaxis occurred.[73]

Despite our intensive efforts over several years, the mechanism of action of PRL on immune phenomena has not yet been clarified. PRL receptors are not easily demon-

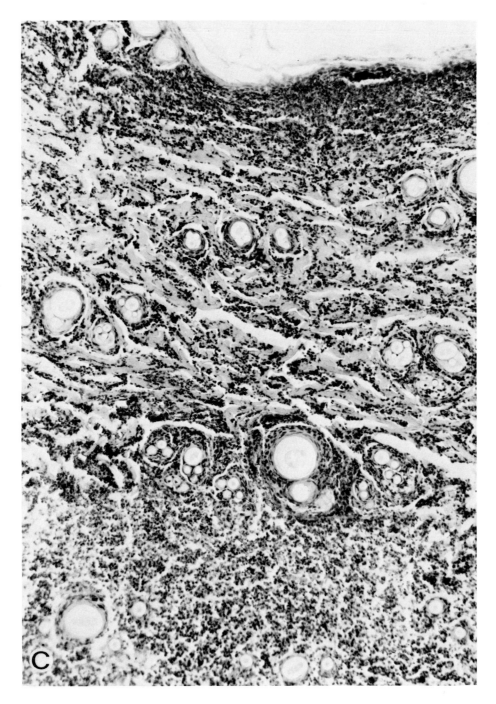

FIGURE 3(C).   Photomicrograph showing DNCB skin reaction in Hypo-X rat given PRL therapy: a severe lesion is evident with an ulcer covered by fibrin, necrotic debris, polymorphonuclear, and mononuclear leukocytes. The underlying dermis is also infiltrated by inflammatory cells. (Hematoxylin-eosin stain; original magnification × 32.)

strable on lymphoid cells and there is no clear-cut documentation of a direct effect of PRL on lymphocytes. Therefore, it is possible that PRL does not influence immune reactions by acting directly on lymphocytes, but rather, through some as yet unidentified intermediate factors. Our recent observations that ectopic pituitary grafts have a thymotropic effect both in hypophysectomized and in normal recipients (Figures 8 and

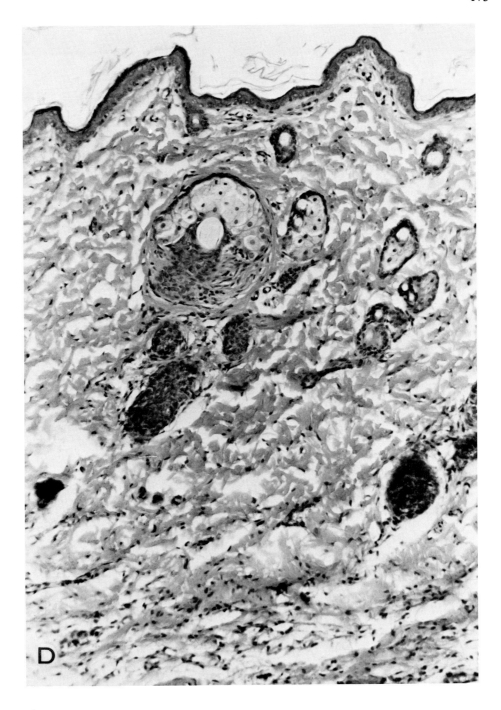

FIGURE 3(D). Photomicrograph of DNCB skin reaction in an intact rat given bromocriptine therapy reveals a minimal lesion. The site of DNCB application shows slight dermal edema and occasional mononuclear inflammatory cells in a perivascular and periappendageal distribution. (Hematoxylin-eosin stain; original magnification × 32.) (This histological material was kindly provided by Drs. K. Kovacs and S. L. Asa, Department of Pathology, University of Toronto.)

9) is compatible with this idea. Body, spleen, and thymus weights are decreased signif-icantly in Hypox animals. SPG, given to Hypox animals increases body and spleen weights modestly, but the thymus weight is increased dramatically and disproportion-

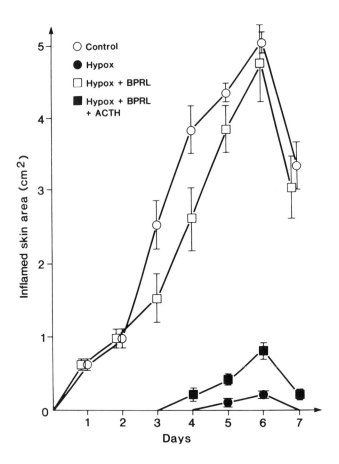

FIGURE 4.   The antagonistic effect of prolactin and ACTH on
DNCB contact sensitivity. Female Wistar Furth rats were hypophysectomized (Hypo-X) and 21 days later groups of five Hypo-X animals
were treated with bovine prolactin (BPRL, 40 μg daily s.c.) or BPRL
+ porcine ACTH (40 μg/day s.c.), commencing on the day of painting
the dorsal skin with dinitrochlorobenzene (DNCB), and maintained
for 5 days. *Statistics:* Control group was significantly different
$p < 0.01$, from Hypo-X, Hypo-X + BPRL + ACTH on days 1 to 7,
from Hypo-X + BPRL on days 3 to 4 ($P < 0.01$) and on day 5 ($P <
0.02$). Hypo-X compared to Hypo-X + BPRL: $P < 0.01$ on days 1 to
7; Hypo-X compared to Hypo-X + BPRL + ACTH: $P < 0.01$ on days
4 to 7; Hypo-X + BPRL compared to Hypo-X + BPRL + ACTH: $P
< 0.01$ on days 1 to 7.[62]

ately to the body weight. This suggests that SPG has a selective stimulatory influence
on the thymus. This conclusion is further supported by the fact that SPG is also capable of selectively increasing thymus weights in nonhypophysectomized recipients, although less dramatically, possibly because of the moderating effect of additional hormonal regulatory mechanisms. Corticosteroids and sex hormones are known to
decrease thymus weight, and these hormones may well be involved in the moderation
of SPG induced-thymus growth in normal recipients. Histologically, the hyperplastic
thymus glands and spleens were found to be normal. Flow cytometric analyses of lymphocytes (T cells, helper and suppressor-cytotoxic subsets of T cells, and B lymphocytes), with the aid of antibodies to specific surface markers, revealed no aberrations
from normal values in thymus, spleen, and mesenteric lymph nodes. Therefore, it appears that SPG stimulates a balanced (physiological) growth in the thymus and to a

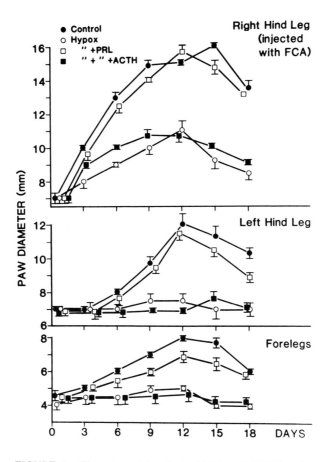

FIGURE 5.   The antagonistic effect of PRL and ACTH on the
development of adjuvant arthritis. Groups of ten female Fisher
animals were used. Final evaluation included eight to ten from
each group. Hypophysectomy was carried out 3 weeks prior to the
initiation of arthritis (by injecting the right hind paw with 0.1 mg
of Freund's complete adjuvant containing 5 mg/mℓ of *Mycobacterium tuberculosis)*. Treatment with bovine prolactin (PRL; 40
μg/day s.c.) and with porcine ACTH (0.02 IU daily s.c.) was initiated on the day of arthritis induction and maintained until the
end of the experiment. Mean paw diameters + SE are plotted in
the Figure. *Statistics:* For the forelegs and right hind legs, the control and Hypox + PRL groups were significantly different
($P < 0.01$) from the Hypox and Hypox + PRL + ACTH groups
on days 6 to 18. For the left hind legs, the above groups differed
significantly on days 9 to 18. Controls differed from Hypox +
PRL occasionally, but not regularly. (See Figure 1 for abbreviations.)[63]

lesser extent in the spleen.[74] Additional experiments are underway to clarify whether
or not PRL is responsible for the lymphotropic effect of SPG.

Singh and Owen[75] studied the effect of catecholamines, histamine, and peptide hormones on the maturation of thymocytes in mice. When thymocytes from 14-day mouse
embryos were exposed in vitro to PRL, the expression of the Thy-1 and TL antigens
was stimulated. Glucagon also had a significant stimulatory effect, whereas parathyroid hormone, calcitonin, and insulin did not influence the expression of these two
antigens. The effect of glucagon could be inhibited by propranolol, but the effect of
PRL was only marginally altered by this β adrenergic antagonist. Bhat et al.[76] demonstrated recently that bovine PRL increased mitotic activity of the bursa of Fabricius in

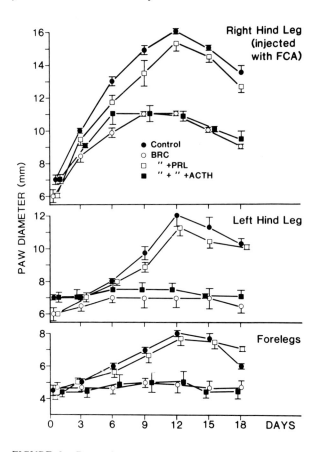

FIGURE 6.   Prevention of adjuvant arthritis by bromocriptine (BRC), restoration by prolactin (PRL), and inhibition of restoration by ACTH. Groups of ten female Fischer animals were used. Treatment with bromocriptine (BRC, 5 mg/kg/day s.c.) was started 1 week before the induction of arthritis and continued throughout the experiment. Prolactin was given at 100 μg/rat/day and ACTH at 0.02 IU/rat/day, both subcutaneously, starting on the day of arthritis induction and continuing until termination of the experiment. *Statistics:* for the forelegs and right hind legs, controls and BRC + PRL differed significantly from BRC and from BRC + PRL + ACTH on days 6 to 18, and for the left hind legs, on days 9 to 18. Only occasional differences occurred between control and BRC and BRC + PRL + ACTH.[63]

chicks. At the same time, PRL inhibited histologically demonstrable bursal secretory activity. These observations, although preliminary in nature, indicate that PRL stimulates the primary lymphoid organs, which could explain most of its immunomodulatory effect.

IV. PLACENTAL LACTOGEN

In our studies, human placental lactogen (HPL) was capable of restoring antibody formation and contact sensitivity reaction to DNCB in Hypox rats, although HPL seemed to be somewhat less potent than PRL or GH. However, no significant difference in potency was evident in other experiments (Figures 1 and 2).

Arezzini et al.[77] investigated the effect of HPL on body and thymus growth in Snell-Bagg pituitary dwarf mice. Body weight gain was lower than that observed by the same

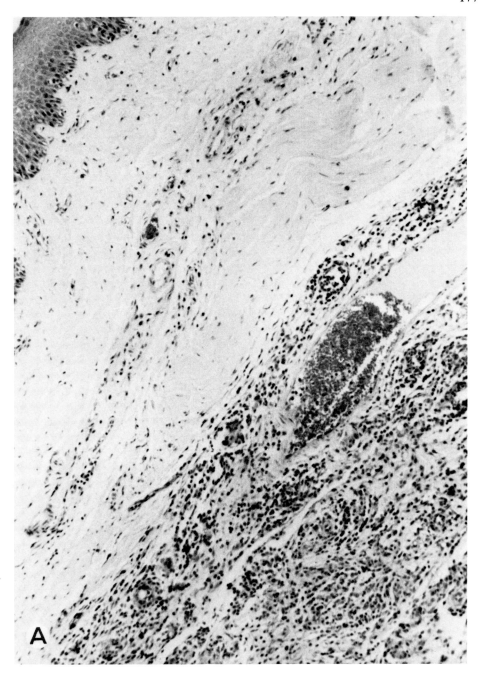

FIGURE 7. Histology of arthritis lesions in hormonally manipulated rats. (A) Histology of adjuvant arthritis in a hypophysectomized rat given PRL treatment. There is an infiltrate of mononuclear inflammatory cells involving subcutaneous tissue and muscle overlying bone of one limb. (Hematoxylin-eosin stain; original magnification × 32.) (B) In an intact rat given bromocriptine treatment, histologic examination reveals no evidence of adjuvant arthritis. The subcutaneous tissue and muscle overlying bone shows mild edema and minimal infiltration with occasional mononuclear inflammatory cells. (Hematoxylin-eosin stain; original magnification × 32.) (Courtesy of Drs. S. L. Asa and K. Kovacs, Department of Pathology, University of Toronto.)

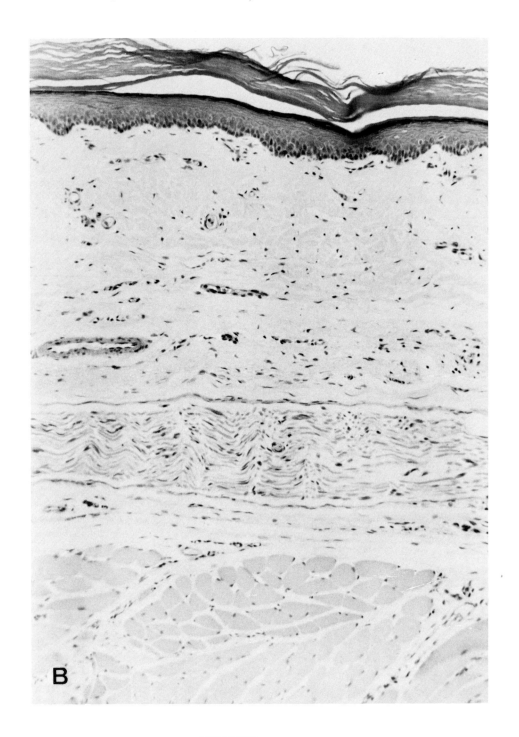

FIGURE 7 B

dose of human GH. However, the hyperplasia of the thymus and spleen was comparable to that induced by human GH.

Plasma levels of human PL in pregnancies complicated by Rhesus isoimmunization
showed that in mild and moderately affected cases the levels were normal, while in
severely affected cases they were raised.[78]

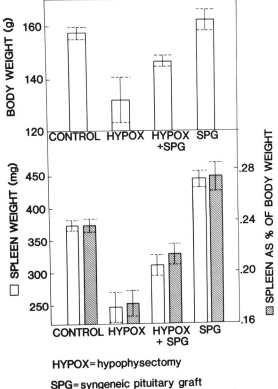

FIGURE 8. Body and spleen weights in control and in hormonally altered rats. The following groups were created from female Fischer animals: five controls; seven hypophysectomized; seven Hypox given two syngeneic pituitary grafts each under the kidney capsule; five normal animals grafted with two syngeneic pituitaries each under their kidney capsule. Hypophysectomy was performed on day 0, SPG were given on day 15 and body and organ weights were taken on day 22.

A dose-dependent suppression of sheep peripheral blood lymphocytes to PHA and Con A was observed when the cultures were supplemented with a soluble extract of fetal membranes. HPL, ovine PRL, GH, and luteinizing hormone were inactive in the same system.[79]

HPL was found to suppress the PHA induced stimulation of human lymphocytes. Suppression was strongest when the lymphocytes have been preincubated for 24 hr with the hormone.[80]

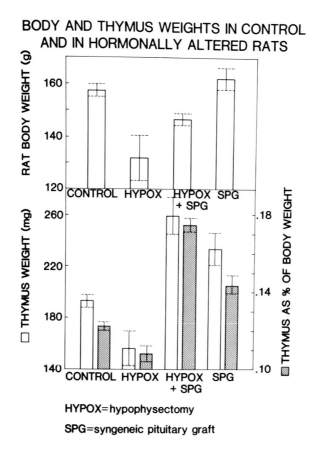

FIGURE 9.   Body and thymus weights in control and in hormonally altered rats. Groups of female Fischer rats were as-
sembled and treated as described in the legend to Figure 8.

REFERENCES

1. Nicoll, C. S., Ontogeny and evolution of prolactin's functions, *Fed. Proc. Fed. Am. Soc. Exp. Biol.*, 39, 2563, 1980.
2. Nicoll, C. S., Prolactin and growth hormone: specialists on one hand and mutual mimicks on the other, *Perspect. Biol. Med.*, 25, 369, 1982.
3. Posner, B. I., Kelly, P. A., Shiu, R. P. C., and Friesen, H. G., Studies of insulin, growth hormone and prolactin binding: tissue distribution, species variation and characterization, *Endocrinology*, 95, 521, 1974.
4. Dube, D., Kelly, P. A., and Pelletier, Comparative localization of prolactin-binding sites in different rat tissues by immunohistochemistry, radioautography and radioreceptor assay, *Mol. Cell. Endocrinol.*, 18, 109, 1980.
5. Nagy, E., Berczi, I., and Friesen, H. G., Regulation of immunity in rats by lactogenic and growth hormones, *Acta Endocrinol.*, 102, 351, 1983.
6. Gout, P. W., Beer, C. T., and Noble, R. L., Prolactin-stimulated growth of cell cultures established from malignant Nb rat lymphomas, *Cancer Res.*, 40, 2433, 1980.
7. Tanaka, T., Shiu, R. P. C., Gout, P. W., Beer, C. T., Noble, R. L., and Friesen, H. G., A new sensitive and specific bioassay for lactogenic hormones: measurement of prolactin and growth hormone in human serum, *J. Clin. Endocrinol. Metab.*, 51, 1058, 1980.

8. Shiu, R. P. C., Elsholtz, H. P., Tanaka, T., Friesen, H. G., Gout, P. W., Beer, C. T., and Noble, R. L., Receptor-mediated mitogenic action of prolactin in a rat lymphoma cell line, *Endocrinology,* 113, 159, 1983.

9. Fleming, W. H., Pettigrew, N. M., Matusik, R. J., and Friesen, H. G., Thymic origin of the prolactin-dependent Nb2-lymphoma cell line, *Cancer Res.,* 42, 3138, 1982.

10. Russell, D. H., Matrisian, L., Kibler, R., Larson, D. F., Poulos, B., and Magun, B. E., Prolactin receptors on human lymphocytes and their modulation by cyclosporine, *Biochem. Biophys. Res. Commun.,* 121, 899, 1984.

11. Brambell, F. W. R., *The Transmission of Passive Immunity from Mother to Young,* North Holland, Amsterdam, 1970.

12. Rose, M. E., Orlans, E., and Buttress, N., Immunoglobulin class in hen's egg: their segregation in yolk and white, *Eur. J. Immunol.,* 4, 521, 1974.

13. Sterzl, J. and Silverstein, A. M., Developmental aspects of immunity, *Adv. Immunol.,* 6, 337, 1967.

14. Berczi, I., Stipkovits, L., Bereznai, T., and Antal, T., The role of immunological conditions in *E. coli*-disease of newborn calves, *Zentralbl. Veterinaermed. B,* 14, 408, 1967.

15. Brambell, F. W. R., The transmission of immunity from mother to young and the catabolism of immunoglobulins, *Lancet,* 2, 1087, 1966.

16. Rodewald, R., Intestinal transport of antibodies in the newborn rat, *J. Cell Biol.,* 58, 189, 1973.

17. Pittard, W. B., Breast milk immunology: a frontier in infant nutrition, *Am. J. Dis. Child.,* 133, 83, 1979.

18. Kleinman, R. E. and Walker, W. A., Enteromammary immune system: important new concept in breast milk host defense, *Dig. Dis. Sci.,* 24, 876, 1979.

19. McClelland, D. B. L., Antibodies in milk, *J. Reprod. Fert.,* 65, 537, 1982.

20. Ogra, P. L., Losonsky, G. A., and Fishaut, M., Colostrum-derived immunity and maternal-neonatal interaction, in *The Secretory Immune System,* McGhee, J. R. and Mestecky, J., Eds.; *Ann. N.Y. Acad. Sci.,* 409, 82, 1983.

21. Keller, M. A., Heiner, D. C., Kidd, R. M., and Myers, A. S., Local production of IgG4 in human colostrum, *J. Immunol.,* 130, 1654, 1983.

22. Goldblum, R. M., Ahlstedt, S., Carlsson, B., Hanson, L. A., Jodal, U., Lindin-Janson, G., and Sohl-Akerlund, A., Antibody forming cells in human colostrum after oral immunization, *Nature (London),* 257, 797, 1975.

23. Allardyce, R. A., Shearman, D. J. C., Simpson, D. B. L., Marwick, K., Simpson, A. J., and Laidlow, R. B., Appearance of specific colostrum antibodies after clinical infection with *Salmonella typhimurium, Br. Med. J.,* 3, 307, 1974.

24. Bienenstock, J., Befus, D., McDermott, M., Mirski, S., and Rosenthal, K., Regulation of lymphoblast traffic and localization in mucosal tissues, with emphasis on IgA, *Fed. Proc. Fed. Am. Soc. Exp. Biol.,* 42, 3213, 1983.

25. Mohr, J. A., Lymphocyte sensitization passed to the child from the mother, *Lancet,* I, 688, 1972.

26. Schlesinger, J. J. and Covelli, H. D., Evidence for transmission of lymphocyte responses to tuberculin by breast-feeding, *Lancet,* II, 529, 1977.

27. Gendre, F., Huart, B., Binder, P., Deschaux, P., and Fontanges, R., Study of the transmission of the immunostimulation from mother to offspring in mice by two immunostimulants and by the direct PFC technique, *C. R. Acad. Sci. Ser. C,* 296, 15, 1983.

28. Roberts, S. A. and Turner, M. W., Specific suppression of rat IgE responses with milk from immunized females and with feeds of serum antibody, *Immunology,* 48, 195, 1983.

29. Cramer, D. V., Gill, T. J., III, and Knauer, G., The influence of maternal immunization on the antibody response of the offspring in genetically high-responding rats, *Am. J. Pathol.,* 90, 317, 1978.

30. Weiler, I. J., Weiler, E., Sprenger, R., and Cosenza, H., Idiotype suppression by maternal influence, *Eur. J. Immunol.,* 7, 591, 1977.

31. Kresina, T. F. and Nisonoff, A., Passive transfer of the idiotypically suppressed state by serum from suppressed mice and transfer of suppression from mothers to offspring, *J. Exp. Med.,* 157, 15, 1983.

32. Ceriani, R. L., Fetal mammary gland differentiation *in vitro* in response to hormones. I. Morphological findings, *Dev. Biol.,* 21, 506, 1970.

33. Ceriani, R. L., Fetal mammary gland differentiation in vitro in response to hormones. II. Biochemical findings, *Dev. Biol.,* 21, 530, 1970.

34. Anderson, R. R., Brookreson, A. D., and Turner, C. W., Experimental growth of mammary gland in male and female mice, *Proc. Soc. Exp. Biol. Med.,* 106, 567, 1961.

35. Clifton, K. H. and Furth, J., Ducto-alveolar growth in mammary glands of adreno-gonadectomized male rats bearing mammotropic pituitary tumors, *Endocrinology,* 66, 893, 1960.

36. Furth, J., Clifton, K. H., Gadsen, E. L., and Buffett, R. F., Dependent and autonomous mammotropic pituitary tumors in rats; their somatotropic features, *Cancer Res.,* 16, 608, 1956.

37. Weisz-Carrington, P., Roux, M. E., and Lamm, M. E., Plasma cells and epithelial immunoglobulins in the mouse mammary gland during pregnancy and lactation, *J. Immunol.,* 119, 1306, 1977.

38. Weisz-Carrington, P., Roux, M. E., McWilliams, M., Phillips-Quagliata, J. M., and Lamm, M. E., Hormonal induction of the secretory immune system in the mammary gland, *Proc. Natl. Acad. Sci. U.S.A.*, 75, 2928, 1978.

39. Weisz-Carrington, P., Roux, M. E., McWilliams, M., Phillips-Quagliata, J. M., and Lamm, M. E., Organ and isotype distribution of plasma cells producing specific antibody after oral immunization: evidence for a generalized secretory immune system, *J. Immunol.*, 123, 1705, 1979.

40. Weisz-Carrington, P., Emancipator, S., and Lamm, M. E., Binding and uptake of immunoglobulins by mouse mammary gland epithelial cells in hormone-treated cultures, *J. Reprod. Immunol.*, 6, 63, 1984.

41. Klareskog, L., Forsum, U., and Peterson, P. A., Hormonal regulation of the expression of Ia antigens on mammary gland epithelium, *Eur. J. Immunol.*, 10, 958, 1980.

42. McCarty, K. S., Jr., Sasso, R., Budwit, D., Georgiade, G. S., and Seigler, H. F., Immunoglobulin localization in the normal human mammary gland: variation with the menstrual cycle, *Am. J. Pathol.*, 107, 322, 1982.

43. Seelig, L. L., Jr., Dynamics of leukocytes in rat mammary epithelium during pregnancy and lactation, *Biol. Reprod.*, 22, 1211, 1980.

44. Gala, R. R. and Westphal, V., Corticosteroid-binding globulin in the rat: possible role in the initiation of lactation, *Endocrinology*, 76, 1079, 1965.

45. Sasaki, K. and Ito, T., Effects of pregnancy and lactation on lymphocytes in the bone marrow of the mouse: a quantitative electron microscopic study, *Arch. Histol. Jpn.*, 43, 211, 1980.

46. Sasaki, K. and Ito, T., Effects of pregnancy and lactation on the peripheral lymphatic tissue in the mouse: qualitative and quantitative morphology, *Arch. Histol. Jpn.*, 43, 423, 1980.

47. Iversen, B. M. and Ofstad, J., Suppressed development of experimental glomerulonephritis in lactating rats, *Scand. J. Immunol.*, 10, 237, 1979.

48. Kim, Y. -W. and Halsey, J. F., Metabolism and clearance of antibody-excess immune complexes in lactating mice, *J. Immunol.*, 129, 619, 1982.

49. Gambel, P. I., Cleland, A. W., and Ferguson, F. G., Alterations in thymus and spleen cell populations and immune reactivity during syngeneic pregnancy and lactation, *J. Clin. Lab. Immunol.*, 3, 115, 1980.

50. Connan, R. M., The effect of host lactation of the ''self-cure'' of *Nippostrongylus brasiliensis* in rats, *Parasitology*, 61, 27, 1970.

51. Dineen, J. K. and Kelly, J. D., The suppression of rejection of *Nippostrongylus brasiliensis* in lactating rats: the nature of the immunological defect, *Immunology*, 22, 1, 1972.

52. Kelly, J. D. and Dineen, J. K., The suppression of rejection of *Nippostrongylus brasiliensis* in Lewis strain rats treated with ovine prolactin. The site of immunological defect, *Immunology*, 24, 551, 1973.

53. Ngwenya, B. Z., Effect of lactation on cell-mediated immunity of Swiss mice to *Trichinella spiralis*, *Cell. Immunol.*, 24, 116, 1976.

54. Clarkson, A. B., Jr. and Mellow, G. H., Rheumatoid factor-like immunoglobulin M protects previously uninfected rat pups and dams from *Trypanosoma lewisi*, *Science*, 214, 186, 1981.

55. Mellow, G. H. and Clarkson, A. B., Jr., *Trypanosoma lewisi*: enhanced resistance in naive lactating rats and their suckling pups, *Exp. Parasitol.*, 53, 217, 1982.

56. Herrick, C. A. and Cross, S. X., The development of natural and artificial resistance of young rats to the pathogenic effects of the parasite *Trypanosoma lewisi*, *J. Parasitol.*, 22, 126, 1936.

57. Asa, S. L., Bilbao, J. M., Kovacs, K., Josse, R. G., and Kreines, K., Lymphocytic hypophysitis of pregnancy resulting in hypopituitarism: a distinct clinicopathologic entity, *Ann. Intern. Med.*, 95, 166, 1981.

58. Chen, C. L., Amenomori, Y., Lu, K. H., Voogt, J. L., and Meites, J., Serum prolactin levels in rats with pituitary transplants or hypothalamic lesions, *Neuroendocrinology*, 6, 220, 1970.

59. Berczi, I., Nagy, E., Kovacs, K., and Horvath, E., Regulation of humoral immunity in rats by pituitary hormones, *Acta Endocrinol.*, 98, 506, 1981.

60. Nagy, E. and Berczi, I., Prolactin and contact sensitivity, *Allergy*, 36, 429, 1981.

61. Berczi, I. and Nagy, E., A possible role of prolactin in adjuvant arthritis, *Arthritis Rheum.*, 25, 591, 1982.

62. Berczi, I., Nagy, E., Asa, S. L., and Kovacs, K., Pituitary hormones and contact sensitivity in rats, *Allergy*, 38, 325, 1983.

63. Berczi, I., Nagy, E., Asa, S. L., and Kovacs, K., The influence of pituitary hormones on adjuvant arthritis, *Arthritis Rheum.*, 27, 682, 1984.

64. Meites, J. and Clemens, J. A., Hypothalamic control of prolactin secretion, *Vitam. Horm.*, 30, 165, 1972.

65. Parkes, D., Drug therapy: bromocriptine. *N. Engl. J. Med.*, 301, 873, 1979.

66. Nagy, E., Berczi, I., Wren, G. E., Asa, S. L., and Kovacs, K., Immunomodulation by bromocriptine, *Immunopharmacology*, 6, 231, 1983.

67. Spangelo, B. L., Hall, N. R., NcGillis, J. P., and Goldstein, A. L., Evidence for an interaction between prolactin and the primary immune response, *Fed. Proc. Fed. Am. Soc. Exp. Biol.*, 43 (Abstr. 1131), 1610, 1984.

68. Stevens, F. M., McCarthy, C. F., and Craig, A., Is prolactin trophic to the intestine in coeliac disease, *Gut*, 19, A992, 1978.

69. Ferrari, C., Boghen, M., Paracchi, A., Rampini, P., Raiteri, F., Benco, R., Romussi, M., Codecasa, F., Mucci, M., and Bianco, M., Thyroid autoimmunity in hyperprolactinaemic disorders, *Acta Endocrinol.*, 104, 35, 1983.

70. Holck, S. and Laursen, H., Prolactinoma coexistent with granulomatous hypophysitis, *Acta Neuropathol.*, 61, 253, 1983.

71. Karmali, R. A. and Horrobin, D. F., The effect of prolactin on the response of human lymphocytes to phytohaemagglutinin, *Br. J. Obstet. Gynaecol.*, 83, 904, 1976.

72. Berczi, I., unpublished results, 1982.

73. Harris, R. D., Kay, N. E., Seljeskog, E. L., Murray, K. J., and Douglas, S. D., Prolactin suppression of leukocyte chemotaxis *in vitro*, *J. Neurosurg.*, 50, 462, 1979.

74. Houston, G., Hormone Induced Changes in Lymphoid Organs, Proc. B.Sc. (Med.) Presentations, University of Manitoba, 1984, 43.

75. Singh, U. and Owen, J. J. T., Studies on the maturation of thymus stem cells. The effects of catecholamines, histamine and peptide hormones on the expression of T cell alloantigens, *Eur. J. Immunol.*, 6, 59, 1976.

76. Bhat, G., Gupta, S. K., and Maiti, B. R., Influence of prolactin on mitotic activity of the bursa of Fabricius of the chick, *Gen. Comp. Endocrinol.*, 52, 452, 1983.

77. Arezzini, C., De Gori, V., Tarli, P., and Neri, P., Weight increase of body and lymphatic tissues in dwarf mice treated with human chorionic somatomammotropin (HCS), *Proc. Soc. Exp. Biol. Med.*, 141, 98, 1972.

78. Ward, R. H. T., Letchworth, A. T., Niven, P. A. R., and Chard, T., Placental lactogen levels in rhesus isoimmunization, *Br. Med. J.*, 1, 347, 1974.

79. Staples, L. D., Brown, D., Binns, R. M., and Heap, R. B., The influence of protein hormones and conceptus extracts on sheep lymphocyte transformation induced in vitro, *Placenta*, 4, 125, 1983.

80. Contractor, S. F. and Davies, H., Effect of human chorionic somatomammotrophin and human chorionic gonadotrophin on phytohaemagglutinin-induced lymphocyte transformation, *Nature (London) New Biol.*, 243, 284, 1973.

Chapter 7

GONADOTROPINS AND SEX HORMONES

I. Berczi

TABLE OF CONTENTS

I. INTRODUCTION

The effect of sex hormones on lymphoid tissue has been recognized since the early studies on the influence of glucocorticoids on the immune system. Selye[1] pointed out that all hormonally active steroids will produce thymic involution, if they are administered for a sufficiently long period. Early investigations revealed that both androgens and estrogens, and even large amounts of progesterone or gonadotropic hormone, produce thymic atrophy. Other studies showed that gonadal secretions exert a constant moderating influence on the growth of lymphatic organs through life.[2] The finding of Herrick and Cross[3] that young rats, weaned at 20 days of age, could be protected by oestrin injections from an otherwise lethal infection of *Trypanosoma lewisi,* revealed the importance of hormones on host resistance to parasites. Numerous investigators studied the influence of a variety of hormones on immunity to parasites during the 1940s and 1950s. It is beyond the scope of this book to review these often controversial early studies. Instead the reader is referred to a monograph on the subject.[4]

As sex hormones are concerned with reproduction, their influence on the immune system is likely to be connected with this primary function. The transmission of immunity to the young through the colostrum and milk and the regulatory influence of sex hormones and prolactin on mammary immune function is discussed in the previous chapter. Medawar and Sparrow[5] recognized immediately, after the discovery of histocompatibility antigens in the mid 1940s, that the conceptus in mammals is the equivalent of a homograft and therefore, it should not survive. One of Medawar's colleagues, Billingham, pursued this problem and pointed out in a recent overview that presently there is no satisfactory explanation for the remarkable success of mammalian reproduction, although many possibilities have been proposed.[6] The possible role of hormones in the immunobiology of gestation is reviewed by Clark in Chapter 13.

II. THE EFFECT OF GONADOTROPINS ON IMMUNE REACTIONS

A. Chorionic Gonadotropin

Treatment of mice with human chorionic gonadotropin (HCG) was reported to depress delayed-type hypersensitivity reactions, which were dependent on the presence of the gonads.[7,8] HCG treatment of female BALB/c mice resulted in enhanced natural killer (NK) cell activity, similar to that seen in pregnant animals.[9] In vitro treatment of mouse lymphocytes with HCG led to the induction of suppressor cells capable of depressing the polyclonal activation of B lymphocytes.[10]

The i.p. administration of HCG to adult female rats failed to prolong the survival of intrauterine skin allografts when compared with saline treated controls.[11] Studies conducted in our laboratory showed no influence of HCG on the antibody response of intact, or hypophysectomized (Hypox) rats. There was no apparent influence, when HCG was given to Hypox animals as part of a combined treatment with ACTH, growth hormone (GH), and thyroid stimulating hormone (TSH) during experiments on contact sensitivity reactions and adjuvant arthritis.[12-14]

The treatment of guinea pigs with 4000 IU of HCG i.p. 1 to 7 days prior to skin testing inhibited the development of delayed hypersensitivity skin responses for 3 weeks. Furthermore, lymphocytes from HCG treated guinea pigs exhibited depressed response to phytohemagglutinin (PHA) and PPD.[15] Several investigators reported that the response of human peripheral blood lymphocytes to PHA and to other mitogens was depressed by HCG, due to the generation of suppressor cells.[16-19] The mixed lymphocyte reaction was also suppressed by HCG.[20]

However, a number of other investigators pointed out that these in vitro effects of commercial HCG preparations are due to impurities rather than HCG itself.[21-25] Therefore, the direct effect of HCG on lymphocyte reactions is, at best, questionable.

B. Luteinizing and Follicle Stimulating Hormones (LH, FSH)

The injection of mice with 5-hydroxytryptophan, phentolamine, and haloperidol before, or together with sheep red blood cells (SRBC), induced a complete and longlasting inhibition of antibody production. Treatment with LH, FSH, and ACTH, before the administration of the inhibitory drugs and antigen, prevented the immune blockage. The injection of SRBC induced an early elevation of serum LH.[26]

Macrophages isolated from rat testes, but not peritoneal macrophages, responded to FSH with the secretion of lactate in a dose-dependent manner.[27] The response of sheep peripheral blood lymphocytes to PHA, Con A, and pokeweed mitogen (PWM) was not influenced by ovine LH.[28]

During our experiments, Hypox rats were treated with LH and FSH either alone, or in combination with other pituitary hormones, to test their possible role in restoration of immunocompetence. These experiments revealed no influence of LH and FSH on contact sensitivity reactions and on adjuvant arthritis.[29,30]

III. RECEPTORS FOR SEX STEROID HORMONES IN LYMPHOID TISSUE

Specific, high affinity estrogen receptors have been found in thymuses of rat, mouse, man, and cattle. The cytoplasmic receptors bound estradiol and similar estrogenic compounds, such as diethylstilbestrol, but this receptor had no affinity to other steroid hormones: progesterone, testosterone, or cortisol. A dissociation constant of 2×10^{-10} M was reported by several investigators. Autoradiographic studies showed that the radioactive label was confined in single cells, which may be identical with thymic reticuloepithelial cells.[31-36]

Specific androgen receptors were also found in mouse and rat thymuses. The dissociation constant was estimated to be 1.34×10^{-8} M, when cytosol preparations from whole thymus glands were used. However, binding was markedly lower when cytosols were prepared from isolated thymocytes. Neither whole lymphocytes isolated from intact thymus nor their nuclei exhibited specific androgen binding. Nonlymphoid cells isolated from the thymus exhibited high levels of androgen binding.[37,38]

Progesterone was found to compete effectively for triamcinolone acetonide (TA) binding sites in rat thymocytes, as well as to inhibit the biochemical effects of TA. In competitive binding experiments with cytosolic receptors, progesterone was more effective than the antiglucocorticoid, cortexolone, in inhibiting TA binding. However, progesterone was less efficient than cortisol, or TA, in depleting the cytosol receptors. Additional binding of progesterone was observed in cells presaturated with TA, suggesting that in rat thymocytes, progesterone binding components, other than glucocorticoid receptors, are also present.[39]

The bursa of Fabricius in the chicken has receptors for estradiol, testosterone, progesterone, and glucocorticoids. Cytosol preparations from predominantly lymphoid bursal cells bound glucocorticoids, but not estrogen, androgen, or progesterone. This observation suggests that estrogen, androgen, and progestin receptors are present in the epithelial cells of the bursa.[40-42] Treatment of sexually immature chicks with dihydrotestosterone induced a significant decrease in the cytosolic glucocorticoid hormone receptor levels in both the thymus and bursa tissues and decreased the blastogenesis index in the bursa, but not in the thymus.[43] Human peripheral blood T lymphocytes had no androgen receptors, but specific estrogen receptors could be demonstrated in the suppressor/cytotoxic (OKT8-positive) subset of T lymphocytes.[44] Normal human peripheral blood mononuclear cells and axillary lymph node cells were found to have a cytosolic progestin binding protein. Whole cell assay and/or a cell free preparation technique were employed with different natural and synthetic progestin and glucocorticoid tracers.[45]

Cell nuclei, prepared from the rat uterus, contained two types of estrogen receptors: type I was high affinity, low capacity translocatable estrogen receptor, whereas type II was a lower affinity, nontranslocatable binding site. This latter type was shown to be characteristic of eosinophils. Autoradiographic studies revealed that eosinophilic granules have the capacity of binding estradiol.[46,47]

IV. SEX DIFFERENCE IN THE IMMUNE RESPONSE

Numerous observations proved that sex differences exist both in experimental animals and man with regard to various immune parameters and functions. Thus, sex differences have been detected in the morphology of the bone marrow, in immunoglobulin levels and humoral immunocompetence, in serum concentrations of complement components, in various parameters of cell mediated immunity, and in the susceptibility to develop autoimmune disease, infectious diseases, and cancer. The possible role of sex hormones and of hormones in general in infectious disease, autoimmune disease, and cancer are discussed in detail in Chapters 14, 15, and 16 of this monograph and for this reason will be mentioned only briefly here.

The factors responsible for sex differences in the immune response remain poorly understood. In a number of cases, clear indications were obtained for the influence of estrogens and androgens on various immune phenomena, and these hormones were proposed as being responsible for the sex difference observed. However, in other cases genetic factors are responsible, as exemplified by X-linked agammaglobulinemias. Even when sex hormones are responsible for the alteration of immune parameters, differences in hormone levels, in target organ sensitivity to the hormones,[48] and even in hormone metabolism (please see Chapter 15), or possibly, some combination of the above, may be responsible for the immune changes observed.

Women were found to have significantly higher IgM serum levels than men, both as adults and children older than 6 years. Although the mean IgG level was found to be markedly higher and the mean IgA concentration was slightly higher in blacks than in whites, in the younger adults of both races mean IgM values were markedly higher in females than in males.[49,50] Concentrations of either complement components were determined in sera of 419 healthy children aged 1 to 19 years. A significant correlation between concentration and age for all components (Clq, cls, C4, C3, C5, factor B, properdin, and C1 inhibitor) was observed for girls. However, in boys a significant correlation was present only for Clq, C1, C3, C5, and properdin.[51] The polymorphism of complement factor B was analyzed in six different mouse strains. Females of each strain had only three bands compared with the four or five found in males. However, no differences were found in the serum level between males and females.[52]

Female Swiss mice were more responsive to bovine serum albumin and developed a stronger and longer-lasting immune response.[53] The alloantibody response of male and female C57BL/6J and C3H mice against H-2^b and H-2^k histocompatibility antigen haplotypes were studied after transplantation of F_1 fetal bone marrow, or F_1 spleen cells. Female mice produced much more IgG_1 than males, although they produced comparable amounts of IgG_2 when fetal allografts were used.[54]

The ABO and Lewis blood groups, secretor status, and serum agglutinins against O red blood cells (the antibody was presumed to be auto-anti-I) were determined in 546 normal individuals. Among non-A secretors of both sexes, female donors had a higher score than did males.[55]

The clearance of lymphocytes, sensitized with IgG antibodies, was studied in MRL/Mp-1pr (MRL-1pr) and NEp-+/+ (MRL-+/+) mice, which develop spontaneously autoimmune disease. An age-dependent decline in clearance was detected in both strains, which occurred earlier in the MRL-1pr strain and corresponded with the relative severity of autoimmune disease in these strains. Androgen treatment improved clearance in the MRL-+/+, but not in the MRL-1pr strain. Even though autoantibody levels, renal function, and survival were improved, castration, followed by estrogen administration, did not influence immune clearance, or autoimmune disease, in MRL-1pr mice.[56] Both New Zealand white (NZW) and black (NZB) mice develop clinically silent glomerulonephritis. In the NZW strain, the renal lesion is more pronounced in females and is caused by the deposition of immune complexes in the glomeruli. By contrast, NZB mice show only minimal sex differences, and their lesions are less advanced than those of NZW females.[57]

Rats bearing the nude (rnu) mutation developed their killer (K) and natural killer (NK) cytotoxic potential at 3 months of age, which was comparable in rnu/rnu athymic animals with their normal rnu/+ litter mates. These cytotoxic activities did not decrease in old male rats, but they did so in female rnu/rnu animals.[58]

Lymphocytes from female mice, or from male mice that cannot produce and respond to testosterone (Tfm/y), were more reactive than male lymphocytes to alloantigens in mixed lymphocyte reactions. Spleen cells from Tfm/y mice with estrogen implants showed higher responsiveness to alloantigens than did control Tfm/y animals. Thymocytes of female animals reacted more effectively than male cells, in mixed lymphocyte reactions, in the presence of T cell growth factor. Furthermore, Con A stimulated female spleen cells produced more interleukin 2 than did spleen cells from males, or from testosterone treated females. Lymphocytes from preimmunized females responded more vigorously to soluble antigens in vitro than did lymphocytes from preimmunized males, or from preimmunized testosterone treated females. Antigen presenting cells from female spleen were more efficient than their male counterparts in initiating a secondary response in primed lymphocytes from either male or female mice. Moreover, castration of male mice enhanced and androgen treatment of females reduced, the efficiency of antigen presentation in this system.[59] Immunity and tolerance to guanosine were studied in male and female BALB/c and SJL mice and in their hybrid and backcross offspring. SJL mice were higher responders and BALB/c mice were more susceptible to tolerance induction by guanosine-isologous IgG treatment. Males were more easily tolerized than females in both strains, which was best seen in the secondary immune response of animals tolerized before primary immunization. Both male and female F_1 mice were high responders; nevertheless, both sexes were easily tolerized. Experiments on backcross animals revealed that the genetic control of immune reactivity was complex and that it was linked neither to immunoglobulin heavy chain genes nor to the H-2 haplotype. Females were more resistant than males to tolerance induction in backcross animals as well.[60]

It has long been recognized in medicine that women are more prone to autoimmune disease than are men.[61] In systemic lupus erythematosus (SLE) approximately 90% of the patients are female.[62] Women are affected two to three times more frequently by rheumatoid arthritis than men.[63] Recent findings suggest that hormonal factors are responsible, at least in part, for this notable sex difference. Patients affected by SLE appear to have abnormal sex hormone metabolism that leads to a net increase in estrogens and/or decrease of androgens.[64-68] Oral contraceptive therapy with estrogens, even at low doses, often induces exacerbation of SLE activity. Progesterone oral contraceptives were devoid of such unfavorable effects.[69] Furthermore, a case controlled study showed that the incidence rate of rheumatoid arthritis among oral contraceptive users was halved,[70] which indicates that this disease is also influenced by sex hormones.

In murine models of SLE, where an increased susceptibility of females could be demonstrated, estrogens were responsible for the exacerbation of the disease, whereas androgens had a suppressive effect.[71] However, a similar autoimmune syndrome that develops spontaneously in BXSB mice has an early onset in males, and females develop symptoms at a much slower rate. The defect in this form of murine SLE was demonstrated to be due to a Y chromosome-linked gene, though the participation of one or more additional genes was also suggested.[72-74] Autoimmune hemolytic anemia was induced in various strains of mice by immunization with rat erythrocytes. In five of seven responding strains, a higher frequency of female mice developed erythrocyte autoantibodies than did males. Female mice also showed a more rapid onset of antibody formation, requiring fewer immunizations and accompanied by a more severe anemia. Gonadectomy and treatment with opposite sex hormone abolished this sex difference in autoantibody formation. No evidence could be obtained for an X-chromosome-linked mechanism.[75] Male and female mouse spleen cells were compared for their ability to develop cytotoxicity to autologous embryo fibroblasts in vitro. Male cells developed significantly greater reactivity than did female cells. The cytotoxicity of male cells was totally abolished by treatment with a mouse anti-T cell antiserum, but such an antiserum had less effect on female effector cells.[76]

Experimental allergic encephalomyelitis recurred in 45% of female Lewis rats, which was as severe as the first attack, whereas all the males had one episode with subsequent recovery at about 20 days post immunization.[77]

V. THE INFLUENCE OF GONADECTOMY ON THE IMMUNE SYSTEM

Prepubertal orchidectomy of mice delayed the normal rate of thymic involution, leading to a relative hypertrophy of the thymus, which was maximal 1 month after operation. Lymph nodes and spleens were also enlarged 6 weeks after orchidectomy. The enlarged peripheral lymph nodes showed widening of the paracortical area, which is thymus dependent. Synchronous thymectomy and orchidectomy prevented the lymph node enlargement, but it did not affect the increase of spleen size until 3 months after surgery. Postpubertal orchidectomy, performed at 10 to 12 weeks of age, also led to increased thymic size and peripheral lymph node and spleen mass. However, lymph nodes of orchidectomized mice were significantly greater than that of controls at 3 months after operation. Changes in spleen size were apparent only after correction for changes in body mass.[78] Castration of adult male B10 mice led to a marked decrease in the expression of Thy-1^b antigen, which is present on all thymocytes and mature T lymphocytes. The effect of castration was substantially weaker in the congenic B10.A strain.[79] Thymic estrogen receptor concentrations were significantly higher in female BDF$_1$ mice than in males. Castration elevated the thymic estrogen receptor expression in males to levels nearly equivalent to that of females. Therefore, androgenic hormones may suppress estrogen receptor expression in the thymus.[80] Female, but not male, (NZBxSJL) F$_1$ hybrid mice develop thymic abnormalities during aging. Prepubertal orchidectomy performed from 3 weeks to 3 months of age resulted in thymic alterations (dull staining for Thy-1 and Lyt-1.2 antigens, weak reaction with peanut agglutinin and the emergence of surface immunoglobulin bearing cells) when examined at 12 months of age. However, when orchidectomy was performed between 6 and 9 months of age, there was an increase of all thymocyte subsets, without major qualitative abnormality at either 12 or 18 months of age. Therefore, the lack of thymic disease in intact males may be due to a suppressive effect of androgens that can be reversed by early, but not by late, orchidectomy.[81,82]

Skin grafts were rejected by a higher percentage of female mice and in shorter time than did males. Combined gonadectomy and adrenalectomy increased rejection more in males than in females, so that the sex difference was abolished. Oophorectomy also increased the proportion of rejections in females, but females with transplanted testes showed a significantly smaller rejection percentage than oophorectomized animals without transplants. Orchidectomized males receiving transplanted ovaries showed no change in percentage, but the rejection rate was accelerated. Reactivity to oxazolone, to SRBC, and the development of graft-vs.-host disease (GVH), which are mediated by T cells, were increased in orchidectomized mice.[83] Orchidectomy had no influence on the production of antibodies to bovine serum albumin, to skin allografts, and to pneumococcal polysaccharide.[84]

VI. THE EFFECT OF ESTROGENS ON THE IMMUNE SYSTEM

A. Mouse

There is little difference between male and female bone marrow with regard to the number of hemopoietic stem cells. However, the female spleen has on the average 20% more cells and about 300% more stem cells. Spleen of female mice in proestrous contained up to three times as many hemopoietic stem cells as during the estrous and postestrous stage of the cycle.[85] Mice treated with pharmacologic doses of estrone (50 μg, 3 times weekly for 4 weeks) became leukopenic, but not anemic. Bone marrow cellularity, ^{59}Fe uptake, and granulocyte progenitor cell concentration and total content declined markedly in the females by the 1st week of treatment. Only granulocyte progenitors began to recuperate during 2 weeks after cessation of estrone therapy. Splenic weight, ^{59}Fe uptake, and granulocyte progenitor cells increased during estrone therapy about twofold and tenfold, respectively, by day 17 after cessation of treatment. It was suggested that estrone directly suppresses granulocyte progenitor cell production, or proliferation, in addition to altering the hemopoietic supportive microenvironment.[86] In newborn mice up to 2 weeks of age, androgen and estrogen receptors were barely detectable in the thymus. No effect was apparent when estradiol and dihydrotestosterone were used in thymic organ cultures at concentrations up to 10^{-6} M. These results indicate that thymic sensitivity to sex hormones develops postnatally.[87]

Mesenteric lymph nodes were labeled with ^{3}H-thymidine and transferred to syngeneic female mice at various stages of their estrous cycle. When given to proestrus and estrous animals, a significant number of IgA and IgG containing cells localized in the cervices and vaginae. During metestrus and diestrus, however, few labeled cells localized in the genital tract. The estrous cycle did not influence the localization of IgA containing cells in the small intestine.[88]

Spleen cells from young adult female BALB/c mice responded better than those of males to mitogens and to particulate antigens. Newborn mice did not demonstrate the sex associated immune difference, which began to appear at weaning. The blastogenic responsiveness to PHA, Con A, and lipopolysaccharide (LPS) of female animals was greater at proestrus and metaestrus, as compared to estrus and diestrus. Similar differences were observed in IgM plaque-forming proestrus and metestrus. The peak of responsiveness corresponded to reported elevated levels of estrogen and pregnenolone during these phases of the cycle.[89,90]

Estrogen was found to enhance significantly the production of hemolytic antibodies to SRBC in C57BL mice, whereas in C3H mice a moderate inhibition of hemolysin titers was noted. Furthermore, normal C57BL females showed significantly higher hemolysin titers than did C57BL males. No such difference was found in the C3H strain.[91] Treatment of mice with stilbestrol decreased the hemolytic and agglutinating antibody formation to SRBC, which was dependent on the dose and the route of administration of the antigen. Higher doses of antigen could compensate for the effect of stilbestrol.[92]

Diethylstilbestrol (DES) treatment (0.22 and 8 mg/kg) of adult female mice caused a decrease in thymus weight and bone marrow cellularity. Histologically, a progressive loss of cortical thymic lymphocytes and splenic white pulp was noticed. Pluripotent hemopoietic stem cells and macrophage granulocyte progenitors were also decreased in the bone marrow in a dose related manner. On the other hand, circulating lymphocytes, blood monocytes, splenic weight, and spleen cellularity showed a dose-dependent increase, as did the number of peritoneal macrophages and their phagocytic, proliferative, and tumor cell cytolytic capacity. A dose related depression of antibody response, cutaneous delayed hypersensitivity, and in vitro lymphoproliferative responses to mitogens and to allogeneic leukocytes was also demonstrated. Co-culture experiments indicated that the immunosuppressive effect of DES is due, at least in part, to the induction of suppressor cells that reside in the adherent cell population.[93,94]

The treatment of male mice with DES increased the intravascular clearance rate of a lipid emulsion in a dose-dependent fashion. The enhancement of vascular clearance was associated with a concomitant increase in hepatic phagocytosis.[95] Mice, pretreated with estrogens, showed an increased hepatic and decreased splenic uptake of ^{51}Cr-labeled SRBC. The antibody response to SRBC was proportional to the amount of red cells localizing in the spleen. Antibody formation could be enhanced by blockage of the phagocytic activity of liver macrophages.[96]

Treatment of neonatal female mice with DES resulted in a decreased number of antibody forming cells in spleens, when immunized as adult animals with SRBC, or LPS. Ovariectomy, or ovariectomy plus subsequent estradiol treatment, did not influence the altered response of such DES treated animals. Ovariectomy of normal animals reduced the response to LPS to the level of DES treated females, which could be increased again to the level of normal controls by additional estradiol treatment. In vitro mixing experiments of purified T and B lymphocytes from control and DES treated females indicated that the diminished antibody response, induced by neonatal exposure to DES, was due to a defect in the T lymphocyte population. T cells from DES treated females were deficient in their ability to support a primary anti-SRBC response in vitro and contained a reduced number of Lyt-1$^+$ cells. No difference was observed in suppressor cell activity.[97] Neonatal treatment of mice with DES diminished also the delayed hypersensitivity response to oxazolone.[98] Mouse fetuses were exposed to DES through maternal dosing (0.1 mg/kg) on day 16 of gestation. DES slightly suppressed cell mediated immune function in both males and females, whereas a sex specific difference occurred in the humoral immune function. There was an enhanced antibody response to a T independent antigen in males and either no effect or slight depression in females.[99]

Estrogens were reported to prolong skin graft survival in mice.[100] In mixed lymphocyte reactions, estradiol (1 to 5 μg/mℓ) reduced markedly DNA synthesis and blocked the generation of cytotoxic lymphocytes. The cytotoxic activity of mature effector cells generated in vitro was not influenced by estradiol.[101] Treatment of mice with estradiol reduced NK cell activity and eliminated the genetic resistance to bone marrow transplantation. Androgen treatment had no effect. Estradiol did not affect natural killing in vitro and the loss of NK activity was not due to a soluble or a cellular suppressor and was not dependent on the thymus. Estrogen induced osteoproliferation and some undefined deficiency of marrow dependent cells were suggested as the mechanism of reduced NK activity.[102-104] Splenocytes from estradiol treated mice suppressed the NK activity of splenocytes from untreated animals, when the two cell populations were mixed during cytotoxicity assays. Additional treatment of mice with the interferon inducer, polyinosinic-polycytidylic acid (poly-I:C), resulted in moderate restoration of NK activity, but had no effect on the suppressor activity. The suppressor cells had the properties of the monocyte-macrophage lineage.[105] Estradiol treatment of mice did not reduce NK cell activity against YAC-1 lymphoma and UV-2237 fibrosarcoma target cells, but it was associated with a higher incidence of experimental and spontaneous pulmonary metastasis of the syngeneic UV-2237 fibrosarcoma, K1735 and B16 melanoma tumors. Athymic nude mice, treated with estradiol, also showed a low level of NK cell activity and an enhanced susceptibility to metastasis of allogeneic tumor cells. The activity of NK cells by poly-I:C and *Corynebacterium parvum,* was also impaired in estradiol treated animals, whereas the activation of tumoricidal macrophages was not.[106]

Treatment of neonatal female mice with DES reduced their NK activity. Cellular or humoral suppressors of natural killing could not be detected, and poly-I:C failed to increase the level of NK activity in DES treated animals. The cytotoxic activity of spleen cells from neonatally treated female animals against the I-51 target was not reduced in comparison with controls. However, the DES injected females had only about half the cytotoxic activity against the I-522 and YAC-1 cells as did controls. Furthermore, control animals eliminated intravenously injected radioactive YAC-1 and I-522 target cells faster than did DES treated females, whereas there was no difference in the elimination of I-51 cells. DES treated females showed a higher cumulative mortality after the inoculation of low numbers of I-522 cells, but again no difference was observed with I-51 cells. The incidence of females developing methylcholanthrene induced sarcomas was higher among DES injected animals than among controls. It was concluded that female mice treated neonatally with DES have a functionally defective NK cell population, which leads to increased tumor susceptibility.[107-109]

Spleen lymphocytes, taken at the age of 4 to 6 months from neonatally DES treated females, had about half the percentage of cells undergoing capping after exposure to Con A than controls. In addition, the response to Con A, or LPS, of spleen cells of DES treated females was reduced when tested at 6, 10, and 18 weeks or 17 months of age. DES injection from day 6 through day 10 did not cause such changes in the mitogen response.[107,110]

B. Rat

Estradiol treatment of ovariectomized, or prepubertal intact, female rats caused a significant decrease in thymus weight. In sexually mature females, but not in prepubertal animals, the weight of the adrenal increased parallel with thymus involution.[111] Estradiol inhibited calcium- but not magnesium-induced mitogenesis of rat thymocytes in vitro.[112] Gonadectomy enhanced the Con A and PHA response of rat thymic lymphocytes, which was further enhanced by additional adrenalectomy. Estradiol treatment of gonadectomized animals suppressed the responsiveness back to normal. Direct placement of estradiol into the tissue culture medium, containing castrate sera at physiological concentrations, failed to depress thymocyte blastogenesis to noncastrate levels. On the other hand, sera prepared from castrate animals, treated with estradiol at physiological concentrations, was successful in depressing the blastogenic response to noncastrate levels. Sera from thymectomized animals did not enhance Con A induced blastogenesis, but the PHA response was significantly increased. This effect was lost if sera from thymectomized animals treated with estradiol was utilized.[113]

The treatment of rats with stilbestrol, prior to immunization, decreased the hemolytic and agglutinating antibody titers, which were dependent on the dose and the route of administration of SRBC.[92]

Wira and co-workers[114-120] studied the effect of estradiol on uterine secretion of immunoglobulins in rats. IgG was maximal at proestrus, but barely detectable at estrus, diestrus, and following ovariectomy. IgA was also highest at proestrus, but remained elevated at estrus and dropped to low levels at diestrus and following ovariectomy. The increased uterine immunoglobulin secretion at proestrus could be reproduced readily by the treatment of ovariectomized rats with physiological amounts of estradiol. IgA that was secreted against the concentration gradient was always in a dimeric form, whereas IgG accumulated in the lumen of the uterus down a concentration gradient. No IgA increase was observed when progesterone was given along with estradiol. Within 3 hr after a single injection of 1 μg of estradiol to ovariectomized rats, both IgA and IgG levels increased significantly in uterine tissue, remained elevated at 6 hr and declined by 22 hr after drug treatment. Under these conditions estradiol also increased the levels of luminal IgG, but had no effect on either IgA or IgM. Treatment with other steroid hormones (progesterone, cortisol, dihydrotestosterone, and estriol), when injected at doses known to elicit *physiological* effects in their respective target tissues, had no effect on uterine secretions of immunoglobulins. Estradiol had a marked effect on the association of IgA with uterine epithelial cells, as revealed by immunofluorescence. Furthermore, the levels of secretory component produced by uterine tissues in culture were highest at proestrus and lowest at diestrus, showing parallel variation with IgA secretion. No indication for the involvement of uterine epithelial cells in the secretion of IgG was revealed. Changes in uterine vasculature that results in increased uterine permeability within the first few hours after hormone exposure were proposed as the mechanism of IgG secretion. An accumulation of IgA+ cells in the uteri of ovariectomized rats was also observed after estradiol treatment. In thymectomized rats luminal levels of both IgA and IgG were significantly reduced, but the estradiol induced movement of IgA from tissue to lumen against a concentration gradient was still present.[114-120]

Our recent studies indicate that the usual dose of prolactin (PRL), sufficient to reconstitute the immune reactivity of Hypox rats, gives rise to only partial reconstitution, if the ovaries are also removed (Figure 1). Furthermore, ovariectomy alone is able to induce a significant decrease in the reactivity of the animals to DNCB. The response of ovariectomized animals can be fully reconstituted by estradiol treatment, but Hypox + OV animals need both PRL and estradiol for full reconstitution, at least at the dose level used. Nevertheless, PRL was able to restore a significant degree of immunocompetence in Hypox animals, even when both the gonads and the adrenals were removed. It is somewhat surprising that neither LH, nor FSH showed any restoring activity in Hypox female animals, yet estradiol seems to be a very potent steroid hormone for restoring the immune reactivity of such rats. However, there are indications that PRL may be an important pituitary hormone for regulation of the secretion of sex steroid hormones. The ovary, testicles, and adrenals all have PRL receptors.[121-123] Moreover, PRL has an influence on ovarian estrogen, androgen, and progesterone synthesis.[124,125] High amounts of PRL are known to inhibit ovarian function in women, whereas physiological levels may in fact be necessary for normal ovarian function.[126] Finally, estrogens are known to stimulate PRL release both in experimental animals and man.[127-129] Therefore, there is a compelling body of evidence indicating that sex hormones and PRL regulate each other. The synergism of estrogens and PRL during the development of mammary immune function has been discussed earlier. Our experiments suggest that a similar synergism may exist for all forms of immune reactivity. Further experiments are required to elucidate the interaction of PRL and of sex hormones in immune reactivity.

Autoimmune thyroiditis can be induced in PVG/c rats by thymectomy and irradiation, and female animals are more susceptible than are males. Prepubertal ovariectomy was found to augment further this susceptibility. Estrogen, administered repeatedly (1 or 10 μg/100 g), partially suppressed the development of thyroiditis and the formation of antibodies to thyroglobulin. Estrogen, administered as a single implant, had a similar effect. Estrogen also reduced the incidence of thyroiditis and autoantibody production in orchidectomized male rats.[130]

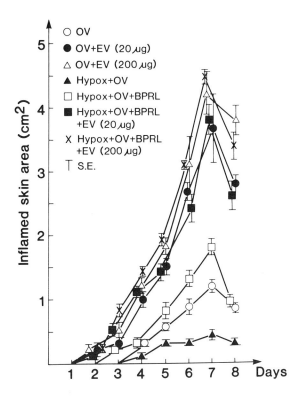

FIGURE 1. The synergism of estradiol and prolactin in the maintenance of contact sensitivity reactions in rats. Groups of five female Fischer rats weighing 150 to 170 g were used. Ovariectomy (OV) and hypophysectomy (Hypox) were performed on day 0, treatment with estradiol valerate (EV; 20 and 200 µg/day/animal s.c.) was started on day 14 and maintained until the end of the experiment. Treatment with bovine prolactin (BPRL; 40 µg/day/animal s.c.) was started on day 21 and maintained until the end of the experiment. Contact dermatitis was induced on day 21 by dinitrochlorobenzene (DNCB), dissolved in acetone at 200 mg/mℓ concentration and 20 µℓ of this solution were applied to an area measuring approximately 1 cm² on the shaved dorsal skin. The diameters of the inflamed skin lesions were measured daily in diagonal directions, and the mean affected skin areas ± SE were calculated and are shown in the figure. *Statistical evaluation:* The reactivity of OV animals was significantly lower ($P < 0.01$) than those of OV treated with EV throughout the experiment. OV animals reacted significantly better than OV + Hypox animals from days 4 to 8. Treatment with BPRL improved significantly the reactivity of OV + Hypox animals throughout the experiment. Additional treatment with EV resulted in further significant improvements (days 3 to 8), and the reactivity of such animals was restored to the level of those of OV + EV treated groups.

The rate of regeneration of tissue mast cells, after depletion by Polymyxin B in normal and thymectomized rats, was increased by estrogen treatment.[131] The subplantar injection of 1 mℓ of carrageenan induces a hyperthermic response in rats, which is more dramatic in females than in males. The lower reactivity of males can be reversed by estradiol treatment.[132]

C. Guinea Pig

High affinity estrogen receptors ($K_d = 0.18$ nM) were present in the cytosol of guinea pig fetal thymus. The levels of available cytoplasmic receptors increased during fetal development from 9.7 fmol/mg protein at 36 days of gestation to 31 fmol/mg protein by the end of gestation. Estradiol treatment of pregnant animals (1 mg/kg) decreased the number of large thymocytes in the outer cortex of the fetal thymus, without affecting the total number of cortical lymphocytes. This led to a significant decrease in the weight of the thymus. The in vitro incorporation of ^{3}H-thymidine by fetal thymocytes was also reduced by 50% after such treatment. Cytoplasmic estrogen receptors of thymocytes were reduced and nuclear estrogen receptors were increased at the same time. If estrogen treatment was maintained for 2 to 6 days, a further reduction occurred in cortical thymocytes with decreased numbers, but without affecting medullary thymocytes in the fetuses. If the animals were treated simultaneously with estradiol and with the anti-estrogen, tamoxifen (2 mg/kg), the changes induced by estradiol alone could be prevented. The susceptibility of fetal thymus to estrogen treatment increased progressively from 42 days of gestation until birth.[133,134]

A lymphoid cell peculiar to guinea pigs, called the Kurloff cell, resembles mononuclear lymphocytes and possesses a characteristic proteoglycan containing inclusion body. The function of these cells is obscure. Their number increases in the blood and organs of guinea pigs during pregnancy, and it has been suggested that Kurloff cells may play some role in the protection of trophoblast from immunological damage. A transient rise in Kurloff cells was observed in the blood after a single injection of estrogen, whereas a sustained increase occurred when estrogen was administered in oil suspension.[135]

Daily treatment of guinea pigs with estradiol (75 μg/kg) for 23 days reduced their antibody response to penicilloyl-coupled guinea pig gammaglobulin and also delayed the rate of titer decay.[136,137] Uterine tissues, and ileum strips, taken from immunized guinea pigs, displayed greater contractility in the Schultz-Dale test during estrous, when exposed to the specific antigen, than tissues from similarly sensitized nonestrous guinea pigs. Excised ileum strips, taken from similarly sensitized, estrogen treated male guinea pigs, revealed no significant difference from the ileum of sensitized male controls.[138]

Estradiol (1 to 50 μg/mℓ) did not affect normal macrophage migrations and failed to suppress the production of migration inhibitory factor by lymphocytes from immunized guinea pigs, when stimulated by antigen.[139]

D. Man

Peripheral blood lymphocyte counts reached a minimum in 18 female volunteers during midcycle, which coincided with the maximum level of estradiol in the serum. Active T cells did not show cyclic variations. Monocyte and granulocyte counts were significantly higher in the luteal than in the follicular phase; their variation was closely related to progesterone, but not to estradiol.[140] The formation of early E rosettes by normal human peripheral blood T lymphocytes was increased by incubation with physiological concentrations of estradiol, which was hormone specific.[141] Exposure of human lymphocytes to DES in vitro led to the induction of sister chromatid exchanges. The natural estrogens, estradiol and estriol, did not induce such changes. Estradiol and DES inhibited strongly the PHA induced proliferation of lymphocytes. Estriol was a weak inhibitor.[142]

The IgG and IgA content of cervical mucus in relation to ovulatory cycles was assessed in 32 healthy women. A minimum concentration of immunoglobulins was present at midcycle.[143] The serum levels of IgE were not influenced significantly by the follicular and luteal phases of menstrual cycle, or by pregnancy. Nor were IgE levels different in man with gonadal disgenesis, indicating that sex steroid hormones have little or no effect on IgE levels.[144]

Several investigators observed that the response of human peripheral blood lymphocytes to mitogens (PHA, Con A, PPD) and in the mixed lymphocyte culture is inhibited by estradiol and DES.[145-149] However, physiological concentrations of estradiol were found to enhance the PWM stimulated immunoglobulin secretion of human lymphocytes. Additional experiments revealed that this enhancing effect was due to the inhibition of suppressor T lymphocytes by estradiol.[150] Others found that the suppressive effect of sex steroids on mitogen responses and on the mixed lymphocyte reaction was either very weak or nonexistent, and it has been postulated that sex hormones exert their inhibitory effects by suboptimal binding to glucocorticoid receptors in lymphocytes. The relative immunosuppressive potency of a given hormone is related to its affinity for the glucocorticoid receptor.[151,152]

Fifty-eight postmenopausal women were followed during 6 months of treatment with various synthetic and natural estrogens. Sera of these women inhibited the mixed lymphocyte reaction. Although the levels of two immunosuppressive factors, namely cortisone and pregnancy zone protein, were increased during treatment, the individual values of these factors were not correlated to depressed lymphocyte reactivity. A direct effect of estrogen on lymphocytes was suggested.[153]

Serum from rats, treated with estradiol, contained a low molecular weight factor, capable of reducing the spontaneous binding of SRBC to lymphocytes, suppressing the antigen induced inhibition of leukocyte migration, and partially blocking the PHA response. At the same time, this factor increased the number of lymphocytes with receptors for C3b and IgM, and increased the number of direct plaque forming cells (PFC) following in vitro sensitization. All these effects were abolished if the rats were thymectomized before estradiol treatment.[154]

Estradiol inhibited weakly the expression of IgG and complement receptors by human monocytes.[155] Estradiol binds covalently to normal human neutrophils, eosinophils, and monocytes. This reaction involves the peroxidase enzyme of neutrophils and monocytes and possibly also eosinophils and catalase.[156]

E. Other Species

In beagle dogs and stump-tail monkeys (Macaca speciosa), the degranulation of mast cells induced by the agent 48/80 was inhibited by the injection of estrogens (premarin).[157]

Seven female calves were injected with 80 mg of DES at 8 weeks of age and four animals were immunized 1 week later with alum-adsorbed tetanus toxoid. A booster injection was given 2 weeks later. Estrogen treatment did not influence the immune response.[158]

VII. THE INFLUENCE OF ANDROGENS ON THE IMMUNE SYSTEM

The effect of androgens on erythropoiesis has been studied extensively, and androgens are in use in clinical practice for the enhancement of erythropoiesis. It is beyond the scope of this book to survey the biological effect of androgens on the hemopoietic system. Instead, the interested reader is referred to a recent review.[159]

It has been mentioned briefly already that androgens have a moderating effect on autoimmune reactions in various animal models and possibly also in patients with autoimmune disease. This aspect of the effects of androgens on immune reactions is discussed in Chapter 15.

A. Mouse

Treatment of various strains of mice with testosterone and with a variety of anabolic androgens caused a marked reduction in thymus cell number and an increase in the responsiveness of thymus cells to Con A and PHA. The number of large cells expressing 20α-steroid dehydrogenase was increased in the bone marrow.[160] The T/B lymphocyte ratio was significantly higher in the spleens of adult female than in adult male mice. Neonatal administration of androgen to females decreased the T/B ratio, whereas neonatal castration of males resulted in a permanent increase of this ratio.[161] Female mice, treated with testosterone immediately after irradiation and bone marrow reconstitution, showed no suppressive effect on the recovery of thymus and spleen weight 30 days later. Testosterone treatment had no effect on GVH reaction and the survival of skin homografts. However, the PFC response to SRBC in the spleen was dramatically suppressed by such treatment, suggesting that testosterone inhibits the differentiation of stem cells towards mature B lymphocytes. The anti-SRBC response recovered completely 90 days after testosterone administration. Testosterone had a similar immunosuppressive effect in adult mice 30 days after a single i.p. injection.[162] Immunoglobulin levels were determined in two strains of mice, previously classified by seminal vesicle bioassay as high (C57L/J) and low (A/J) responders to androgen. Among C57L/J mice, males had lower values of IgM and IgG2 than females of the strain and lower values than male mice of the A/J strain, in which no sex related difference was observed in immunoglobulin levels. Neonatal gonadectomy did not change immunoglobulin levels in either strain, indicating that the concentration of androgen in mature animals was not responsible for their low immunoglobulin levels.[163]

Although no sex difference was apparent in the primary IgM PFC response to SRBC in pre- and postpubertal NZB, DBA/2, and BALB/c mice, orchidectomy increased, and testosterone implants reduced the antibody response, if followed by sublethal irradiation. This suggests that androgens may affect rapidly regenerating stem cells and/or their differentiating progeny. Strain differences in target organ sensitivity to androgen were not found.[164]

Five α derivatives of testosterone, which are present in the placenta, decreased significantly the contact sensitivity reaction of mice to oxazolone and decreased slightly the number of PFC. However, 5 β-androstane-3,17-dione, which is not found in the placenta, did not affect contact sensitivity, but enhanced significantly the PFC number. All the androstane derivatives tested decreased thymus weight and cellularity and all androgens tested, except the most suppressive 5 α-androstane-17-dione, caused a significant increase of spleen weight.[165] Castration decreased, and testosterone replacement therapy increased the activity of splenic suppressor T cells in a variety of mouse strains.[166] Nonautoimmune strains of mice are easily made tolerant to bovine gammaglobulin (BGG) by the injection of large amounts of deaggregated BGG. On the other hand, the autoimmune-prone NZB and (NZB × NZW)F₁, MLR/Mp-Ipr/Ipr and BXSB/Mp strains failed to become tolerant. Experiments performed in neonatally thymectomized (NZB × DBA/2)F₁ mice that were lethally irradiated at 3 months of age and reconstituted with parental bone marrow and thymocytes revealed that the development of tolerance was dependent on the strain of the donor cells and the sex of the recipient mice. Thymocytes of NZB were necessary for the manifestation of tolerance defect. Androgens protected against the tolerance defect imposed by NZB thymocytes and promoted tolerance in the presence of normal marrow. NZB marrow did not prevent tolerance in association with normal thymocytes. However, NZB marrow prevented androgen mediated tolerance in the presence of NZB thymocytes. Therefore, the thymic defect was sufficient to prevent tolerance in female animals, whereas an additional marrow defect was necessary to prevent tolerance in males.[167]

C57BL/6 mice, given ten doses of cyproterone acetate (0.5 mg/mouse/day), had involuted thymuses, a reduced capacity to produce antibodies, and delayed rejection of skin allografts.[168] The injection of 300 mg/kg cyclophosphamide i.p. into female AKR mice caused a reversible neutropenia, which could be prevented by transfusion and androgen administration.[169]

The expression of the sex-linked protein (Slp) locus within the major histocompatibility complex of mice is controlled by testosterone. Males of Slp positive strains begin to produce this serum protein at 5 to 6 weeks of age with the onset of sexual maturity. Production can be prevented by castration of immature males and initiated by testosterone treatment. Females of Slp positive strain develop normal male levels, if treated with testosterone. Castration of mature males of Slp positive strains leads to a sharp decrease in the serum level of Slp protein within 3 weeks and complete disappearance by 200 days. Treatment of such males with testosterone can normalize Slp levels again. Males of Slp positive mouse strains have higher levels of endogenous testosterone than males of Slp negative strains.[170] The serum levels of C4-binding protein is also regulated by testosterone. It decreases in castrated males and increases in testosterone treated castrated females.[171]

B. Rat

Rat thymuses were shown to contain steroidal 5α-reductase, which can convert testosterone to androgenic metabolites.[172] Treatment of X-irradiated (400 R) rats with testosterone or mesterolone accelerated the recovery of leukocytes.[173] Testosterone administration to normal male and female rats caused an increased erythropoiesis and granulopoiesis. At the same time the bone marrow and thymus lymphocytic cellularity was diminished. Peripheral lymphoid tissue was not affected. Humoral immune responsiveness was increased and normal inflammatory response was retained.[174]

Male rats had approximately fivefold greater concentration of secretory component (SC) in tears than did females. Castration of male, but not of female, rats reduced the SC content of tears. Administration of testosterone to orchidectomized rats reversed this decline, but progesterone, estradiol, and cortisol had no effect. Thus, androgens may influence the production and/or secretion of SC by ocular tissues and play a role in the ocular secretory immune system of the rat.[175]

Testosterone antagonized the rate of regeneration of tissue mast cells in normal and thymectomized rats after depletion by polymixin B.[131] The higher hyperthermic response of female rats to carrageenan could be reversed by testosterone treatment.[132]

C. Chicken

Selye[176] was the first to notice that the bursa of Fabricius is under the influence of steroid hormones and that the morphological development of this organ was most actively inhibited by large doses of folliculoids and testoids. Subsequent investigations revealed that 0.63 mg of 19-nortestosterone in 0.1 mℓ of corn oil, injected into eggs on the 5th day of incubation, inhibits completely the development of the bursa of Fabricius.[177] Reduction in the size of the spleen and thymus was also noted. Furthermore, such hormonally bursectomized chicken were unable to produce antibodies against ovine serum albumin. The immunodeficient birds weighed less than controls and were generally in poor health.[178] The serious impairment of the humoral immune response in chicks lacking the bursa because of testosterone treatment during embryonic life, was confirmed by others.[179,180] If chicken embryos are treated with 4 mg of testosterone propionate on the 12th day of embryonic life, small bursa remnants will remain, but without follicles. Such animals form almost exclusively IgM antibodies to SRBC and influenza virus, though there is no response to some other antigens. Surgical removal of bursal remnants did not affect significantly the anti-SRBC response. In adoptive cell transfer experiments, the impaired B cell function of testosterone treated chickens could not be improved by the addition of T cells. Finally, B lymphocytes of such testosterone treated chicks were lacking a cell surface antigen specific for bursa-derived cells.[181,182]

D. Man

Human lymphocytes and alveolar macrophages have the capacity to metabolize androstenedione.[183,184] Testosterone was found, by several investigators, to inhibit the response of human peripheral blood lymphocytes to various mitogens (PHA, Con A, PPD, PWM) and to alloantigens in mixed lymphocyte reactions. Marked variations from individual to individual was noted. It was suggested that sex hormones affect lymphocyte function through suboptimal binding to glucocorticoid receptors.[152,147-149]

Preincubation of human lymphocytes with testosterone, but not estradiol or progesterone, resulted in the generation of modest, but significant, suppressor cell activity.[185] The expression of receptors for IgG and complement by human monocyte was inhibited by testosterone, but less effectively than glucocorticoids.[155] It may be relevant to note here that an anabolic synthetic steroid, danazol, was found to be effective in the treatment of hereditary and angioneurotic edema, and might also prove useful in the treatment of idiopathic thrombocytic purpura and systemic lupus erythematosus.[186,187]

E. Guinea Pig

Guinea pigs were treated with an antiandrogenic agent, cyproterone acetate, s.c. with 5 mg/100 g doses for 10 days. The animals were immunized immediately after the last dose of drug with a single i.p. injection of 1 mℓ of 20% SRBC. Cyproterone acetate reduced thymus weight, induced a significant lymphopenia and reduced hemolysin formation in both sexes of animals.[188]

VIII. THE EFFECT OF PROGESTERONE ON THE IMMUNE SYSTEM

A. Mouse

Progesterone, 1 to 10 μg/mℓ, added to mixed lymphocyte culture at the time of initiation, diminished the ability of both alloantigen specific and nonspecific suppressor cells to inhibit the proliferative response of homologous lymphocytes in response to alloantigens. Progesterone had a direct inhibitor effect on suppressor cell function.[189] DNA synthesis was markedly reduced in murine mixed lymphocyte cultures by progesterone and the generation of cytotoxic lymphocytes was blocked. Progesterone did not suppress the cytotoxic activity of mature effector cells generated previously in vitro.[101]

B. Rat

The estradiol stimulated accumulation of IgA and IgG in the rat uterus was inhibited when the animals were also treated with progesterone.[119] PVG/c rats developed autoimmune thyroiditis after thymectomy and X-irradiation. The repeated administration of progesterone at doses of 250 ng and 1500 μg/100 g body weight augmented the level of autoimmunity.[130]

C. Man

The cyclic variations of circulating monocytes and granulocytes in 18 female volunteers correlated closely with changes of progesterone levels during the menstrual cycle.[140]

Progesterone, in concentrations comparable to those present in pregnancy serum, inhibited the cytotoxic effect of nonpregnant women's lymphocytes on human embryonic fibroblast cells. Pregnancy sera exerted a similar inhibition, which could be reduced by 80%, after progesterone was depleted to 5% of its original concentration.[190] The response of human peripheral blood lymphocytes to mitogens (PHA, Con A, PWM) and in mixed lymphocyte culture was shown to be inhibited by progesterone in a number of laboratories. In general, high concentrations were required, and the inhibitory effect was much weaker than the one achieved with cortisol. Furthermore, cortisol inhibited irreversibly lymphocyte thymidine incorporation if added during the first 12 hr of culture, whereas the progesterone-mediated inhibition was reversible.[149,151,191,192] Addition of progesterone, but not estradiol or testosterone, to Con A stimulated cultures of human lymphocytes, increased significantly the generation of suppressor T lymphocytes.[185] The expression of Fc receptors for IgM and receptors for complement by human monocytes was inhibited significantly by progesterone, but less effectively than by glucocorticoids.[155]

D. Other Species

Treatment of monkeys with progesterone and other progestoids rendered them susceptible to oncogenesis by the Rous chicken sarcoma virus. Skin homografts were also prolonged in such animals.[193,194] Treatment of dogs and rabbits with medorxyprogesterone or melengestrol prolonged significantly the survival of renal and skin allografts, respectively. Progesterone treatment alone did not prolong allograft survival, possibly because it is metabolized rapidly.[195]

IX. THE INFLUENCE OF ORAL CONTRACEPTIVES ON THE IMMUNE SYSTEM OF WOMEN

Users of oral contraceptives may develop antibodies to the synthetic hormone ingredients, which will lead to immune complexes. Such complexes are indicated in the pathogenesis of thrombosis, but apparently do not cause renal lesions.[196] Immune complexes are able to trigger a variety of reactions within the immune system, which could lead to altered responsiveness, to abnormal regulation, or even to pathological changes. It remains to be seen whether or not the persistence of immune complexes in users of oral contraceptives have consequences other than thrombosis. Furthermore, when considering the effect of oral contraceptives on immune reactions, one should keep in mind, in addition to the possibility of altered immune reactivity due to complexes, that these are not natural hormones and their effect may not be comparable to the physiological counterparts.

Women using oral contraceptives or during pregnancy, have a high serum level of pregnancy associated alpha macroglobulin. A high percentage of peripheral T lymphocytes and monocytes with surface bound pregnancy associated alpha macroglobulin can also be identified.[197] Oral contraception with combined estrogen/progestogen pills caused a significant increase in mean IgA and IgG levels in the cervical mucus.[198] Delayed-type hypersensitivity responses to recall antigens (*Candida albicans*, mumps, tetanus toxoid), as well as the in vitro responsiveness of lymphocytes to mitogens, was found to be normal in 20 healthy women taking oral contraceptives.[199] Forty-five women taking oral contraceptives of combined estrogen/progestogen type, 27 receiving injections of medroxyprogesterone acetate and 15 women using the sequential pill method, were sensitized with dinitrochlorobenzene. Women taking the combined pill, or receiving i.m. progesterone, showed a significantly increased responsiveness, whereas women using the sequential pill method had a decreased skin reactivity in the estrogenic phase.[200,201]

Although Gerretsen et al.[202] found no difference between the response of lymphocytes from users of oral contraceptives and from normal individuals, to Con A and PHA, several other investigators observed that the PHA response was impaired, especially in long-term users of oral contraceptives.[203-206] The magnitude of depression of lymphocyte responsiveness was inversely related to the progestagenic potency of the contraceptives used. Depression persisted even 1 year after cessation of oral contraception. Experiments performed in autologous, as compared to homologus serum, suggested that that serum inhibitory factors may be important. No evidence for a direct suppressive effect of synthetic estrogens and gestagens on lymphocytes could be obtained.[205] In contrast, others found that a significant suppression of the PHA response was associated with the use of progestogen pills for 12-18 months. Short-term therapy did not effect responsiveness. Estradiol and progesterone, at concentrations of 1 μg/mℓ, suppressed PHA induced lymphocyte transformation in vitro.[206]

The effect of widely-employed steroid contraceptive agents on the immune reactivity of mice and rats was evaluated. Three different progesterone (lynestrenol, norethindrone, or norethynodrel) were administered in combination with estrogen (mestranol) in minimal antifertility doses. All the steroid contraceptive agents reduced significantly the severity of allergic encephalomyelitis in rats, but had variable effects on the antibody response of mice to SRBC and on anti mouse erythrocyte autoantibody formation. There was no effect on the anti-SRBC response of rats. Treatments with contraceptive steroids, which were otherwise immunosuppressive, did not modify the response of mice to T-independent antigen.[207]

X. THE EFFECT OF LYMPHOID FACTORS ON SEX HORMONE SECRETION AND ON THE GONADS

Several lines of evidence indicate a relationship between the development and function of the thymus and the ovary. Athymic female nude mice have an atrophic ovary, whereas in their normal heterozygous counterparts with normal thymus the development of the ovary is very similar, if not identical, to that of other mouse strains. The ovaries of athymic females, at three weeks of age, contain more atretic follicles, than those osf their heterozygous littermates. At 5 to 7 weeks of age the ovaries contained no, or very few, corpora lutea in nude animals. This ovarial immaturity may persist throughout life and can be reversed by treatment with exogenous gonadotropin.[208-210] Athymic male mice had significantly reduced concentrations of LH and FSH in comparison to heterozygous animals, which persisted in adult life, and was associated with markedly reduced circulating testosterone levels. Histologically, the number of Leydig cells appeared to be reduced in the testes from 20-day-old animals, but was normal at 40 days of age, with spermatogenesis. Therefore, in contrast with athymic females, athymic male mice have normal reproductive capacity, despite the hormonal abnormalities.[211]

In a variety of mouse strains, neonatal thymectomy leads to ovarian disgenesis, characterized by the abscence of follicles and corpora lutea. Ovarian disgenesis could be prevented with thymus grafts, given within 14 days of birth, or by grafting with adult spleen at 7 days of age. Thymocytes or spleen cells injected i.p. are also effective, whether from male or female donors.[212-214] Rats injected i.p. with antithymocyte serum for two weeks showed altered ovarian function. During such treatment, unovulation with the persistence of corpora lutea and a tendency toward a permanent diestrus state was evident.[215] Neonatal thymectomy of female Wistar rats reportedly disrupts the size distribution and number of ovarian follicles by the 10th day of life, culminating in ovarian disgenesis at 130 days of age.[216] Thymectomy of female rat pups at 5 days of age ameliorated the adrogenizing effect of a syngeneic testis transplant on ovarian morphology at 90 days of age.[217] Thymic hormones (thymosin fraction five and thymosin β4) stimulated the secretion of luteinizing hormone releasing factor from superfused medial basal hypothalami of cycling female rats. Furthermore, LH was released from pituitary gland superfused in sequence with the hypothalamus.[218] Treatment of female mice with thymic hormone (thymosin fraction 5) elevated estrogen levels and advanced the tissue of vaginal opening. Single injections of estradiol benzoate decreased thymus weight and caused a transient reduction in circulating plasma levels of thymic hormone (thymosin αl), indicating an inverse relationship between estrogen and thymic hormone. Additionally, thymectomy at 30 days of age had no effect on reproductive maturation.[219]

The number of Leydig cells and testosterone production were increased in the testes of chick embryos submitted to early surgical bursectomy. Bursal grafts normalized these changes.[220,221] Macrophage homogenates stimulated primary cultures of mouse granulosa cells to secrete more progesterone. Treatment of macrophages with Con A caused the release of luteotropic factors with apparent molecular weights of 26,000 and 41,000 daltons.[222] Human trophoblasts, co-cultured with neonatal human lymphocytes, increased their production of HCG. Lymphocytes from normal donors and from patients with gynecological cancer caused a reduction in trophoblast HCG production, while maternal lymphocytes had no significant effect.[223]

These and other observations suggest that there is a developmental relationship between the primary lymphoid organs and the gonads that continues in functional interaction during adult life.

REFERENCES

1. Selye, H., The pharmacology of steroid hormones and their derivatives, *Rev. Can. Biol.*, 1, 577, 1942.
2. Dougherty, T. F., Effect of hormones on lymphatic tissue, *Physiol. Rev.*, 32, 379, 1952.
3. Herrick, C. A. and Cross, S. X., The development of natural and artificial resistance of young rats to the pathogenic effects of the parasite *Trypanosoma lewisi*, *J. Parasitol.*, 22, 126, 1936.
4. Jackson, G. J., Herman, R., and Singer, I., Eds., *Immunity to Parasitic Animals*, Appleton-Century-Crofts, New York, 1970.
5. Medawar, P. P. and Sparrow, E. M., Effect of adrenocortical hormones, adrenocorticotropic hormone and pregnancy on skin transplantation immunity, *J. Endocrinol.*, 14, 240, 1956.
6. Billingham, R. E. and Head, J. R., Immunology of reproduction: present status, *Ann. Immunol. (Paris)*, D131, 125, 1980.
7. Bartocci, A., Papademetriou, V., Schlick, E., Nisula, B. C., and Chirigos, M. A., Effect of crude and purified human chorionic gonadotropin on murine delayed-type hypersensitivity: a role for prostaglandins, *Cell. Immunol.*, 71, 326, 1982.
8. Bartocci, A., Welker, R. D., Schlock, E., Chirigos, M. A., and Nisula, B. C., Immunosuppressive activity of human chorionic gonadotrophin preparations in vivo: evidence for gonadal dependence, *Cell Immunol.*, 82, 334, 1983.
9. Papademetriou, V., Bartocci, A., Stylos, W. A., and Chirigos, M. A., Augmentation of cytotoxicity by splenic cells of pregnant or human chorionic gonadotropin-treated normal mice, *J. Immunopharmacol.*, 2, 309, 1980.
10. Fuchs, T., Hammarström, L., Smith, C. I. E., and Brundin, J., In vitro induction of murine suppressor T-cells by human chorionic gonadotropin, *Acta Obstet. Gynecol. Scand.*, 59, 355, 1980.
11. Kaye, M. D., Jones, W. R., Ing, R. M. Y., and Markham, R., Effect of human chorionic gonadotropin on intrauterine skin allograft survival in rats, *Am. J. Obstet. Gynecol.*, 110, 640, 1971.
12. Berczi, I., Nagy, E., Kovacs, K., and Horvath, E., Regulation of humoral immunity in rats by pituitary hormones, *Acta Endocrinol.*, 98, 506, 1981.
13. Nagy, E. and Berczi, I., Prolactin and contact sensitivity, *Allergy*, 36, 429, 1981.
14. Berczi, I. and Nagy, E., A possible role of prolactin in adjuvant arthritis, *Arthritis Rheum.*, 25, 591, 1982.
15. Han, T., Human chorionic gonadotropin: its inhibitory effect on cell-mediated immunity in vivo and in vitro, *Immunology*, 29, 509, 1975.
16. Contractor, S. F. and Davies, H., Effect of human chorionic sommatomammotrophin and human chorionic gonadotrophin on phytohaemagglutinin-induced lymphocyte transformation, *Nature (London) New Biol.*, 243, 284, 1973.
17. Adcock, E. W., III, Teasdale, F., August, C. S., Cox, S., Meschia, G., Battaglia, F. C., and Naughton, M. A., Human chorionic gonadotropin: its possible role in maternal lymphocyte suppression, *Science*, 181, 845, 1973.

18. Fuchs, T., Hammarström, L., Smith, C. I. E., and Brundin, J., In vitro induction of human suppressor T cells by a chorionic gonadotropin preparation, *J. Reprod. Immunol.,* 3, 75, 1981.

19. Fuchs, T., Hammarström, L., Smith, C. I. E., and Brundin, J., Sex-dependent induction of human suppressor T cells by chorionic gonadotropin, *J. Reprod. Immunol.,* 4, 185, 1982.

20. Beling, C. B. and Weksler, M. E., Suppression of mixed lymphocyte reactivity by human chorionic gonadotropin, *Clin. Exp. Immunol.,* 18, 537, 1974.

21. Caldwell, J. L., Stites, D. P., and Fudenberg, H. H., Human chorionic gonadotropin: effects of crude and purified preparations on lymphocyte responses to phytohemagglutinin and allogeneic stimulation, *J. Immunol.,* 115, 1249, 1975.

22. Morse, J. H., The effect of human chorionic gonadotropin and placental lactogen on lymphocyte transformation in vitro, *Scand. J. Immunol.,* 5, 779, 1976.

23. Morse, J. H., Stearns, G., Arden, J., Agosto, G. M., and Canfield, R. E., The effects of crude and purified human gonadotropin on in vitro stimulated human lymphocyte cultures, *Cell. Immunol.,* 25, 178, 1976.

24. Bean, M. A., Salser, J. S., Newman, M., Stahl, K., and Balis, M. E., Human chorionic gonadotropin: doubtful role as an inhibitor of cell-mediated immunity, *Cancer Immunol. Immunother.,* 2, 85, 1977.

25. Rolfe, B. E., Morton, H., and Clarke, F. M., Early pregnancy factor is an immunosuppressive contaminant of commercial preparations of human chorionic gonadotrophin, *Clin. Exp. Immunol.,* 51, 45, 1983.

26. Pierpaoli, W. and Maestroni, G. J. M., Pharmacological control of the hormonally modulated immune response. II. Blockade of antibody production by a combination of drugs acting on neuroendocrine functions. Its prevention by gonadotropins and corticotrophin, *Immunology,* 34, 419, 1978.

27. Yee, J. B. and Hutson, J. C., Testicular macrophages: isolation, characterization and hormonal responsiveness, *Biol. Reprod.,* 29, 1319, 1983.

28. Staples, L. D., Brown, D., Binns, R. M., and Heap, R. B., The influence of protein hormones and conceptus extracts on sheep lymphocyte transformation induced in vitro, *Placenta,* 4, 125, 1983.

29. Berczi, I., Nagy, E., Asa, S. L., and Kovacs, K., Pituitary hormones and contact sensitivity in rats, *Allergy,* 38, 325, 1983.

30. Berczi, I., Nagy, E., Asa, S. L., and Kovacs, K., The influence of pituitary hormones on adjuvant arthritis, *Arthritis Rheum.,* 27, 682, 1984.

31. Grossman, C. J., Sholiton, L. J., and Nathan, P., Rat thymic estrogen receptor. I. Preparation, location and physiochemical properties, *J. Steroid Biochem.,* 11, 1233, 1979.

32. Grossman, C. J., Sholiton, L. J., Blaha, G. C., and Nathan, P., Rat thymic estrogen receptor. II. Physiological properties, *J. Steroid Biochem.,* 11, 1233, 1979.

33. Ranelletti, F. O., Carmignani, M., Marchetti, P., Natoli, C., and Ianobelli, S., Estrogen binding by neoplastic human thymus cytosol, *Eur. J. Cancer,* 16, 951, 1980.

34. Malacarne, P., Piffanelli, A., Indelli, M., Fumero, S., Mondino, A., Gionchiglia, E., and Silvestri, S., Estradiol binding in rat thymus cells, *Hormone Res.,* 12, 224, 1980.

35. Imanishi, Y., Seiki, K., and Haruki, Y., Cytoplasmic estrogen receptor in castrated rat thymus, *Endocrinol. Jpn.,* 27, 395, 1980.

36. Barr, I. G., Khalid, B. A. K., Pearce, P., Toh, B.-H., Bartlett, P. F., Scollary, R. G., and Funder, J. W., Dihydrotestosterone and estradiol deplete corticosensitive thymocytes lacking in receptors for these hormones, *J. Immunol.,* 128, 2825, 1982.

37. Raveche, E. S., Vigersky, R. A., Rice, M. K., and Steinberg, A. D., Murine thymic androgen receptors, *J. Immunopharmacol.,* 2, 425, 1980.

38. Sasson, S. and Mayer, M., Effect of androgenic steroids on rat thymus and thymocytes in suspension, *J. Steroid Biochem.,* 14, 509, 1981.

39. Kaiser, N., Mayer, M., Miholland, R. J., and Rosen, F., Studies of the antiglucocorticoid action of progesterone in rat thymocytes: early *in vitro* effects, *J. Steroid Biochem.,* 10, 379, 1979.

40. Szenberg, A., Influence of testosterone on the primary lymphoid organs of the chicken, in *Hormones and the Immune Response,* CIBA Study Group No. 36, Wolstenholme, G. E. and Knight, J., Eds., Churchill Livingstone, London, 1970, 42.

41. Glick, B. and Schwarz, M. R., Thymidine and testosterone incorporation by bursal and thymic lymphocytes, *Immunol. Commun.,* 4, 123, 1975.

42. Sullivan, D. A. and Wira, C. R., Sex hormone and glucocorticoid receptors in the bursa of Fabricius of immature chicks, *J. Immunol.,* 122, 2617, 1979.

43. Coulson, P. B., Thornthwaite, J. T., Skafar, D. F., and Seaver, S. S., Modulation of glucocorticoid hormone receptor levels in chicken lymphoid tissue following treatment with androgens *in vivo, J. Steroid Biochem.,* 17, 1, 1982.

44. Cohen, J. H. M., Danel, L., Cordier, G., Saez, S., and Revillard, J.-P., Sex steriod receptors in peripheral T cells: absence of androgen receptors and restriction of estrogen receptors to OKT8-positive cells, *J. Immunol.,* 131, 2767, 1983.

45. Nicoletti, G., Nanni, P., De Giovanni, C., Galli, M. C., Lollini, P. L. Prodi, G., Gobbi, M., Bartolis, M. S., and Grilli, S., Evidence of a progestin binding protein in mononuclear cells from peripheral blood of patients with leukaemia or normal donors, *J. Exp. Clin. Cancer Res.,* 2, 423, 1983.

46. Geuskens, M. and Uriel, J., *In Vitro* binding of oestradiol and notadrenaline to rat tissue eosinophils. Combined ultrastructural localization of tritiated oestradiol and peroxidase activity in their specific granules, *Biol. Cell,* 34, 237, 1979.

47. Lyttle, C. R., Medlock, K. L., and Sheehan, D. M., Eosinophils as the source of uterine nuclear type II estrogen binding sites, *J. Biol. Chem.,* 259, 2697, 1984.

48. Cohn, D. A., High sensitivity to androgen as a contributing factor in sex differences in the immune response, *Arthritis Rheum.,* 22, 1218, 1979.

49. Butterworth, M., MacClellan, B., and Allansmith, M., Influence of sex on immunoglobulin levels, *Nature (London),* 214, 1224, 1967.

50. Stewart, C. C., Farshy, C. E., and Reimer, C. B., The relationship of race, sex and age to concentrations of serum immunoglobulins expressed in international units in healthy adults in the USA, *Bull. WHO* 52, 179, 1975.

51. Roach, B., Kim, Y., Jerone, E., and Michael, A. F., Influence of age and sex on serum complement components in children, *Am. J. Dis. Child.,* 135, 918, 1981.

52. Roos, M. H. and Demant, P., Murine complement factor B (BF): sexual dimorphism and H-2-linked polymorphism, *Immunogenetics,* 15, 23, 1982.

53. Terres, G., Morrison, S. L., and Habricht, G. S., A quantitative difference in the immune response between male and female mice, *Proc. Soc. Exp. Biol. Med.,* 127, 664, 1968.

54. Tartakovsky, P., De Baetselier, P., Feldman, M., and Segal, S., Sex-associated differences in the immune response against fetal major histocompatibility antigens, *Transplantation,* 32, 395, 1981.

55. Dube, V. E., Tanaka, M., Chmiel, J., and Anderson, B., Effect of ABO group, secretor status and sex on cold hemagglutinins in normal adults, *Vox Sang.,* 46, 75, 1984.

56. Shear, H. L., Wofsy, D., and Talal, N., Effects of castration and sex hormones on immune clearance and autoimmune disease in MRL/Mp-1pr/1pr and MRL/Mp-+/+ mice, *Clin. Immunol. Immunopathol.,* 26, 361, 1983.

57. Kelley, V. E. and Winkelstein, A., Age and sex-related glomerulonephritis in New Zealand white mice, *Clin. Immunol. Immunopathol.,* 16, 142, 1980.

58. Chassoux, D., Dokhelar, M. C., Tursz, T., and Salomon, J. C., Antibody-dependent cellular cytotoxicity and natural killing in nude rats: quantitative study according to age and sex, *Ann. Immunol. Inst. Pasteur,* D134, 309, 1983.

59. Weinstein, Y., Ran, S., and Segal, S., Sex associated differences in the regulation of immune responses controlled by the MHC of the mouse, *J. Immunol.,* 132, 656, 1984.

60. Borel, Y. and Stollar, B. D., Strain and sex dependence of carrier-determined immunologic tolerance to guanosine, *Eur. J. Immunol.,* 9, 166, 1979.

61. Anderson, J. R., Buchanan, W. W., and Goudie, R. B., *Autoimmunity. Clinical and Experimental,* Charles C Thomas, Springfield, Ill., 1967.

62. Dubois, A. L., *Lupus Erythematosus,* 2nd ed., Dubois, E. L., Ed., University of Southern California Press, Los Angeles, 1974, 232.

63. Zvaifler, N. J., Rheumatoid arthritis, in *Autoimmunity. Genetic, Immunologic, Virological and Clinical Aspects,* Talal, N., Ed., Academic Press, New York, 1977, 569.

64. Stern, R., Fishman, J., Brusman, H., and Kunkel, H. G., Systemic lupus erythematosus associated with Klinefelter's syndrome, *Arthritis Rheum.,* 20, 18, 1977.

65. Lahita, R. G., Bradlow, H. L., Fishman, J., and Kunkel, H. G., Estogen metabolism in systemic lupus erythematosus: patients and family members, *Arthritis Rheum.,* 25, 843, 1982.

66. Lahita, R. G., Kunkel, H. G., and Bradlow, H. L., Increased oxidation of testosterone in systemic lupus erythematosus, *Arthritis Rheum.,* 26, 1517, 1983.

67. Inman, R. D., Jovanovic, L., Markenson, J. A., Longcope, C., Dawood, M. Y., and Lockshin, M. D., Systemic lupus erythematosus in men: genetic and endocrine features, *Arch Intern. Med.,* 142, 1813, 1982.

68. Jungers, P., Nahoul, K., Pelissier, C., Dougados, M., Tron, F., and Bach, J.-F., Low plasma androgens in women with active or quiescent systemic lupus erythematosus, *Arthritis Rheum.,* 25, 454, 1982.

69. Jungers, P., Dougados, M., Pelissier, C., Kuttenn, F., Tron, F., Lesavre, P., and Bach, J.-F., Influence of oral contraceptive therapy on the activity of systemic lupus erythematosus, *Arthritis Rheum.,* 25, 618, 1982.

70. Vandenbroucke, J. P., Valkenburg, H. A., Boersma, J. W., Cats, A., Festen, J. J. M., Huber-Bruning, O., and Rasker, J. J., Oral contraceptives and rheumatoid arthritis: further evidence for a preventive effect, *Lancet,* II, 839, 1982.

71. Talal, N., Sex steroid hormones and systemic lupus erythematosus, *Arthritis Rheum.,* 24, 1054, 1981.

72. Eisenberg, R. A., Izui, S., McConahey, P. J., Hang, L., Peters, C. J., Theofilopoulos, A. N., and Dixon, F. J., Male determined accelerated autoimmune disease in BXSB mice: transfer by bone marrow and spleen cells, *J. Immunol.*, 125, 1032, 1980.

73. Golding, B., Golding, H., Foiles, P. G., and Morton, J. I., CBA/N X-Linked defect delays expression of the Y-linked accelerated autoimmune disease in BXSB mice, *J. Immunol.*, 130, 1043, 1983.

74. Rosenberg, Y. J. and Steinberg, A. D., Influence of Y and X chromosomes on B cell responses in autoimmune prone mice, *J. Immunol.*, 132, 1261, 1984.

75. Milich, D. R. and Gershwin, M. E., Murine autoimmune hemolytic anemia induced via xenogenic erythrocyte immunization. III. Influences of sex, *Clin. Immunol. Immunopathol.*, 18, 1, 1981.

76. Gorczynski, R. M., Autoreactivity developing spontaneously in cultured mouse spleen cells. II. Comparison of cytotoxicity of cultured male and female spleen cells, *Immunology*, 31, 615, 1976.

77. Keith, A. B., Sex difference in Lewis rats in the incidence of recurrent experimental allergic encephalomyelitis, *Nature (London)*, 272, 824, 1978.

78. Castro, J. E., Orchidectomy and the immune response. I. Effect of orchidectomy on lymphoid tissues of mice, *Proc. R. Soc. London Ser. B*, 185, 425, 1974.

79. Mickova, M., The effect of orchiectomy on the manifestation of Thy-1^b (θ-C3H) antigen in H62 congenic mouse strains, *Folia Biol. (Prague)*, 20, 343, 1974.

80. Gillette, S. and Gillette, R. W., Changes in thymic estrogen receptor expression following orchidectomy, *Cell. Immunol.*, 42, 194, 1979.

81. Dumont, F., Barrois, R., and Habbersett, R. S., Prepubertal orchidectomy induces thymic abnormalities in aging (NZB X SJL)F$_1$ male mice, *J. Immunol.*, 129, 1642, 1982.

82. Dumont, F., Habbersett, R. C., and Monier, J.-C., Thymic abnormalities induced by castration in aged (NZB X SJL)F$_1$ male mice: distinct effects of early and late castration, *Clin. Immunol. Immunopathol.*, 27, 56, 1983.

83. Graff, R. J., Lappé, M. A., and Snell, G. D., The influence of the gonads and adrenal glands on the immune response to skin grafts, *Transplantation*, 1, 105, 1969.

84. Castro, J. E., Orchidectomy and the immune response. II. Response of orchidectomized mice to antigens, *Proc. R. Soc. London Ser. B*, 185, 437, 1974.

85. Lord, B. I. and Murphy, M. J., Jr., The estrous cycle and the hemopoietic stem cell in the mouse, *Blood*, 40, 390, 1972.

86. Adler, S. S., and Trobaugh, F. E., Effects of estrogen on erythropoiesis and granuloid progenitor cell (CFU-C) proliferation in mice, *J. Lab. Clin. Med.*, 91, 960, 1978.

87. Barr, I. G., Pyke, K. W., Pearce, P., Toh, B. -H., and Funder, J. W., Thymic sensitivity to sex hormones develops post-natally; an *in vivo* and an *in vitro* study, *J. Immunol.*, 132, 1095, 1984.

88. McDermott, M. R., Clark, D. A., and Bienenstock, J., Evidence for a common mucosal immunologic system. II. Influence of the estrous cycle on B immunoblast migration into genital and intestinal tissues, *J. Immunol.*, 124, 2536, 1980.

89. Krzych, U., Strausser, H. R., Bressler, J. P., and Goldstein, A. L., Quantitative differences in immune responses during the various stages of the estrous cycle in female BALB/c mice, *J. Immunol.*, 121, 1603, 1978.

90. Krzych, U., Strausser, H. R., Bressler, J. P., and Goldstein, A. L., Effects of sex hormones on some T and B cell functions, evidenced by differential immune expression between male and female mice and cyclic pattern of immune responsiveness during the estrous cycle in female mice, *Am. J. Reprod. Immunol.*, 1, 73, 1981.

91. Stern, K. and Davidsohn, I., Effect of estrogen and cortisone on immune hemoantibodies in mice of inbred strains, *J. Immunol.*, 75, 479, 1955.

92. Warr, G. W. and Šljivić, V., Stilbestrol-induced depression of the antibody response, *Experientia*, 28, 1356, 1972.

93. Boorman, G. A., Luster, M. I., Dean, J. H., and Wilson, R. E., The effect of adult exposure to diethylstilbestrol in the mouse on macrophage function and numbers, *J. Reticuloendothel. Soc.*, 28, 547, 1980.

94. Luster, M. I., Boorman, G. A., Dean, J. H., Luebke, R. W., and Lawson, L. D., The effect of adult exposure to diethylstilbestrol in the mouse: alterations in immunological functions, *J. Reticuloendothel. Soc.*, 28, 561, 1980.

95. Loose, L. D. and Di Luzio, N. R., Dose-related reticuloendothelial system stimulation by diethylstilbestrol, *J. Reticuloendothel. Soc.*, 20, 457, 1976.

96. Šljivić, V. A., Clark, D. W., and Warr, G. W., Effects of oestrogens and pregnancy on the distribution of sheep erythrocytes and the antibody response in mice, *Clin. Exp. Immunol.*, 20, 179, 1975.

97. Kalland, T., Alterations of antibody response in female mice after neonatal exposure to diethylstilbestrol, *J. Immunol.*, 124, 194, 1980.

98. Kalland, T. and Forsberg, J.-G., Delayed hypersensitivity to oxazolone in neonatally estrogenized mice, *Cancer Lett.*, 4, 141, 1978.

99. Luster, M. I., Faith, R. E., McLachlan, J., and Clark, G. C., Effect of in utero exposure to diethyl-stilbestrol on the immune response in mice, *Toxicol. Appl. Pharmacol.*, 47, 279, 1979.

100. Simmons, R. L., Price, A. L., and Ozerkis, A. L., The immunologic problem of pregnancy. V. The effect of estrogen and progesterone on allograft survival, *Am. J. Obstet. Gynecol.*, 100, 908, 1968.

101. Pavia, C. S., Siiteri, P. K., Perman, J. D., and Stites, D. P., Suppression of murine allogeneic cell interactions by sex hormones, *J. Reprod. Immunol.*, 1, 33, 1979.

102. Seaman, W. E. and Gindhart, T. D., Effect of estrogen on natural killer cells, *Arthritis Rheum.*, 22, 1234, 1979.

103. Seaman, W. E., Blackman, M. A., Gindhart, T. D., Roubinian, J. R., Loeb, J. M., and Talal, N., β-Estradiol reduces natural killer cells in mice, *J. Immunol.*, 121, 2193, 1978.

104. Seaman, W. E., Gindhart, T. D., Greenspan, J. S., Blackman, M. A., and Talal, N., Natural killer cells, bone, and the bone marrow: studies in estrogen-treated mice and in congenitally osteopetrotic (mi/mi) mice, *J. Immunol.*, 122, 2541, 1979.

105. Milisauskas, V. K., Cudkowicz, G., and Nakamura, I., Role of suppressor cells in the decline of natural killer cell activity in estrogen-treated mice, *Cancer Res.*, 43, 5240, 1983.

106. Hanna, N. and Schneider, M., Enhancement of tumor metastasis and suppression of natural killer cell activity by β-estradiol treatment, *J. Immunol.*, 130, 974, 1983.

107. Kalland, T. and Forsberg, J.-G., Permanent inhibition of capping of spleen lymphocytes from neo-natally oestrogen-treated female mice, *Immunology*, 39, 281, 1980.

108. Kalland, T. and Forsberg, J.-G., Natural killer cell activity and tumor susceptibilty in female mice treated neonatally with diethylstilbestrol, *Cancer Res.*, 41, 5134, 1981.

109. Kalland, T., Reduced natural killer activity in female mice after neonatal exposure to diethylstilbes-trol, *J. Immunol.*, 124, 1297, 1980.

110. Kalland, T., Strand, O., and Forsberg, J.-G., Long-term effects of neonatal estrogen treatment on mitogen responsiveness of mouse spleen lymphocystes, *J. Natl. Cancer Inst.*, 63, 413, 1979.

111. Sfikakis, A., Sfikakis, P., and Varonos, D., Oestradiol induced interaction between adrenals and thymus in the female rat, *Acta Endocrinol.*, 98, 41, 1981.

112. Morgan, J. I. and Perris, A. D., The influence of sex steroids on calcium- and magnesium-induced mitogenesis in isolated rat thymic lymphocytes, *J. Cell. Physiol.*, 83, 287, 1974.

113. Grossman, C. J., Sholition, L. J., and Roselle, G. A., Estradiol regulation of thymic lymphocyte function in the rat: mediation by serum thymic factors, *J. Steroid Biochem.*, 16, 683, 1982.

114. Wira, C. R. and Sandoe, C. P., Sex steroid hormone regulation of IgA and IgG in rat uterine secre-tions, *Nature (London)*, 268, 534, 1977.

115. Wira, C. R. and Sandoe, C. P., Hormonal regulation and immunoglobulins — influence of estradiol on immunoglobulin-A and immunoglobulin-G in the rat uterus, *Endocrinology*, 106, 1020, 1980.

116. Sullivan, D. A. and Wira, C. R., Hormonal regulation of immunoglobulins in the rat uterus: uterine response to a single estradiol treatment, *Endocrinology*, 112, 260, 1983.

117. Sullivan, D. A. and Wira, C. R., Estradiol regulation of secretory component in the rat uterus, in *The Secretory Immune System*, McGhee, J. R. and Mestecky, J., Eds., *Ann. N.Y. Acad. Sci.*, 409, 882, 1983.

118. Sullivan, D. A. and Wira, C. R., Hormonal regulation of immunoglobulins in the rat uterus: uterine response to multiple estradiol treatments, *Endocrinology*, 114, 650, 1984.

119. Wira, C. R., Sullivan, D. A., and Dandoe, C. P., Epithelial cell involvement in the estradiol-stimu-lated accumulation of IgA in the rat uterus, *J. Steroid Biochem.*, 19, 469, 1983.

120. Wira, C. R., Sullivan, D. A., and Sandoe, C. P., Estrogen-mediated control of the secretory immune system in the uterus of the rat, in *The Secretory Immune System*, McGhee, J. R., and Mestecky, J., Eds., *Ann. N.Y. Acad. Sci.*, 409, 534, 1983.

121. Posner, B. I., Kelly, P. A., Shiu, R. P. C., and Friesen, H. G., Studies of insulin, growth hormone and prolactin binding: tissue distribution, species variation and characterization, *Endocrinology*, 95, 521, 1974.

122. Aragona, C., Bohnet, H. G., and Friesen, H. G., Localization of prolactin binding in prostate and testis: the role of serum, prolactin concentration on the testicular LH receptor, *Acta Endocrinol.*, 84, 402, 1977.

123. Dunaif, A. E., Zimmerman, E. A., Friesen, H. G., and Frantz, A. G., Intracellular localization of prolactin receptor and prolactin in the rat ovary by immunocytochemistry, *Endocrinology*, 110, 1465, 1982.

124. Dorrington, J. and Gore-Langton, R. E., Prolactin inhibits oestrogen synthesis in the ovary, *Nature (London)*, 290, 600, 1981.

125. Veldhuis, J. D. and Hammond, J. M., Oestrogens regulate divergent effects of prolactin in the ovary, *Nature (London)*, 284, 262, 1980.

126. Seppälä, M., Prolactin and female reproduction, *Ann. Clin. Res.*, 10, 164, 1978.

127. Amenomori, Y., Chen, C. L., and Meites, J., Serum prolactin levels in rats during different repro-ductive states, *Endocrinology*, 86, 506, 1970.

128. Gooren, J. E., van der Veen, E. A., van Kessel, H., Harmsen-Louman, W., and Wiegel, A. R., Prolactin secretion in the human male is increased by endogenous oestrogens and decreased by exogenous/endogenous androgens, *Int. J. Androl.,* 7, 53, 1984.
129. Barbarino, A., De Marinis, L., Mancini, A., and Farabegoli, C., Estrogen-dependent plasma prolactin response to gonadotropin-releasing hormone in intact and castrated men, *J. Clin. Endocrinol. Metab.,* 55, 1212, 1982.
130. Ahmed, S. A., Young, P. R., and Penhale, W. J., The effects of female sex steroids on the development of autoimmune thyroiditis in thymectomized and irradiated rats, *Clin. Exp. Immunol.,* 54, 351, 1983.
131. Kameswaran, L., Krishna, N. M., Gopal, N. N., Nareshkumar, M. P., Parvathavarthini, S., and Subramanian, C. N., Study of hormonal influences on mast cells in rats, *Indian J. Med. Res.,* 67, 795, 1978.
132. Trottier, R. W., Moore, E., McMillan, J., and Evans, N., Hormonal manipulation of carrageenin-induced pyresis in rats, *Experientia,* 33, 639, 1977.
133. Screpanti, I., Gulino, A., and Pasqualini, J. R., The fetal thymus of guinea pig as an estrogen target organ, *Endocrinology,* 111, 1552, 1982.
134. Gulino, A., Screpanti, I., and Pasqualini, J. R., Estrogen and antiestrogen effects on different lymphoid cell populations in the developing fetal thymus of guinea pig, *Endocrinology,* 113, 1754, 1983.
135. Revell, P. A., Kurloff cell levels in peripheral blood of normal and oestrogen treated guinea pigs, *Br. J. Exp. Pathol.,* 55, 525, 1974.
136. Feigen, G. A., Fraser, R. C., Peterson, N. S., and Dandliker, W. B., Sex hormones and the immune response. I. Host factors in the production of penicillin-specific antibodies in the female guinea pig, *Int. Arch. Allergy Appl. Immunol.,* 57, 385, 1978.
137. Feigen, G. A., Fraser, R. C., and Peterson, N. S., Sex hormones and the immune response. II. Perturbation of antibody production by estradiol 17β, *Int. Arch. Allergy Appl. Immunol.,* 57, 488, 1978.
138. Ozkaragoz, I., Quantitative experiments on the effect of estrogen on the response of guinea pig ileum and uterus to specific antigens, *Acta Allergol.,* 25, 271, 1970.
139. Kitzmiller, J. L. and Rocklin, R. E., Lack of suppression of lymphocyte MIF production by estradiol, progesterone and human chorionic gonadotropin, *J. Reprod. Immunol.,* 1, 97, 1980.
140. Mathur, S., Mathur, R. S., Goust, J. M., Williamson, H. O., and Fudenberg, H. H., Cyclic variations in white cell subpopulations in the human menstrual cycle: correlations with progesterone and estradiol, *Clin. Immunol. Immunopathol.,* 13, 246, 1979.
141. Souweine, G., Danel, L., Costa, O., Tubiana, N., Martin, P., Monier, M. C., and Saez, S., Effect of physiological concentrations of sex hormones on the formation of early sheep red blood cell rosettes by human lymphocytes: possible relations with the presence of sex-hormone-cytosol-receptors in lymphocytes, *Biomed. Express,* 33, 150, 1980.
142. Hill, A. and Wolff, S., Sister chromatid exchanges and cell division delays induced by diethylstilbestrol, estradiol and estriol in human lymphocytes, *Cancer Res.,* 43, 4114, 1983.
143. Davis, K. P., Maciulla, G. J., Yannone, M. E., Gooch, G. T., Lox, C. D., and Whetstone, M. R., Cervical mucus immunoglobulins as an indicator of ovulation, *Obstet. Gynecol.,* 62, 388, 1983.
144. Mathur, S., Mathur, R. S., Goust, J. M., Williamson, H. O., and Fudenberg, H. H., Sex steroid hormones and circulating IgE levels, *Clin. Exp. Immunol.,* 30, 403, 1977.
145. Ablin, R. J., Bruns, G. R., Guinan, P., and Bush, I. M., Antiandrogenic suppression of lymphocytic blastogenesis: in vitro and in vivo observations, *Experientia,* 30, 1351, 1974.
146. Ablin, R. J., Bruns, G. R., Guinan, P., and Bush, I. M., The effect of estrogen on the incorporation of ³H-thymidine by PHA-stimulated human peripheral blood lymphocytes, *J. Immunol.,* 113, 705, 1974.
147. Mendelsohn, J., Multer, M. M., and Bernheim, J. L., Inhibition of human lymphocyte stimulation by steroid hormones: cytokinetic mechanisms, *Clin. Exp. Immunol.,* 27, 127, 1977.
148. Wyle, F. A. and Kent, J. R., Immunosuppression by sex steroid hormones. I. The effect upon PHA- and PPD-stimulated lymphocytes, *Clin. Exp. Immunol.,* 27, 407, 1977.
149. Clemens, L. E., Siiteri, P. K., and Stites, D. P., Mechanism of immunosuppression of progesterone on maternal lymphocyte activation during pregnancy, *J. Immunol.,* 122, 1978, 1979.
150. Paavonen, T., Andersson, L. C., and Adlercruetz, H., Sex hormone regulation of in vitro immune response: estradiol enhances human B cell maturation via inhibition of suppressor T cells in pokeweed mitogen-stimulated cultures, *J. Exp. Med.,* 154, 1935, 1981.
151. Schiff, R. I., Mercier, D., and Buckley, R. H., Inability of gestational hormones to account for the inhibitory effects of pregnancy plasmas on lymphocyte responses in vitro, *Cell. Immunol.,* 20, 69, 1975.
152. Harty, J. I., Catalona, W. J., and Gomolka, D. M., Modification of lymphocyte responsiveness by hormones used in treatment of urologic malignancies, *J. Urol.,* 116, 484, 1976.

153. Helgason, S. and Vonschoultz, B., Estrogen replacement therapy and the mixed lymphocyte reaction, *Am. J. Obstet. Gynecol.,* 141, 393, 1981.

154. Stimson, W. H. and Hunter, I. C., Oestrogen-induced immunoregulation mediated through the thymus, *J. Clin. Lab. Immunol.,* 4, 27, 1980.

155. Schreiber, A. D., Parsons, J., McDermott, P., and Cooper, R. A., Effect of corticosteroids on human monocyte IgG and complement receptors, *J. Clin. Invest.,* 56, 1189, 1975.

156. Klebanoff, S. J., Estrogen binding by leukocytes during phagocytosis, *J. Exp. Med.,* 145, 983, 1977.

157. Ambrus, M. S. and Ambrus, J. L., Effect of estrogens on the mast cell degranulating action of compound 48/80, *J. Med.,* 3, 321, 1972.

158. Peetoom, J., Ruitenberg, E. J., Kroes, R., and Berkvens, J. M., Influence of estrogens on the immune response, *Zentralbl. Veterinaermed. B.,* 17, 989, 1970.

159. Molinari, P. F., Erythropoietic mechanisms of androgens: a critical review and clinical implications, *Haematologica,* 67, 442, 1982.

160. Weinstein, Y. and Isakov, Y., Effects of testosterone metabolites and of anabolic androgens on the bone marrow and thymus in castrated female mice, *Immunopharmacology,* 5, 229, 1983.

161. Dorner, G., Eckert, R., and Hinz, G., Androgen-dependent sexual dimorphism of the immune system, *Endocrinologie,* 76, 112, 1980.

162. Fujii, H., Nawa, Y., Tsuchiya, H., Matsuno, K., Fukumoto, T., Fukuda, S., and Kotani, M., Effect of a single administration of testosterone on the immune response and lymphoid tissues in mice, *Cell. Immunol.,* 20, 315, 1975.

163. Cohn, D. A. and Hamilton, J. B., Sensitivity to androgen and the immune response: immunoglobulin levels in two strains of mice, one with high and one with low target organ responses to androgen, *J. Reticuloendothel. Soc.,* 20, 1, 1976.

164. Morton, J. I., Weyant, D. A., Siegel, B. V., and Golding, B., Androgen sensitivity and autoimmune disease. I. Influence of sex and testosterone on the humoral immune response of autoimmune and non-immune mouse strains to sheep erythrocytes, *Immunology,* 44, 661, 1981.

165. Rembiesa, R., Ptak, W., and Bubak, M., The immunosuppressive effects of mouse placental steroids, *Experientia,* 30, 82, 1974.

166. Weinstein, Y. and Berkovich, Z., Testosterone effect on bone marrow, thymus and suppressor T cells in the (NZB X NZW)F$_1$ mice: its relevance to autoimmunity, *J. Immunol.,* 126, 998, 1981.

167. Laskin, C. A., Taurog, J. D., Smathers, P. A., and Steinberg, A. D., Studies of defective tolerance in murine lupus, *J. Immunol.,* 127, 1743, 1981.

168. Viklický, V., Polačková, M., Vojtíšková, M., Dráber, P., and Khoda, M. E., Immunosuppressive effect of an antiandrogenic steroid (cyproterone acetate) in mice, *Folia Biol.(Prague),* 23, 145, 1977.

169. DiBenedetto, J., Jr., Higby, D. J., Chester, S. J., and Albala, M. M., Reversal of cyclophosphamide induced neutropenia by hypertransfusion and androgen therapy, *J. Med.,* 11, 385, 1980.

170. Klein, J., *Biology of Mouse Histocompatibility-2 Complex,* Springer-Verlag, Basel, 1975.

171. Ferreira, A., Weisz-Carrington, P., and Nussenzweig, V., Testosterone control of serum levels of C4-binding protein in mice, *J. Immunol.,* 121, 1213, 1978.

172. Sholiton, L. J., Grossman, C. J., and Taylor, B. B., Rat thymic homogenates convert testosterone to androgenic metabolites, *J. Steroid Biochem.,* 13, 1365, 1980.

173. Horn, Y., A comparison of two androgenic hormones as leukopoietic agents in irradiated rats, *Oncology,* 26, 16, 1972.

174. Frey-Wettstein, M. and Craddock, C. G., Testosterone-induced depletion of thymus and marrow lymphocytes as related to lymphopoieis and hematopoiesis, *Blood,* 35, 257, 1970.

175. Sullivan, D. A., Bloch, K. J., and Allansmith, M. R., Hormonal influence on the secretory immune system of the eye: androgen regulation of secretory component levels in rat tears, *J. Immunol.,* 132, 1130, 1984.

176. Selye, H., Morphological changes in the fowl following chronic overdosage with various steroids, *J. Morphol.,* 73, 401, 1943.

177. Meyer, R. K., Rao, M. A., and Aspinall, R. L., Inhibition of the development of the bursa of Fabricius in the embryos of the common fowl by 19-nortestosterone, *Endocrinology,* 64, 890, 1959.

178. Mueller, A. P., Wolfe, H. R., and Meyer, R. K., Hormonal bursectomy in chickens, *J. Immunol.,* 85, 172, 1960.

179. Szenberg, A. and Warner, N. L., Dissociation of immunological responsiveness in fowls with hormonally arrested development of lymphoid tissue, *Nature (London),* 194, 146, 1962.

180. Warner, N. L., Uhr, J. W., Thorbecke, G. J., and Ovary, Z., Immunoglobulins, antibodies and the bursa of Fabricius: induction of agammaglobulinemia and the loss of all antibody forming capacity by hormonal bursectomy, *J. Immunol.,* 103, 1317, 1969.

181. Hirota, Y., Suzuki, T., and Bito, Y., The development of unusual B-cell functions in the testosterone-propionate-treated chicken, *Immunology,* 39, 29, 1980.

182. Hirota, Y., Suzuki, T., and Bito, Y., The B-cell development independent of the bursa of Fabricius but dependent upon the thymus in chickens treated with testosterone propionate, *Immunology*, 39, 37, 1980.

183. Milewich, L., Whisenant, M. G., and Sawyer, M. K., Androstenedione metabolism by human lymphocytes, *J. Steroid Biochem.*, 16, 81, 1982.

184. Milewich, L., Kaimal, V., and Toews, G. B., Androstenedione metabolism in human alveolar macrophages, *J. Clin. Endocrinol. Metab.*, 56, 920, 1983.

185. Holdstock, G., Chastenay, B. F., and Krawitt, E. L., Effects of testosterone, oestradiol and progesterone on immune regulation, *Clin. Exp. Immunol.*, 47, 449, 1982.

186. Rosen F. S., Hormonal treatment of hereditary angioneurotic oedema: an important use of anabolic steroids, *Clin. Immunol. Allergy*, 3, 259, 1983.

187. Ahn, Y. S., Harrington, W. J., Simon, S. R., Mylvaganam, R., Pall, L. M., and So, A. G., Danazol for the treatment of idiopathic thrombocytopenic purpura, *N. Engl. J. Med.*, 308, 1396, 1983.

188. Vojtíšková, M., Polačková, M., Viklický, V., and Pokorná, Z., Immunosuppressive and contraceptive effects of testosterone and cyproterone acetate in guinea pigs, *Immunol. Lett.*, 1, 53, 1979. *Lett.*, 1, 53, 1979.

189. O'Hearn, M. and Stites, D. P., Inhibition of murine suppressor cell function by progesterone, *Cell. Immunol.*, 76, 340, 1983.

190. Szekeres, J., Csernus, V., Pejtsik, S., Emody, L., and Pacsa, A. S., Progesterone as an immunologic blocking factor in human pregnancy serum, *J. Reprod. Immunol.*, 3, 333, 1981.

191. Mori, T., Kobayashi, H., Nishimura, T., Mori, T. S., Fujii, G., and Inou, T., Inhibitory effect of progesterone on the phytohaemagglutinin-induced transformation of human peripheral lymphocytes, *Immunol. Commun.*, 4, 519, 1975.

192. Neifeld, J. P. and Tormey, D. C., Effects of steroid hormones on phytohemagglutinin-stimulated human peripheral blood lymphocytes, *Transplantation*, 27, 309, 1979.

193. Munroe, J. S. and Windle, W. F., Tumors induced by chicken sarcoma in monkeys conditioned with progesterone, *Nature (London)*, 216, 811, 1967.

194. Munroe, J. S., Progesteroids as immunosuppressive agents, *J. Reticuloendothel. Soc.*, 9, 361, 1971.

195. Turcotte, J. G., Haines, R. F., Niederhuber, J. E., and Gikas, P. W., Allograft prolongation with synthetic progestins, *Transplant. Proc.*, 3, 814, 1971.

196. Beaumont, J. L. and Beaumont, V., Immune reactivity and the vascular risk in oral contraceptive users, *Am. J. Reprod. Immunol.*, 1, 119, 1981.

197. Stimson, W. H., Identification of pregnancy-associated α-macroglobulin on the surface of peripheral blood leucocyte populations, *Clin. Exp. Immunol.*, 28, 445, 1977.

198. Chipperfield, E. J. and Evans, B. A., Effect of local infection and oral contraception on immunoglobulin levels in cervical mucus, *Infect. Immunity*, 11, 215, 1975.

199. Dwyer, J. M., Knox, G. E., and Mangi, R. J., Cell mediated immunity in healthy women taking oral contraceptives, *Yale J. Biol. Med.*, 48, 91, 1975.

200. Gerretsen, G., Kremer, J., Bleumink, E., and Nater, J. P., Dinitrochlorobenzene sensitization test in women on hormonal contraceptives, *Lancet*, II, 347, 1975.

201. Gerretsen, G., Kremer, J., Nater, J. P., Bleumink, E., de Gast, G. C., and The, T. H., Immune reactivity of women on hormonal contraceptives: dinitrochlorobenzene sensitization test and skin reactivity to irritants, *Contraception*, 19, 83, 1979.

202. Gerretsen, G., Kremer, J., Bleumink, E., Nater, J. P., de Gast, G. C., and The, T. H., Immune reactivity of women on hormonal contraceptives: phytohemagglutinin and concanavalin-A induced lymphocyte response, *Contraception*, 22, 25, 1980.

203. Fitzgerald, P. H., Pickering, A. F., and Ferguson, D. N., Depressed lymphocyte response to PHA in long-term users of oral contraceptives, *Lancet*, I, 615, 1973.

204. Barnes, E. W., MacCuish, A. C., Loudon, N. B., Jordan, J., and Irvine, W. J., Phytohaemagglutinin-induced lymphocyte transformation and circulating autoantibodies in women taking oral contraceptives, *Lancet*, I, 898, 1974.

205. Keller, A. J., Irvine, W. J., Jordan, J., and Loudon, N. B., Phytohemagglutin-induced lymphocyte transformation in oral contraceptive users, *Obstet. Gynecol.*, 49, 83, 1977.

206. Tezabwala, B. U., Hegde, U. C., Joshi, J. V., Jaswaney, V. L., and Rao, S. S., Studies on cell-mediated immunity in women using different fertility regulating methods, *J. Clin. Lab. Immunol.*, 10, 199, 1983.

207. Vecchi, A., Tagliabue, A., Mantovani, A., Anaclerio, A., Barale, C., and Spreafico, F., Steroid contraceptive agents and immunological reactivity in experimental animals, *Biomedicine*, 24, 231, 1976.

208. Alten, H. E. and Groscurth, P., The postnatal development of the ovary in the "nude" mouse, *Anat. Embryol.*, 148, 35, 1975.

209. Lintern-Moore, S. and Pantelouris, E. M., Ovarian development in athymic nude mice. I. The size and composition of the follicle population, *Mech. Age. Dev.*, 4, 385, 1975.

210. Lintern-Moore, S. and Pantelouris, E. M., Ovarian development in athymic nude mice. V. The effects of PMSG upon the numbers and growth of follicles in the early juvenile ovary, *Mech. Age. Dev.,* 5, 259, 1976.

211. Rebar, R. W., Morandini, I. C., Petze, J. E., and Erickson, G. F., Hormonal basis of reproductive defects in athymic mice: reduced gonadotropins and testosterone in males, *Biol. Reprod.,* 27, 1267, 1982.

212. Nishizuka, Y. and Sakakura, T., Thymus and reproduction: sex-linked dysgenesia of the gonad after neonatal thymectomy in mice, *Science,* 166, 753, 1969.

213. Nishizuka, Y. and Sakakura, T., Ovarian dysgenesis induced by neonatal thymectomy in the mouse, *Endocrinology,* 89, 886, 1971.

214. Sakakura, T. and Nishizuka, Y., Thymic control mechanism in ovarian development: reconstitution of ovarian dysgenesis in thymectomized mice by replacement with thymic and other lymphoid tissues, *Endocrinology,* 90, 431, 1972.

215. Bukovsky, A., Presl, J., Krabec, Z., and Bednarik, T., Ovarian function in adult rats treated with antithymocyte serum, *Experientia,* 33, 280, 1977.

216. Lintern-Moore, S., Effect of athymia on the initiation of follicular growth in the rat ovary, *Biol. Reprod.,* 17, 155, 1977.

217. Lipscomb, H. L. and Sharp, J. G., Thymectomy modifies androgenizing effects of a testis transplant during critical period for neuroprogramming, *Experientia,* 35, 842, 1979.

218. Rebar, R. W., Miyake, A., Low, T. L. K., and Goldstein, A. L., Thymosin stimulates secretion of luteinizing hormone-releasing factor, *Science,* 214, 669, 1981.

219. Allen, L. S., McClure, J. E., Goldstein, A. L., Barkley, M. S., and Michael, S. D., Estrogen and thymic hormone interactions in the female mouse, *J. Reprod. Immunol.,* 6, 25, 1984.

220. Pedernera, E. A., Romano, M., Besedovsky, H. O., and Del Carmen Aguilar, M., The bursa of Fabricius is required for normal endocrine development in chicken, *Gen. Comp. Endocrinol.,* 42, 413, 1980.

221. Romano, M., Aguilar, M. C., Mendez, M. C., and Pedernera, E., Bursa of Fabricius produces *in vitro,* a factor which inhibits the chorionic gonadotropin response of the newly hatched chick testis, *J. Steroid Biochem.,* 15, 429, 1981.

222. Kirsch, T. M., Vogel, R. L., and Flickinger, G. L., Macrophages: a source of luteotropic cybernins, *Endocrinology,* 113, 1910, 1983.

223. Dickman, W. J. and Cauchi, M. N., Lymphocyte induced stimulation of human chorionic gonadotrophin production by trophoblastic cells *in vitro, Nature (London),* 271, 377, 1978.

Chapter 8

THE PITUITARY THYROID AXIS

I. Berczi

TABLE OF CONTENTS

I. INTRODUCTION

The thyroid gland produces thyroxin (3,5,3′,5′-tetraiodo-L-thyronine or T_4), which is metabolized to triiodothyronine (3,5,,3′-triodo-L-thyronine or T_3), which is considered to be the biologically active form of thyroxin. Although thyroid hormones are very important for the normal maintenance of a variety of body functions, their mechanism of action is still in debate. In a recent review, Sterling[1] lists six different pathways of thyroid hormone action, for which at least some supportive experimental evidence exists. These are

1. Acting on nuclear transcription
2. Mitochondrial activation
3. Regulation of the sodium pump
4. Incorporation of thyroid hormones into thyrosin pathways
5. Acting through adrenergic receptors
6. Acting on the plasma membrane

Naturally, combinations of the above effects are also possible. More recently, Mariash and Oppenheimer[2] suggested that the primary action of T_3 at the molecular level is the multiplication of other nuclear signals.

In target tissues of thyroid hormone, cytoplasmic receptors of extremely high number (there are more than 20 million primary sites in the cytosol of rat liver cells) exist that interact with T_3 after the hormone is diffused or transported into the cell. However, these complexes are not translocated into the nucleus, but rather, the association is readily reversible, and a minute amount of intracellular T_3 remains unbound, which can interact with effector loci in the nucleus or in mitochondria. In addition to cytoplasmic receptors, there are indications that plasma membrane T_3 receptors also exist.

The liver, kidney, myocardium, skeletal muscle, lung, intestine, and adipose tissue do have mitochondrial receptors for thyroid hormones, and therefore, are classified as thyroid reactive tissues. On the other hand, the brain, spleen, and the testes are the so-called thyroid hormone unresponsive tissues, because they do not have such receptors and their oxygen consumption is unaffected by thyroid hormones.[1] To date, there is no compelling evidence for the existence of thyroid hormone receptors in lymphoid tissue.

II. THE EFFECT OF THYROID HORMONES ON IMMUNE PHENOMENA

A. Mouse

A significant hyperplasia of the thymus was observed in mice treated with T_3 during the 1st month of life. The number of thymic epithelial cells increased twofold after treatment, along with a similar increment of cortical volume and a 50% increase of medullar volume. Cortical epithelial cells increased at the same rate as the cortex, but medullary epithelial cells grew more rapidly and were mostly responsible for volume enlargement.[3] Young mice treated with T_3 had increased serum levels of thymic hormone (thymulin) and an increased number of thymulin containing cells in their thymuses.[4]

The immunodeficiency of pituitary dwarf Snell-Bagg mice could be reconstituted by injections of growth hormone and thyroxin. Neonatal thymectomy prevented such reconstitution.[5] Similar observations were made by Pierpaoli and co-workers.[6] Furthermore, these investigators treated mice with propyl-thiouracil, which caused changes in lymphoid tissues and impairment of the immune response. These effects could be reversed by growth hormone (GH) and thyroxin treatment.[6]

Mice were treated with thyroxin in order to accelerate their catabolism of antigen. Immune-type elimination was not observed during primary exposure, but treatment with the hormone predisposed the animals to immune elimination on second and third exposure to the antigen (^{131}I-bovine gammaglobulin). When the catabolism of the animals was slowed down by raising the ambient temperature, or by providing a high carbohydrate diet, less antibody was formed against BCG after the use of mycobacterial adjuvants, suggesting that these adjuvants are maximally effective when the antigen is catabolized rapidly.[7]

Both the peripheral lymphocyte counts and T cells were increased in mice treated with thyroxin for 3 months. Thymic incorporation of tritiated thymidine was also significantly increased. Furthermore, the rejection of Ehrlich carcinoma was significantly accelerated in such T-cell rich mice.[8] Thyroxin treated mice did not show a consistent increase in splenic anti-SRBC (sheep red blood cells) plaque-forming cells (PFC). However, the total number of spleen cells in thyroxin treated animals was decreased, and for this reason, the number of PFC/10^6 lymphocytes was higher than those of controls. In spite of this, spleen cells of thyroxin treated animals generated more PFC during the primary response to SRBC in vitro, than did control cells, and the calculated PFC/spleen was also higher. Moreover, the addition of thyroxin to normal splenic cell cultures enhanced their response to SRBC. The optimum concentration of thyroxin for in vitro immune response was found to be 10^{-8} M.[9] Triiodothyronine (5×10^{-9} M) augmented the response of murine lymphocytes to phytohemaglutinin (PHA). Higher concentrations were suppressive.[10] The antibody response (measured by PFC assay) was significantly suppressed in C57BL/6J mice treated with thyroxin (40 μg 5 times per week) for 30 days. Mitogenic responses of lymphocytes from treated animals to PHA and Con A were also suppressed. Mitogen responses returned to normal within 14 days after the discontinuation of the treatment. A prolonged survival of allogeneic skin grafts and suppression of delayed-type hypersensitive reactions in thyroxin-treated animals were also apparent.[11]

B. Rat

The administration of thyroxin to young rats resulted in a marked reduction of IgG transport from the gastrointestinal tract to the circulation.[12] Young rats, treated with T_3, had increased serum levels of thymic hormone (thymulin) and an increased number of thymulin containing cells in their thymuses.[4] Thymocytes from weanling rats were exposed to T_3 and their uptake of the glucose analogue, 2-deoxyglucose (2-DG), was measured. Significant stimulation of 2-DG accumulation was produced by T_3 concentrations ranging from 1 nM to 10 μM. Triiodothyronine also stimulated the uptake by thymocytes of the nonmetabolizable glucose analogue, 3-O-methylglucose. Inhibition of protein synthesis did not influence these effects of T_3.[13] Subsequent experiments revealed that T_3 and epinephrine are synergistic in increasing the accumulation of 2-DG in rat thymocytes. The preincubation of rat thymocytes with various catecholamines alone and together with T_3 led to the following conclusions with regards to the effect of these agents on sugar transport: catecholamines stimulate the accumulation of 2-DG through the β receptor; the synergistic interaction between T_3 and epinephrine involves both the β- and α-adrenergic receptors and the two agents act through a common or interrelated mechanism; and the effects of T_3 and epinephrine either alone or together are independent of new protein synthesis.[14]

Rats made hypothyroid (thyroidectomized or treated with 6-propyl-2-thiouracil — PTU) and hyperthyroid (by treatment with T_3 added to PTU in the drinking water) were studied in respect to total, helper, and suppressor T lymphocytes in blood and spleen. The cells and their subsets were identified with the aid of monoclonal antibodies. Hypothyroid rats had a decreased proportion of suppressor T cells in the spleen, but the number of suppressor T cells was increased in the blood. Treatment with T_3 prevented these alterations. No alterations of T cells were evident in animals treated with high doses of T_3 for 17 days.[15] The removal of the thyroid gland from newborn or from young adult rats caused a reduction in the number of peripheral blood lymphocytes and depression of the antibody response to SRBC or to chicken red blood cells and diminished response of spleen cells to PHA. Perinatally thyroidectomized rats exhibited these deficiencies after weaning, whereas in the animals thyroidectomized in young adult age, immunodepression was evident 45 to 60 days after the operation. In both cases daily injections with thyroxin could completely restore the immune system of thyroid deprived animals.[16] Thyroidectomy reduced the development of adjuvant induced-arthritic lesions in rats. The response was restored by treatment with T_3 or T_4.[17]

Our experiments showed that thyroid function is not essential for the reconstitution of immunocompetence in hypophysectomized rats. Treatment of Hypox animals with thyroid stimulating hormone (TSH) either alone, or in combination with various pituitary hormones, did not seem to affect immune reactivity.[18-20] However, our experiments were short-term (4 to 6 weeks duration) and thus, do not contradict the results of Fabris,[16] who observed immunodeficiency in thyroidectomized adult animals 45 to 60 days after surgery.

C. Chicken

Chicken embryos, 9-days old, were given spleen allografts in order to induce graft-vs.-host (GVH) reaction. Eight days after grafting the recipients developed mesenchymatous goiter, which was associated with decreased thyroid activity as revealed by a reduction of follicle numbers and a fall in T_4 levels. The authors suggested that the thyroid is a target organ of this immunological conflict.[21] During the primary response of chicken to SRBC, serum antibody titers and depression of serum T_3 levels were significantly correlated. Drug induced suppression of thyroid function inhibited the production of serum antibodies, both in the primary and secondary response to SRBC. However, serum antibody titers rose dramatically within 48 hr after cessation of treatment.[22]

D. Man

Human peripheral blood lymphocytes are capable of converting thyroxin to triiodothyronine, and there is no sex- or age-related difference in this respect.[23] The response of human T lymphocytes to Con A and PHA was not influenced by T_3, but the number of immunoglobulin containing and secreting cells was increased in pokeweed mitogen (PWM) and *S. aureus* stimulated cultures in the presence of T_3. Maximal enhancement was reached at T_3 concentrations of 10^{-9} to 10^{-7} M. Experiments with purified cell populations revealed that T_3 had a direct stimulatory effect on B cell differentiation.[24] Co-cultures of human monocytes with human thyroid cells enhanced the accumulation of prostaglandin E in the medium. Prostaglandin E synthesis was further stimulated if T lymphocytes were present in the culture.[25] Lysosomal acid lipase activity of mononuclear leukocytes in 31 children with various thyroid conditions was positively correlated with serum T_3 and T_4 levels and was significantly higher in hyperthyroid children than in those with hypothyroidism. Enzyme activity also increased significantly in five adult euthyroid males after treatment with 50 μg L-T_3 every 8 hr for 4 days.[26]

III. AUTOIMMUNE THYROID DISEASE

Autoimmune thyroid disease occurs frequently in man with female predominance. It also develops spontaneously in some strains of animals and it can be induced experimentally in laboratory rodents. Although the pathogenesis of the disease is complex and incompletely understood, pre-existing abnormalities in immunoregulation, controlled by genes of the major histocompatibility complex, appear to play a fundamental role.

Certain strains of mice and rats develop thyroiditis spontaneously after thymectomy, though whole body X-irradiation may also be required for the manifestation of the disease. These and numerous other observations indicate the importance of T cell-mediated immunoregulation in the control of thyroid reactive autoimmune clones. In addition to immune abnormalities, pre-existing thyroid abnormality was also observed in the obese strain of chicken. This strain develops spontaneously autoimmune thyroid disease.

In man, thyroid autoimmunity may be predominantly humoral (Graves') or cell-mediated (Hashimoto's) disease. In Graves' disease, antibodies are frequently directed against the TSH receptor and may cause hyperthyroidism through direct stimulation of hormone production, or may inhibit thyroid function through interference with TSH binding to the receptor. Euthyroidism can also occur, if the antibodies produced against the TSH receptor are neither stimulatory nor TSH-displacing.

There is a voluminous literature on the immune abnormalities of experimental and clinical autoimmune thyroid disease. However, these observations do not reveal the possible role of thyroid hormones in the regulation of immune reactions, because of the pre-existing and complex immunoregulatory and endocrine abnormalities that may be present. For this reason this subject will not be discussed here further, but rather, the interested reader is referred to reviews and book chapters on autoimmune thyroid disease.[27-39]

IV. IMMUNE FACTORS INFLUENCING THE TSH-THYROID AXIS

Daily administration of interferon to patients induced significant decreases in the circulating concentrations of T_3, T_4, and free T_4, whereas serum TSH levels were not affected. Interferon treatment had no effect on T_3 uptake, indicating that the decreased serum levels of thyroid hormones were not due to alterations in their binding to thyroxin binding globulin.[40]

The binding of TSH to human fat cell membranes was inhibited by human IgG. Preparations of IgG from sera of thyrotoxic and euthyroid subjects displaced TSH similarly when human fat cell membranes were used. However, on human thyroid membranes, increased TSH displacement was observed with IgG of thyrotoxic patients. It was suggested that this phenomenon is derived from interactions with Fc receptors associated with fat cell membranes.[41]

REFERENCES

1. Sterling, K., Thyroid hormone action at the cell level. I and II, *N. Engl. J. Med.,* 300, 117, 173, 1979.
2. Mariash, C. N. and Oppenheimer, J. H., Thyroid hormone-carbohydrate interaction at the hepatic nuclear level, *Fed. Proc. Fed. Am. Soc. Exp. Biol.,* 41, 2671, 1982.
3. Scheiff, J. M., Cordier, A. C., and Haumont, S., Epithelial cell proliferation in thymic hyperplasia induced by triiodothyronine, *Clin. Exp. Immunol.,* 27, 516, 1977.
4. Savino, W., Wolf, B., Aratan-Spire, S., and Dardenne, M., Thymic hormone containing cells. IV. Fluctuations in the thyroid hormone levels *in vivo* can modulate the secretion of thymulin by the epithelial cells of young mouse thymus, *Clin. Exp. Immunol.,* 55, 629, 1984.
5. Baroni, C. D., Scelsi, R., Mingazzini, P. L., Cavallero, A., and Uccini, S., Delayed hypersensitivity in the hereditary pituitary dwarf Snell/Bagg mouse, *Nature (London) New Biol.,* 237, 219, 1972.

6. Pierpaoli, W., Fabris, N., and Sorkin, E., Developmental hormones and immunological maturation, in *Hormones and the Immune Response,* CIBA Study Group No. 36, Wolstenholme, G. E. and Knight, J., Eds., Churchill Livingstone, London, 1970, 126.

7. Stark, J. M., Rate of antigen catabolism and immunogenicity of [^{131}I]BCG in mice. II. Immunogenicity of [^{131}I]BCG and adjuvant action after alteration of the metabolic rate by various means, *Immunology,* 19, 457, 1970.

8. Aoki, N., Wakisada, G., and Nagata, I., Effects of thyroxine on T-cell counts and tumour cell rejection in mice, *Acta Endocrinol.,* 81, 104, 1976.

9. Chen, Y., Effect of thyroxine on the immune response of mice in vivo and in vitro, *Immunol. Commun.,* 9, 269, 1980.

10. Keast, D. and Taylor, K., The effect of tri-iodothyronine on the phytohaemagglutinin response of lymphocytes-T, *Clin. Exp. Immunol.,* 47, 217, 1982.

11. Gupta, M. K., Chiang, T., and Deodhar, S. D., Effect of thyroxine on immune response in C57B1/6J mice, *Acta Endocrinol.,* 103, 76, 1983.

12. Jones, R. E., Effects of thyroxine on the transmission of immunoglobulin across the small intestine of young rats, *Biol. Neonat.,* 41, 246, 1982.

13. Segal, J. and Ingbar, S. H., Stimulation by triiodothyronine of the invitro uptake of sugars by rat thymocytes, *J. Clin. Invest.,* 63, 507, 1979.

14. Segal, J. and Ingbar, S. H., Direct and synergistic interactions of 3,5,3′-triiodothyronine and the adrenergic system in stimulating sugar transport by rat thymocytes, *J. Clin. Invest.,* 65, 958, 1980.

15. Pacini, F., Nakamura, H., and Degroot, L. J., Effect of hypo- and hyperthyroidism on the balance between helper and suppressor T-cells in rats, *Acta Endocrinol.,* 103, 528, 1983.

16. Fabris, N., Immunodepression in thyroid-deprived animals, *Clin. Exp. Immunol.,* 15, 601, 1973.

17. Steinetz, B., Giannina, T., Butler, M., and Popick, F., Influence of thyroidectomy and thyroid hormones on adjuvant arthritis in rats, *Proc. Soc. Exp. Biol. Med.,* 133, 401, 1970.

18. Berczi, I., Nagy, E., Kovacs, K., and Horvath, E., Regulation of humoral immunity in rats by pituitary hormones, *Acta Endocrinol.,* 98, 506, 1981.

19. Berczi, I., Nagy, E., Asa, S. L., and Kovacs, K., Pituitary hormones and contact sensitivity in rats, *Allergy,* 38, 325, 1983.

20. Berczi, I., Nagy, E., Asa, S. L., and Kovacs, K., The influence of pituitary hormones on adjuvant arthritis, *Arthritis Rheum.,* 27, 682, 1984.

21. Gerard, A., Leloup, J., and Gerard, H., Effects of the graft versus host reaction on thyroid gland: evidence of correlations between the severity of the immunological conflict and the decrease of thyroid activity in the chick embryo, *C. R. Acad. Sci. Ser. III Vie,* 295, 495, 1982.

22. Keast, D. and Ayre, D. J., Antibody regulation in birds by thyroid hormones, *Dev. Comp. Immunol.,* 4, 323, 1980.

23. Smekens, L., Goldstein, J., and Vanhaelst, L., Measurement of thyroxine conversion to triiodothyronine using human lymphocytes, *J. Endocrinol. Invest.,* 6, 113, 1983.

24. Paavonen, T., Enhancement of human B lymphocyte differentiation in vitro by thyroid hormone, *Scand. J. Immunol.,* 15, 211, 1982.

25. Yamamoto, M., Takai, N. A., Rapoport, B., and Hinds, W. E., Modulation by thymus-derived (T)-cells of thyroid cell-stimulated prostaglandin-E release by human peripheral blood mononuclear cells, *Proc. Natl. Acad. Sci. U.S.A.,* 76, 6627, 1979.

26. Coates, P. M., Hoffman, G. M., and Finegold, D. N., Effect of thyroid hormones on human mononuclear leukocyte lysosomal acid lipase activity, *J. Clin. Endocrinol. Metab.,* 54, 559, 1982.

27. Joasoo, A., Long-acting thyroid stimulator: a review, *Med. J. Aust.,* 1, 595, 1970.

28. Volpé, R., Farid, N. R., Von Westarp, C., and Row, V. V., The pathogenesis of Graves' disease and Hashimoto's thyroiditis, *Clin. Endocrinol.,* 3, 239, 1974.

29. Weigle, W. O., Cellular events in experimental autoimmune thyroiditis, allergic encephalomyelitis, and tolerance to self, in *Autoimmunity. Genetic, Immunologic, Virologic and Clinical Aspects,* Talal, N., Ed., Academic Press, New York, 1977, 141.

30. Doniach, D. and Marshall, N. J., Autoantibodies to the thyrotropin (TSH) receptors on thyroid epithelium and other tissues, in *Autoimmunity. Genetic, Immunologic, Virologic and Clinical Aspects,* Talal, N., Ed., Academic Press, New York, 1977, 621.

31. Volpé, R., Immunological aspects of auto-immune thyroid diseases, *Ann. Endocrinol.,* 42, 169, 1981.

32. Rose, N. R., Kong, Y. -C. M., Okayasu, I., Giraldo, A. A., Beisel, K., and Sundick, R. S., T-cell regulation in autoimmune thyroiditis, *Immunol. Rev.,* 55, 299, 1981.

33. Farid, N. R., Graves' disease, in *HLA in Endocrine and Metabolic Disorders,* Farid, N. R., Ed., Academic Press, New York, 1981, 85.

34. Farid, N. R., Thyroiditis, in *HLA in Endocrine and Metabolic Disorders,* Farid, N. R., Ed., Academic Press, New York, 1981, 145.

35. Bach, J. -F., Boitard, C., and Charreire, J., Bases cellulaires et génétiques des maladies endocriniennes d'origine auto-immune, *Horm. Res.,* 16, 273, 1982.
36. Dessaint, J. P. and Wémeau, J. L., Autoimmunity and hypothyroidism, *Horm. Res.,* 16, 329, 1982.
37. Strakosch, C. R., Wenzel, B. E., Row, V. V., and Volpé, R., Immunology of autoimmune thyroid diseases, *N. Engl. J. Med.,* 307, 1499, 1982.
38. Wick, G., Boyd, R., Hála, K., Thunold, S., and Kofler, H., Pathogenesis of spontaneous autoimmune thyroiditis in obese strain (OS) chickens, *Clin. Exp. Immunol.,* 47, 1, 1982.
39. Bech, K., Immunological aspects of Graves' disease and importance of thyroid stimulating immunoglobulins, *Acta Endocrinol.,* 103, (Suppl. 254), 1, 1983.
40. Orava, M., Cantell, K., Kauppila, A., and Vihko, R., Interferon and serum thyroid hormones, *Int. J. Cancer,* 31, 671, 1983.
41. Gill, D. L., Marshall, N. J., and Eakins, R. P., Effects of immunoglobulins upon the interaction of thyrotropin with receptors in human fat tissue, *Endocrinology,* 107, 1813, 1980.

Chapter 9

THE EFFECT OF MISCELLANEOUS HORMONES AND NEURO-TRANSMITTERS ON THE IMMUNE SYSTEM

I. Berczi

TABLE OF CONTENTS

I. INTRODUCTION

In this chapter, the influence of diverse hormone producing organs, hormones, and/ or neurotransmitters on the immune system is discussed. The significance of most of these observations in relation to neurohormonal immunoregulation is yet to be determined. Some of these factors may yet prove to be important; therefore, a brief overview is given here.

II. PITUITARY HORMONES AND FACTORS

The effect of 8-L-arginine vasopressin (AVP), oxytocin, and deamino-8-D-arginine on the prostaglandin synthesis of human mononuclear phagocytes was examined. The production of prostaglandin E_2 (PGE_2) was stimulated by AVP significantly, whereas oxytocin and deamino-8-D-arginine were much less effective. The capacity of each hormone to stimulate PGE_2 synthesis was proportional to its pressor, but not to its antidiuretic activity.[1] It was found that AVP was also able to change body temperature after central administration, and it was suggested that it functions as an antipyretic hormone.[2]

No direct effect of α-melanocyte stimulating hormone (α-MSH) on immune reactivity has been described to date, but this hormone was capable of reducing fever induced in rabbits by leukocytic pyrogen.[3,4] Therefore, α-MSH may function as a moderator of pyrogenic signals emitted by the immune system towards the central nervous system (CNS).

Although AVP and α-MSH are both produced by the pituitary gland, they have been found also in the CNS,[2,5] which suggests that they also function as neurotransmitters.

III. PARATHYROID HORMONE, CALCITONIN, AND VITAMIN D

Removal of the parathyroid glands from rats induced bone marrow hypoplasia, with strikingly large reductions in the size of the erythroid and lymphoid cell subpopulations.[6] Parathyroidectomy, 24 hr before the injection of sheep red blood cells (SRBC) to rats, impaired lymphocyte DNA synthesis in response to antigen and the development of plaque-forming cells. The removal of parathyroids was without effect after antigen injection.[7]

The human lymphoblastoid cell lines RAN and EB3 express receptors for parathyroid hormone (PTH) and can be used for the detection of antireceptor autoantibodies.[8] Because of the relationship between monocytes and osteoclasts, the effect of PTH, PGE_2, and calcitonin on human monocyte chemiluminescence were studied. Preincubations of monocytes with PTH or PGE_2 for 2 hr, caused a significant decrease in peak chemiluminescence, which occurred during phagocytosis stimulated by latex particles. Salmon calcitonin caused a significant increase in chemiluminescence, whereas preincubation with human calcitonin, at the same molar concentration, had no effect. The production of hydrogen peroxide by phagocytosing monocytes was also significantly affected by parathyroid hormone.[9] The concentration of cAMP increased in human mononuclear leukocytes after treatment with salmon calcitonin, but there was no effect when the cells were separated into adherent (monocytic) and nonadherent (lymphocytic) populations. However, a calcitonin response could be induced in nonadherent cells, by culturing them for 16 hr in medium previously conditioned by the growth of mixed mononuclear leukocytes.[10]

Receptors for 1,25-dihydroxyvitamin D_3 (calcitriol) were detected in human peripheral mononuclear leukocytes. This receptor was present in monocytes, but absent from normal resting peripheral B and T lymphocytes. However, established lines of B, T, non-B and non-T human lymphocytes, as well as in vitro activated T and B lymphocytes obtained from normal humans, did express the receptor.[11] Calcitriol is synthesized by the kidneys. In rats fed with a low calcium and low vitamin D diet, the number of mast cells increased dramatically in the bone marrow. This hormone is known also to act on osteoblasts that express specific receptors for it. Calcitriol, along with the other known regulatory hormones (parathyroid hormone and calcitonin), is an important regulator of bone metabolism. In addition, it was shown to suppress the effect of interleukin 2 on its target cells.[12]

IV. THE INFLUENCE OF THE PINEAL GLAND

Pinealectomy causes an increase in the number of mast cells in the lymph nodes of rats and inhibits the production of antibodies. Calcium uptake by the thymus and spleen is also impaired by pinealectomy, whereas SO_4 uptake was increased.[13] Others found that the removal of the pineal gland from rats had little effect on the degree of immunocompetence in normal and thymectomized animals. However, in some of the immunological tests, an accelerated response was observed.[14] In our laboratory, young adult rats were pinealectomized, and their humoral and cell mediated immune reactivity was studied. Pinealectomy did not influence immune reactivity under our experimental conditions.[15]

Lymphoid tissue can be found within the pineal gland of certain birds. In chicks, lymphocytes begin to accumulate in the pineal stroma 1 week after hatching, reach a maximum at 1 month of age, and disappear almost completely by 4 months of age. The lymphocytes migrating to the pineal gland of chicks are blood borne and composed of 42% B lymphocytes and 51% T lymphocytes at 4 to 5 weeks of age. Intravenous immunization revealed that pineal-established lymphocytes can be stimulated by soluble, but not by particulate, antigens.[16] The pineal gland of rats also undergoes a massive invasion by T lymphocytes.[17]

V. BROWN ADIPOSE TISSUE

The hibernating gland, or in other words, brown adipose tissue, was shown to influence immune reactions by several investigators. Antibody production was inhibited in vitro by chloroform extracts of the brown fat from a variety of animals (hibernating ground squirrel, the nonhibernating winter ground squirrel, the cold-acclimated deer-mouse, and the newborn rabbit). The brown fat from summer ground squirrels, from deer-mice maintained at room temperature, and from nonhibernating winter hamsters was a poor source of inhibitor activity.[18] Brown adipose tissue was taken from rats, homogenized and lyophilized, and then reinjected in normal 8-week-old rats. After six injections, the animals were immunized with bovine serum albumin and 10 to 20 days later were tested for immunity by delayed reaction, Arthus reaction, and the titration of antibody. Delayed and Arthus reactions were significantly impaired in treated animals, particularly 10 days after immunization. The production of circulating antibodies was inhibited to a lesser degree.[19] The removal of brown adipose tissue from rats increased their reactivity to allogeneic lymphocytes, as revealed by the increase of popliteal lymph node weights, and also by their elevated susceptibility to the induction of experimental allergic thyroiditis.[20,21]

VI. SUBSTANCE P

Substance P (SP) is an undecapeptide, which is widely distributed in the nervous system and serves as a neurotransmitter at the central terminals of C-fibers. It is transported from central neurons, where SP is produced, to peripheral terminals, where it can be released by physiologically or electrically stimulated nerves. SP stimulated the proliferative response of human lymphocytes to PHA (10^{-11} to 10^{-7} *M)* and enhanced the proliferative response of human lymphocytes to PHA (10^{-9} to 10^{-7} *M).* An active analogue of SP inhibited these effects.[22] Nontoxic histamine release was elicited by SP from rat peritoneal mast cells in vitro.[23] However, D-amino acid containing analogues of SP, which lack neurostimulatory activity and inhibit the neurologic effects of SP, have greater histamine release potencies than the native mediator.[24]

VII. ANGIOTENSIN

Guinea pig peritoneal exudate macrophages express specific, and saturable, cell surface receptors for angiotensin-II. Two types of receptors were identified: a low number of receptors with high affinity (Ka $\approx 3.5 \times 10^8$ M^{-1}) and a large number of relatively low affinity receptors (Ka $\approx 5 \times 10^8$ M^{-1}). The molecular weight of angiotensin receptors was estimated to be around 50,000 daltons.[25]

Macrophages isolated from liver granulomas of *Schistosoma mansoni* infected mice bound specifically angiotensin-II, as demonstrated by fluorescence and radioligand assays. A total of 526 binding sites were estimated per cell, with a dissociation constant of 0.25 n*M*. Angiotensin-I and III, which are natural analogues of angiotensin-II, competed only weakly for these binding sites. Exposure of macrophages to appropriate concentrations of angiotensin-II resulted in a rapid, dose-dependent increase in intracellular cAMP.[26]

Liver granulomas from mice infected for 8 weeks with *S. mansoni* contained angiotensin-I converting enzyme activity. Angiotensin-II, and to a lesser extent, angiotensin-III, inhibited the migration of mouse peritoneal macrophages in vitro.[27]

VIII. NEUROTENSIN

Neurotensin is a peptide found both centrally and peripherally in the nervous system. Neurotensin stimulated the release of histamine from rat peritoneal mast cells in a dose-dependent manner; 15 to 20% of total cellular histamine was released by 10^{-7} to 10^{-6} *M* concentrations. The release reaction occurred optimally at pH 6.5 to 7.5, at 37°C in the presence of 1 m*M* calcium, and it was complete within 2 min after the addition of neurotensin. The C terminus was identified as the biologically reactive portion of neurotensin.[28]

IX. VASOACTIVE INTESTINAL POLYPEPTIDE

Vasoactive intestinal polypeptide (VIP) was found to be a potent stimulator of lymphocyte adenylate cyclase activity in human peripheral blood lymphocytes, but not in neutrophils, monocytes, or platelets. This stimulation was time-, temperature-, and concentration-dependent. Stimulation by VIP and PGE_1 was additive, whereas somatostatin antagonized the action of VIP. Adenylate cyclase activity was stimulated in both T and B lymphocytes by VIP.[29] Subsequently, specific VIP receptors were detected on human peripheral lymphocytes (1700 sites/cell; Kd = 0.47 ± 0.23 n*M).*[30] In the mouse, T cells, but no B lymphocytes, were found to have specific VIP receptors. Furthermore, VIP inhibited in vitro the response of lymphocytes to T cell mitogens (Con A, PHA) in a dose-dependent fashion, but not to a B cell mitogen (LPS).[31]

REFERENCES

1. Locher, R., Vetter, W., and Block, L. H., Interactions between 8-L-arginine vasopressin and prostaglandin-E2 in human mononuclear phagocytes, *J. Clin. Invest.,* 71, 884, 1983.

2. Ruwe, W. D., Veale, W. L., and Cooper, K. E., Peptide neurohormones: their role in thermoregulation and fever, *Can. J. Biochem. Cell. Biol.,* 61, 579, 1983.

3. Murphy, M. T., Richards, D. B., and Lipton, J. M., Antipyretic potency of centrally administered α-melanocyte stimulating hormone, *Science,* 221, 192, 1983.

4. Glyn-Ballinger, J. R., Bernardini, G. L., and Lipton, J. M., α-MSH injected into the septal region reduces fever in rabbits, *Peptides,* 4, 199, 1983.

5. Samson, W. K., Lipton, J. M., Zimmer, J. A., and Glyn, J. R., The effect of fever on central α-MSH concentrations in the rabbit, *Peptides,* 2, 419, 1981.

6. Rixon, R. H. and Whitfield, J. F., Hypoplasia of the bone marrow in rats following removal of the parathyroid glands, *J. Cell. Physiol.,* 79, 343, 1972.

7. Swierenga, S. H. H., MacManus, J. P., Braceland, B. M., and Youdale, T., Regulation of the primary immune response in vivo by parathyroid hormone, *J. Immunol.,* 117, 1608, 1976.

8. Juppner, H., Bialasiewicz, A. A., and Hesch, R. D., Autoantibodies to parathyroid hormone receptor, *Lancet,* 2, 1222, 1978.

9. Stock, J. L., Coderre, J. A., and Levine, P. H., Effects of calcium-regulating hormones and drugs on human monocyte chemiluminescence, *J. Clin. Endocrinol. Metab.,* 55, 956, 1982.

10. Perry, H. M., III, Kahn, A. J., Chappel, J. C., Kohler, G., Teitelbaum, S. L., and Peck, W. A., Calcitonin response in circulating human lymphocytes, *Endocrinology,* 113, 1568, 1983.

11. Provivedini, D. M., Tsoukas, C. D., Deftos, L. J., and Manolagas, S. C., 1,25-Dihydroxyvitamin D_3 receptors in human leukocytes, *Science,* 221, 1181, 1983.

12. Manolagas, S. C. and Deftos, L. J., The vitamin D endocrine system and the hematolymphopoietic tissue, *Ann. Intern. Med.,* 100, 144, 1984.

13. Csaba, G̅., Kiss, J., and Brodoky, M., The effect of pinealectomy on the Ca and SO_4 turnover of the lymphatic organs, *Experientia,* 23, 148, 1967.

14. Rella, W. and Lapin, V., Immunocompetence of pinealectomized and simultaneously pinealectomized and thymectomized rats, *Oncology,* 33, 3, 1976.

15. Nagy, E. and Berczi, I., unpublished results, 1978.

16. Cogburn, L. A. and Glick, B., Functional lymphocytes in the chicken pineal gland, *J. Immunol.,* 130, 2109, 1983.

17. Uede, T., Ishi, Y., Matsuura, A., Shimogawara, I., and Kikuchi, K., Immunohistochemical study of lymphocytes in rat pineal gland: selective accumulation of T lymphocytes, *Anat. Rec.,* 199, 239, 1981.

18. Sidky, Y. A., Hayward, J. S., and Ruth, R. F., Immunosuppression in vitro by brown fat, *Immunol. Commun.,* 1, 579, 1972.

19. Janković, B. D., Popesković, L., Janežić, A., and Lukić, M. L., Brown adipose tissue: effect on immune reactions in the rat, *Naturwissenschaften,* 61, 36, 1974.

20. Popesković, L., Janežić, A., Lukić, M. L., and Janković, B. D., Brown adipose tissue and immunity: effect of neonatal adipectomy on host-versus-graft and graft-versus-host reactivity in the rat, *Period. Biol.,* 78 (Suppl. 1), 37, 1976.

21. Mitrović, K., Milošević, D., Vujanović, N. L., and Janković, B. D., Brown adipose tissue and immunity: experimental allergic thyroiditis in adipectomized rats, *Period. Biol.,* 78 (Suppl. 1), 38, 1976.

22. Payan, D. G., Brewster, D. R., and Goetzl, E. J., Specific stimulation of human T lymphocytes by substance P, *J. Immunol.,* 131, 1613, 1983.

23. Mazurek, N., Pecht, I., Teichberg, V. I., and Blumberg, S., The role of the N-terminal tetrapeptide in the histamine-releasing action of substance P, *Neuropharmacology,* 20, 1025, 1981.

24. Foreman, J. and Jordan, C., Histamine release and vascular changes induced by neuropeptides, *Agents Actions,* 13, 105, 1983.

25. Thomas, D. W. and Hoffman, M. D., Identification of macrophage receptors for angiotensin: a potential role in antigen uptake for T lymphocyte responses, *J. Immunol.,* 132, 2807, 1984.

26. Weinstock, J. V. and Kassab, J. T., Functional angiotensin II receptors on macrophages from isolated liver granulomas of murine *Schistosoma mansoni, J. Immunol.,* 132, 2598, 1984.

27. Weinstock, J. V. and Blum, A. M., Isolated liver granulomas of murine *Schistosoma mansoni* contain components of the angiotensin system, *J. Immunol.,* 131, 2529, 1983.

28. Rossie, S. S. and Miller, R. J., Regulation of mast cell histamine release by neurotensin, *Life Sci.,* 31, 509, 1982.

29. O'Dorisio, M. S., Hermina, N. S., O'Dorisio, T. M., and Balcerzak, S. P., Vasoactive intestinal polypeptide modulation of lymphocyte adenylate cyclase, *J. Immunol.,* 127, 2551, 1981.

30. Danek, A., O'Dorisio, M. S., O'Dorisio, T. M., and George, J. M., Specific binding sites for vasoactive intestinal polypeptide on nonadherent peripheral blood lymphocytes, *J. Immunol.,* 131, 1173, 1983.

31. Ottaway, C. A. and Greenberg, G. R., Interaction of vasoactive intestinal peptide with mouse lymphocytes: specific binding and the modulation of mitogen responses, *J. Immunol.,* 132, 417, 1984.

Chapter 10

IMMUNOREGULATION BY PITUITARY HORMONES

I. Berczi

TABLE OF CONTENTS

I. INTRODUCTION

This chapter is intended to summarize and interpret the role of pituitary and steroid hormones in immune function. Only certain points will be stressed here, those which are most relevant to the possible immunoregulatory role of the pituitary gland. Some theoretical speculations and predictions will also be made, which reflect the author's opinion, and will need to be tested experimentally.

II. THE ROLE OF THE ACTH-ADRENAL AXIS

A. ACTH

It is clear from experiments conducted on a variety of species that ACTH acts on the immune system through the stimulation of glucocorticoid secretion by the adrenal cortex. Glucocorticoids in turn have an immunosuppressive effect. Although species differences may exist, it seems certain that chronic ACTH treatment leads to the involution of the thymus and other lymphoid organs, and to the suppression of humoral, cell mediated, and autoimmune reactions. ACTH functions as an antagonist to prolactin (PRL) and growth hormone (GH), which have an immunostimulatory effect. Treatment of rats with physiological doses of ACTH had an immunosuppressive effect in normal, in hypophysectomized (Hypox) and hormone reconstituted, and in bromocriptine suppressed and hormone reconstituted rats.[1-5] These observations demonstrate that the physiological stimulation of the adrenal cortex with ACTH generates glucocorticoids in amounts sufficient to elicit an immunosuppressive effect. It is also of relevance that ACTH and a related peptide, α-MSH, were shown to have an antipyretic effect in rabbits.[6-8]

B. Endorphins

Human lymphocytes and platelets have been shown to have opiate receptors of the μ-type. It appears that of the three endorphins (α, β, and γ) secreted by the pituitary gland, only β endorphin affects the immune system, although more studies are required to substantiate this conclusion. Opiate addicts are immunodeficient, and from this it was inferred that opiate peptides have an immunosuppressive effect. However, only in vitro studies have been performed to date in relation to the effect of β endorphin and related peptides on various immune parameters, which may or may not be relevant to their in vivo role in immunoregulation. Furthermore, some of the in vitro results are controversial. For instance, the cytotoxic activity of human natural killer (NK) cells was found to be enhanced significantly by β endorphin and methionine enkephaline, whereas an inhibitory effect was observed on rat NK cell activity.[9,10] Clearly, more experimental data are required for exact delineation of the possible role of opioid peptides in immunoregulation.

C. Glucocorticoids

Glucocorticoid receptors are present in all cell types of the leukocyte series, bone marrow cells having the highest concentration. Receptor numbers increase in stimulated lymphocytes and are regulated also by plasma corticosteroid levels. Thymic hormones and genetic factors also influence the number of glucocorticoid receptors in lymphoid cells.

The lack of adrenal hormones in adrenalectomized animals increases thymus regeneration, leads to an altered distribution of lymphocytes, and enhances humoral and cell mediated immune reactions.

Although glucocorticoids have an influence on all cell types of the leukocyte series, the most dramatic effect is exerted on the thymus, which manifests in profound involution. Apparently, an endonuclease is present in thymocytes, which can be activated by glucocorticoids, and which causes cell lysis after activation.[11-14] The biological significance of this lytic effect of glucocorticoids on thymocytes has not been elucidated, but it appears to be an important regulatory mechanism. It is interesting to note that thymic hormones and genes of the major histocompatibility complex (MHC) have a regulatory influence on the glucocorticoid sensitivity of thymocytes.[15-19] Apparently glucocorticoids have an influence on the thymus in all vertebrates.

It has been established clearly, by a number of investigators, that the circadian rhythm of peripheral blood lymphocytes is regulated by endogenous cortisol.[20,21] Again, the significance of rhythmic changes in leukocyte distribution remains uncertain.

Virtually all immune reactions are regulated by T lymphocytes. Numerous investigations have indicated that glucocorticoids are capable of inhibiting every major T cell function (e.g., helper, suppressor, and killer activities). However, resistance of several T cell functions to glucocorticoid inhibition was also observed under certain conditions. These seemingly contradictory results may be due to the fact that several lymphokines, such as the glucosteroid response modifying factor,[22] or interleukin 2,[23] are capable of abrogating the inhibitory effect of glucocorticoids on T lymphocytes. On the other hand, one of the important effects of glucocorticoids is the inhibition of lymphokine production, especially interleukin 1 by monocytes and interleukin 2 by T lymphocytes, which are indispensible for the initiation of an immune response.

Treatment of mice and rats with glucocorticoids decreases the numbers of B cells in spleen and lymph nodes, but bone marrow B lymphocytes are not affected. Serum immunoglobulin concentrations are also decreased. After the in vivo inhibition of B lymphocytes with glucocorticoids, an overshoot reaction will occur. The application of glucocorticoids to man, in pharmacological doses, decreases serum immunoglobulin levels and the reactivity of B cells to pokeweed mitogen (PWM). However, several investigators observed an enhancement of immunoglobulin secretion by human B cells in vitro in the presence of glucocorticoids. This was true for unstimulated and PWM-stimulated cultures, and the phenomenon was dependent on the use of fetal calf serum in the culture medium. Under these conditions a steroid dependent T cell replacing factor was induced, which was responsible for the augmentation of Ig secretion.

Virtually all functions of the monocyte-macrophage cell lineage are inhibited by glucocorticoids, both in laboratory rodents and man. These include cell metabolism, chemotaxis, phagocytosis, cytotoxic reactions, the capacity to present antigen, and to secrete interleukin 1, as well as the ability to respond to lymphokines. One should caution, however, that there may be a difference between natural and synthetic glucocorticoids in this regard.[24]

The observation by Mishell and co-workers[25-27] that spleen cells, cultured overnight in medium containing fetal bovine serum, became highly resistant to the immunosuppressive effect of hydrocortisone is of major significance. Subsequent experiments revealed that bacterial lipopolysaccharide (LPS), present in fetal calf serum, was the agent responsible for the induction of glucosteroid response modifying factor (GRMF) from macrophage-like cells. During in vitro antibody responses of mouse spleen cells, GRMF provided protection against glucocorticoid mediated immunosuppression in a dose-dependent fashion, leading to the recovery of helper T cell function, which otherwise was suppressed. A similar glucocorticoid antagonizing factor could be induced by the treatment of mice with LPS in vivo.[28] Another lymphokine, polymorphonuclear migration stimulatory factor, was produced also by human monocytes under the influence of cortisol.[29,30] Thus, glucocorticoids do not only seem to regulate the immune system, but it is certain that glucocorticoid related immunoregulatory lymphokines exist (Table 1), which are designed for the modification of the biological effect of corticosteroids on various cell types of the immune system.

Table 1

GLUCOCORTICOID RELATED IMMUNOREGULATORY LYMPHOKINES/
FACTORS

Species	Lymphokine/factor	Biological effect	Ref.
Man	Thymosin fr. 5	Reduction of glucocorticoid binding activity of thymocytes, increase of glucocorticoid resistance	15
Mouse	Thymic humoral factor	Increase of resistance of thymocytes to hydrocortisone	16,17
	Thymosin	Facilitation of recovery from hydrocortisone-induced suppression of the Con-A response of lymphoid cells	18
	Interleukin-1	Restoration of helper cell activity in dexamethasone-inhibited PNA⁻ thymocytes	66
	Interleukin-2	Abrogation of the inhibitory effect of hydrocortisone on Con-A induced activation of thymocytes	67
	Interleukin-2	Reversal of glucocorticoid inhibition of cytotoxic T cells	68
Man	Interleukin-1	Abrogation of the inhibitory effect of dexamethasone on peripheral T cell response to PHA	23
Mouse	GRMF	Glucocorticosteroid response modifying factor derived from Con-A stimulated spleen cells or from LPS stimulated accessory cells, which blocks glucocorticoid mediated suppression of helper T cells and is capable of interfering with the suppressive effect of dexamethasone on the humoral immune response in vitro	22,25
	GAF	Glucocorticoid antagonizing factor present in sera of LPS injected mice	28
Man	SDTCRF	Steroid dependent T cell replacing factor secreted by T cells in the presence of adherent cells	29
	PMSF	Polymorphonuclear migration stimulatory factor produced by monocytes exposed to cortisol in culture	30
	Interferon-A	Abrogates the inhibitory effect of glucocorticoids on NK cells	32
	Interferon or interleukin-2	Reverse prednisone induced inhibition of NK and ADCC activities	33
Mouse	Heparin	Restores the antibody response of cortisol suppressed mice	69

Note: ADCC = antibody dependent cellular cytotoxicity; Con-A = concanavalin A; GAF = glucocorticoid antagonizing factor; GRMF = glucocorticosteroid response modifying factor; LPS = bacterial lipopolysaccharide; NK = natural killer cells; PHA = phytohemagglutinin; PMSF = polymorphonuclear migration stimulatory factor; PNA = peanut agglutinin; SDTCRF = steroid dependent T cell replacing factor; T = thymus derived lymphocytes.

The heterogeneity of killer and NK cells, and the changes in redistribution of these cells after the administration of glucocorticoids to laboratory rodents, and to man, led to controversial results with regards to the effect of corticosteroids on killer cell activity. Nevertheless, it seems certain that some types of NK cells are inhibited by glucocorticoids, both in vivo and in vitro. It is of interest to note that the treatment of mice with cortisol inhibited splenic NK activity, which was mediated by suppressor cells.[31] The in vitro treatment of human peripheral blood leukocytes with *physiological* concentrations of glucocorticoids for 18 to 24 hr reduced markedly their NK activity. On the other hand, human leukocyte *interferon* subtype A enhanced NK activity in the presence of glucocorticoid.[32] In addition to natural killing, the antibody dependent cellular cytotoxicity (ADCC) activity of human lymphocytes was also reduced by preincubation for 24 hr with prednisolone. The NK and ADCC activities of purified T cells, non-T cells, and NK-enriched effector cells was inhibited as well. This prednisolone-induced inhibition could be reversed by the incubation of lymphocytes for 1 hr with interferon, or interleukin 2.[33]

Granulocytes are profoundly affected by glucocorticoids. Immunologically triggered mediator release from mast cells and basophilic leukocytes is inhibited. Moreover, the destruction of mast cells was observed in glucocorticoid treated rats. The chemotactic response of human eosinophils was inhibited by glucocorticoids, both after in vivo treatment, or in vitro exposure. Human neutrophil function is impaired severely by glucocorticoids. Apparently, β-adrenergic receptors are uncoupled from adenylate cyclase; Fc receptors, complement receptors, and chemotactic receptors are rendered nonfunctional in neutrophils by corticosteroids.[34-36]

Studies on immune reactions of several species (mouse, rat, guinea pig, rabbit, man, chicken, frog) revealed the general immunosuppressive effect of these hormones. Immunoglobulin levels, as well as humoral and cell mediated immune reactions are depressed by chronic treatment in vivo, and also in culture systems. However, the cells responsible for the induction of graft-vs.-host (GVH) reaction and immunological memory cells seem to resist the deleterious effect of glucocorticoids.

In contrast with the profound immunosuppressive effect of pharmacological doses/ concentrations of glucocorticoids, it has been shown by several investigators that small physiological concentrations of cortisol, cortisone, and related glucocorticoids are in fact necessary for the humoral immune response by mouse and rabbit lymphocytes in vitro,[37,38] and also for the generation of cytotoxic cells from rat lymphocytes.[39-41] Some of the effects of physiological concentrations of glucocorticoids on the immune system are listed in Table 2. The content of this table illustrates the general immunosuppressive effect of glucocorticoids, which can be overruled by specific stimulation, as indicated by the last three observations listed.

D. Catecholamines and Acetylcholine

Lymphocytes, granulocytes and mast cells have β-$_2$-type catecholamine receptors, whereas platelets express α-type receptors. Catecholamines appear to have major influences on leukocyte recirculation and distribution, some of which is mediated through the ACTH-corticosteroid axis.[42] It is somewhat hazardous to draw conclusions from studies with synthetic catecholamine receptor agonists and antagonists. Nevertheless, it seems reasonably certain that β-adrenergic stimulants stabilize mast cells in several species (mouse, rat, man), inhibit mediator release, and thus, decrease the sensitivity to asthma and allergic reactions. The reaction of murine and human lymphocytes to mitogens (Con A, PHA, PWM, LPS) is also inhibited by catecholamines. Humoral and cell mediated immune reactions in mice are in general inhibited, although some agents seem to cause acceleration and enhancement. Immunoglobulin synthesis by human peripheral blood lymphocytes is enhanced by catecholamines and further amplified by glucocorticoids. The maturation of human neutrophils is inhibited by adrenergic agents. Thus, the effect of β-adrenergic agents on the immune system in general, and on allergic-asthmatic reactions in particular, seems to be inhibitory, although occasional acceleration and enhancement was also observed. Additional observations are needed for further clarification of the effect of catecholamines on the immune system.

Muscarinic-cholinergic receptors have been identified on mouse spleen cells and nicotinic-cholinergic receptors were detected in rabbit thymus. Relatively few studies were performed on the effect of cholinergic agents on various immune parameters. The available evidence seems to indicate that muscarinic agents enhance immune reactivity in general and thus, could act as antagonists to catecholamines. Killer T cell activity, lymphocyte response to phytohemagglutinin (PHA), complement synthesis by macro-

Table 2
SOME PHYSIOLOGICAL EFFECTS OF GLUCOCORTICOIDS ON THE IMMUNE SYSTEM

Species	Glucocorticoid	Biological effect	Ref.
Mouse	Corticosterone	Enhancement of Thy-1.2 antigen expression by thymocytes	59
Man	Cortisol	Stimulation of bone marrow granulocyte/macrophage colonies	60
Mouse	Prednisolone	Depression of circulating lymphocytes in Adrx mice	61
	Cortisone	Circadian rhythm of blood and spleen lymphocytes due to physiological variations in plasma cortisone levels	61
Man	Cortisol	Circadian rhythm of blood T, B, and K cells due to physiological changes in plasma cortisol levels	20,21
Mouse	Glucocorticoid	Inhibition of lymphocyte response to Con-A	62
	Dexamethasone	Abolishment of the activity of antigen primed suppressor T cells	63
	Glucocorticoid	Inhibition of cytotoxic T cells after preincubation in vitro	23
Guinea pig	Glucocorticoids	Inhibition of the production of macrophage mitogenic factor	64
Mouse	Glucocorticoids	Inhibition of the cytotoxic activity of interferon treated macrophages	65
Man	Glucocorticoids	Inhibition of lymphocyte NK activity after preincubation in vitro for 18 to 24 hr	32
Mouse	Cortisol	Small amounts are required for antibody response in vitro	37
Rat	Cortisol	1 μg/mℓ facilitates the generation of killer cells in vitro	39-41
Rabbit	Cortisol, cortisone	Physiological levels are required for the secondary antibody response in vitro	38

Note: Abbreviations: Adrx = adrenalectomy; B = bone marrow derived lymphocytes; Con-A = concanavalin A; K = killer cells; NK = natural killer cells; T = thymus derived lymphocytes; Thy-1.2 = thymus and T cell specific antigen.

phages, and the release of mediators of immediate type hypersensitivity were enhanced by cholinergic agents in several species.

III. GROWTH HORMONE AND INSULIN

Although some lymphocyte cell lines express specific and high affinity receptors for GH, this does not seem to be a general rule for cultured lymphoid cells. Convincing evidence for the presence of GH receptors on normal lymphoid cells is lacking. Despite this uncertainty, a compelling body of observations indicates that GH is necessary for the development of the immune system and for the maintenance of immunocompetence. The immunostimulatory effect of GH appears to be general, including both cell mediated and humoral reactions. GH was shown to antagonize cortisol induced leukopenia in Hypox rats[43] and the immunosuppressive effect of ACTH.[1] A synergistic action of GH with putative thymic hormones has also been suggested.[44,45]

Circulating monocytes express insulin receptors, whereas such receptors in resting lymphocytes are almost undetectable. However, insulin receptors will appear in lymphocytes, if they become stimulated. Insulin is necessary for the maintenance of normal immune function, but it does not seem to act as a primary regulator of the immune system. Further observations are required for the elucidation of the exact role of insulin in immune function.

IV. PROLACTIN

Several attempts failed to reveal PRL receptors in lymphatic tissue. However, a thymus derived rat lymphoma was found to be PRL dependent in growth and to express high affinity receptors for lactogenic hormones.[46] Furthermore, Russell and co-workers[47] suggested recently that normal human lymphocytes do express a low number of PRL receptors. Additional investigations are required to determine whether or not lymphocytes express PRL receptors in vivo. Nevertheless, PRL seems to play an important role in the homing of IgA producing cells to the lactating mammary tissue,[48] and also in the maintenance of general immunocompetence. The evidence available to date suggests that PRL and GH are identical in their effect on the immune system; both hormones are immunostimulatory and are antagonized by ACTH. A related hormone, placental lactogen, affects immune reactions in a manner similar to that of PRL and GH. Further experiments are required for the elucidation of the mechanism of action of PRL on immune phenomena.

V. SEX HORMONES

Up to now there is no hard evidence for a significant influence of gonadotropins on the immune system, despite the fact that the immunomodulatory effect of sex hormones is well established. Estrogen and androgen receptors are present in the thymus and were identified also in the bursa of Fabricius. The epithelial cells, but not the lymphocytes, are receptor positive in both organs. Progesterone seems to act through glucocorticoid receptors, though the existence of specific receptors for this hormone has also been proposed. Apparently, estrogens and androgens also have the capacity to combine with glucocorticoid receptors in lymphocytes and may affect directly certain lymphocyte functions, if present at high concentrations.

There are numerous examples of sex-related difference in the immune reactivity of laboratory animals. In man, susceptibility to autoimmune disease, to certain infections, and some other parameters of immune reactivities also show sex-related differences, which suggest a physiological role for sex hormones in immunoregulation. In animals, this is supported further by castration and hormonal reconstitution experiments. Although our knowledge of the effect of sex hormones on immune reactivity is still very deficient, it appears that estrogens, especially estradiol, enhance immune reactions (with the possible exception of NK cells), whereas androgens, especially testosterone, have a moderating effect. This is very well established in models of autoimmune disease and seems to be supported also by recent clinical studies. The role of progesterone needs further clarification. The available evidence suggests an immunosuppressive effect. Apparently, estradiol regulates the secretion of IgA into the genital tract of females, whereas testosterone controls the secretion of immunoglobulin by the lacrimal gland. Progesterone and estradiol, in addition to PRL, were also shown to play a role in the development of mammary immune function. It remains to be seen whether or not the secretion of immunoglobulin by the mucosal immune system is regulated by steroid hormones and/or PRL.

VI. THYROID HORMONES

The mechanisms of action of thyroid hormones is still a matter of debate, and there is no firm evidence for the presence of hormone receptors in lymphoid tissue. However, human lymphocytes were shown to convert T_4 to T_3, which is the biologically active hormone. Thyroid hormones were also shown, both in vivo and in vitro, to affect some immune functions. Hypothyroidism led to immunodeficiency in several investigations. The fact that thyroid stimulating hormone (TSH) does not play a role in the reconstitution of Hypox rats for immune reactivity suggests that thyroid hormones do not play a primary immunoregulatory role, but rather, affect immune reactions indirectly, possibly through metabolic alterations.

VII. THE POSSIBLE MECHANISM OF IMMUNOREGULATION BY PITUITARY HORMONES

The pituitary gland has the capacity to regulate immune reactions, since it secretes both immunostimulatory (GH, PRL) and immunosuppressive (ACTH) hormones. The possible mechanism of immunoregulation by the pituitary gland is outlined in Figure 1. It is clear that the ACTH-adrenal axis has an immunosuppressive role, and may be named as the suppressor arm of the neurohormonal immunoregulatory system. This suppression is exerted both on the primary (bone marrow, bursa, thymus) and secondary (lymph nodes, spleen) lymphoid organs, and on circulating mononuclear and polymorphonuclear leukocytes. Glucocorticoids are the final mediators of immunosuppression, acting directly on leukocytes through specific glucocorticoid receptors. Physiological levels of glucocorticoids inhibit a number of immune phenomena (Table 2). Thus, one might suggest that glucocorticoids are essential for the maintenance of inhibitory control of the immune system, an idea originally proposed by Jerne.[49] This inhibitory control has been proven already (please see Chapter 1 for details) and is considered fundamental for the prevention of inadvertant lymphocyte activation, which could lead to self destruction by autoimmune clones.

The blood levels of ACTH and of glucocorticoids rise significantly during stressful situations. It is generally considered that these hormonal changes enable the stressed animal, or individual, to cope better with potentially dangerous situations. Stress and trauma are known to be immunosuppressive,[50] which seems to be a meaningless, or possibly even dangerous side effect. However, dangerous situations often result in body injury, which leads to alteration (denaturation) of self antigens. Without a physiological mechanism for immunosuppression, such newly formed and potent immunogens would trigger profound autoimmune reactions in all probability. Autoimmune disease can be induced with relative ease in animals, if immunization is carried out by denatured (by mixing with Freund's complete adjuvant) autoantigens.[51,52] Species-related differences in autoantigens can also be exploited for the induction of autoimmunity.[53] Furthermore, it seems that under normal, nonstressed, conditions the physiological inhibition of the immune system by glucocorticoids actually facilitates the antigen-specific activation of lymphocytes.[37-41] This is made possible by a number of lymphokines that are capable of counteracting the immunosuppressive effect of glucocorticoids (Table 1). The existence of such glucocorticoid-related immunoregulatory lymphokines suggests further that the physiological role of glucocorticoids is indeed the prevention of inadvertent lymphocyte activation.

It has been known for a long time that glucorticoids induce a dramatic involution of the thymus when pharmacologic doses are applied. Thymus involution can be induced also by stressing the animals, or by the administration of ACTH, indicating that the adrenal gland is capable of secreting glucocorticoids in sufficient quantities to have a profound effect on the thymus gland. The extreme sensitivity of the thymus to glucocorticoid-mediated inhibition suggests that this organ plays a crucial role in neurohormonal immunoregulation.

Although the role of β-endorphin and adrenalin in immunoregulation needs further clarification, it appears that both hormones tend to have an immunosuppressive, or moderating, effect. If this can be substantiated, these hormones should be considered as part of the suppressor arm of the neurohormonal immunoregulatory mechanism. It

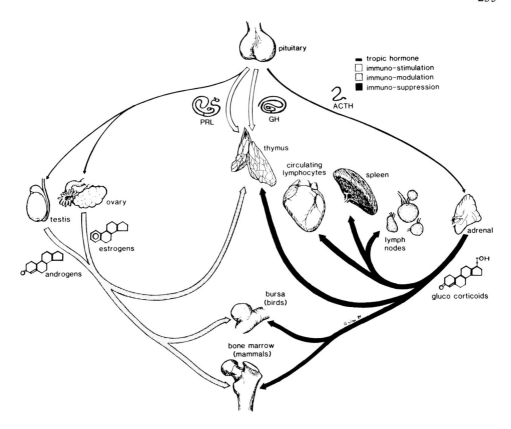

FIGURE 1. The regulatory influence of pituitary hormones on lymphoid organs and cells. (Artwork courtesy of Mr. G. E. Wren, Department of Immunology, University of Manitoba.)

is of interest that the secretion of ACTH and β-endorphin by the pituitary gland is regulated by a common pathway, whereas the synthesis of adrenaline is controlled by glucocorticoids. Thus, the inhibitory control of the immune system may be mediated by several integrated hormones of the ACTH-adrenal axis.

GH has been proposed repeatedly by various investigators as an essential hormone for the development and function of the immune system. However, contradictory findings exist in the literature. The reason for this may be that PRL has not been recognized until recently as a hormone equivalent to GH in the maintenance of immunocompetence. For instance, the various lines and sublines of pituitary dwarf mice may have different PRL status, which could account for the diverging observations on various immune parameters in these animals. Similarly, animals with incomplete hypophysectomy may have significant PRL levels and for this reason, will react immunologically. If, indeed, GH and PRL are essential for the development and maintenance of the immune system, animals and human beings lacking both hormones should not survive. Both the Snell- and Ames-strain of pituitary dwarf mice were found to be deficient in PRL, although minimum concentrations were detectable in males and females of both strains.[53] These animals are also immunodeficient, as discussed in detail in Chapter 3. Pituitary dwarf children were shown to have normal PRL levels.[54,55] Therefore, it is not surprising that such individuals do not show serious deficiencies in immune reactivity.[56]

In Figure 1, both GH and PRL are shown as immunostimulatory hormones acting primarily on the thymus gland. A direct action of these hormones on lymphocytes is not suggested, because of the lack of hard evidence for receptors in lymphoid cells and

Table 3
IMMUNE-DERIVED FACTORS INFLUENCING PITUITARY HORMONE
SECRETION

Species	Factor	Biological effect	Ref.
Man	Endogenous pyrogen	Release of ACTH reserve	70
Mouse, man	Histamine	ACTH release	70-72
Rat	Lymphokine (GIF)	ACTH release	73-75
Monkey	Thymic factor	Elevation of ACTH, β-endorphin	76
Man	Unknown factor(s)	Growth failure in children with immune-inflammatory disease due to deficient growth hormone secretion	77-79
Rat	Thymosin	Stimulation of LHRH and LH release	80

Note: ACTH = adrenocorticotropic hormone; GIF = glucocorticoid increasing factor; LH = luteinizing hormone; LHRH = luteinizing hormone releasing hormone.

because direct effects on in vitro lymphocyte reactions could not be shown convincingly. Since there is evidence for the thymotropic effect of GH in the literature, and we found a similar influence of syngeneic pituitary grafts in rats, one might hypothesize that thymic function is enhanced by these hormones, possibly through the stimulation of thymic hormones. The thymus plays a fundamental role in the regulation of the immune system, and it could suffice for the stimulatory arm of the neurohormonal immunoregulatory mechanism to simply control thymus function. This, however, should serve only as a minimum model for the maintenance of immunocompetence and the situation may turn out to be much more complex in reality.

Interestingly enough, placental lactogen, which is evolutionarily related to GH and PRL, is just as efficient in restoring the immune reactivity of Hypox animals as the above pituitary hormones.[57] The physiological function of placental lactogen is virtually unknown, though it is suspected that this hormone may be involved in osmoregulation during fetal life. However, the mammalian fetus must escape potentially destructive maternal immune reactions, that are triggered by paternal histocompatibility antigens. It is possible that placental lactogen, which is present in large quantities in the amniotic fluid, contributes in some manner to the immunological success of the conceptus. This remains an exciting and largely unexplored area for investigation.

Sex hormones are considered as *immunomodulatory* agents of the neurohormonal regulatory system (Figure 1). Sex hormones do not seem to be essential for the maintenance of immunocompetence, since animals and human beings outside of reproductive age do not show profound immunodeficiency and castration does not result in drastic alteration of the immune response, although some changes are easily detectable. Again, a direct action of sex hormones on lymphocytes cannot be suggested, since clear evidence for the existence of specific receptors in these cells is lacking. However, specific receptors for androgens and estrogens have been identified in the epithelial cells of the thymus and bursa of Fabricius. This supports the hypothesis that sex hormones modulate the production of thymic and bursal hormones, which in turn would influence the immune system. Estrogens, especially estradiol, stimulate most immune reactions, whereas androgens, especially testosterone, have an inhibitory effect. Although this postulate may not apply for all immune reactions, the antagonistic effect of estrogens and androgens has been observed repeatedly. It appears that sex hormones play an important role in the regulation of the immune function of the mammary gland and the female genital tract, which are essential for reproductive success. The possible role of sex hormones in the immunobiology of gestation is discussed by Clark in Chapter 13. Whether or not sex hormones play a more general role in immunoregulation, remains to be seen.

If, indeed, the pituitary gland has an immunoregulatory function, one must assume that immune-derived factors (feedback signals) exist, which are capable of influencing the secretion of regulatory hormones. Only a limited number of studies are available to date, which support the existence of immune-feedback-regulatory signals towards the pituitary gland (Table 3). Nevertheless, these data suggest that both the primary lymphoid organs (thymus) and functional immunocytes emit signals towards the neuroendocrine system, which are able to modify the secretion of various pituitary hormones. These findings, together with the evidence that various pituitary hormones influence immunity, leaves little doubt about the existence of a neurohormonal immunoregulatory mechanism. Further evidence is provided for the regulatory influence of the neurohormonal system on immune phenomena in Chapters 11 and 12.

REFERENCES

1. Hayashida, T. and Li, C.-H., Influence of adrenocorticotropic and growth hormone on antibody formation, *J. Exp. Med.*, 105, 93, 1957.
2. Berczi, I., Nagy, E., Kovacs, K., and Horvath, E., Regulation of humoral immunity in rats by pituitary hormones, *Acta Endocrinol.*, 98, 506, 1981.
3. Berczi, I., Nagy, E., Asa, S. L., and Kovacs, K., Pituitary hormones and contact sensitivity in rats, *Allergy*, 38, 325, 1983.
4. Berczi, I., Nagy, E., Asa, S. L., and Kovacs, K., The influence of pituitary hormones on adjuvant arthritis, *Arthritis Rheum.*, 27, 682, 1984.
5. Nagy, E., Berczi, I., Wren, G. E., Asa, S. L., and Kovacs, K., Immunodulation by bromocriptine, *Immunopharmacology*, 6, 231, 1983.
6. Zimmer, J. A. and Lipton, J. M., Central and peripheral injections of ACTH (1-24) reduce fever in adrenalectomized rabbits, *Peptides*, 2, 413, 1981.
7. Murphy, M. T., Richards, D. B., and Lipton, J. M., Antipyretic potency of centrally administered α-melanocyte stimulating hormone, *Science*, 221, 192, 1983.
8. Glyn-Ballinger, J. R., Bernardini, G. L., and Lipton, J. M., α-MSH injected into the septal region reduces fever in rabbits, *Peptides*, 4, 199, 1983.
9. Mathews, P. M., Froelich, C. J., Sibbitt, W. L., Jr., and Bankhurst, A. D., Enhancement of natural cytotoxicity by β-endorphin, *J. Immunol.*, 130, 1658, 1983.
10. Shavit, Y., Lewis, J. W., Terman, G. W., Gale, R. P., and Liebeskind, J. C., Opioid peptides mediate the suppressive effect of stress on natural killer cell cytotoxicity, *Science*, 223, 188, 1984.
11. Trainin, N., Levo, Y., and Rotter, V., Resistance to hydrocortisone conferred upon thymocytes by a thymic humoral factor, *Eur. J. Immunol.*, 4, 634, 1974.
12. Mayer, M., Galili, U., and Kaiser, N., Intracellular protease activity in glucocorticoid-mediated thymolysis, *Endocrinology*, 110, 2131, 1981.
13. Cidlowski, J. A., Glucocorticoids stimulate ribonucleic acid degradation in isolated rat thymic lymphocytes *in vitro*, *Endocrinology*, 11, 1984, 1982.
14. Voris, B. P., Nicholson, M. L., and Young, D. A., Development of resistance to glucocorticoid hormones during rat thymus cell differentiation: proteins associated with emergence of the resistant state, *Cancer Res.*, 43, 1236, 1983.
15. Ma, D. D. F., Ho, A. H., and Hoffbrand, A. V., Effect of thymosin on glucocorticoid receptor activity and glucocorticoid sensitivity of human thymocytes, *Clin. Exp. Immunol.*, 55, 273, 1984.
16. Karczag, E. and Náray, A., Thymidine kinase activity in murine lymphoid organs following glucocorticoid and heparin administration, *Endokrinologie*, 74, 238, 1979.
17. Karczag, E., Kelemenics, K., Jókay, I., and Földes, I., A kinetic study of glucocorticoid-heparin interaction on the in vivo DNA-synthesis of mouse lymphatic organs, *Immunobiology*, 157, 379, 1980.
18. Cohen, P. L. and Mosier, D. E., Reactivity of steroid-resistant neonatal thymocytes, *Nature (London)*, 251, 233, 1974.
19. Weismann, J. L., Thymus maturation: studies on the origin of cortisone-resistant thymic lymphocytes, *J. Exp. Med.*, 137, 504, 1973.
20. Abo, T., Kawate, T., Itoh, K., and Kumagai, K., Studies on the bioperiodicity of the immune response. I. Circadian rhythms of human T, B and K cell traffic in the peripheral blood, *J. Immunol.*, 126, 1360, 1981.

21. Thomson, S. P., McMahon, L. J., and Nugent, C. A., Endogenous cortisol: a regulator of the number of lymphocytes in peripheral blood, *Clin. Immunol. Immunopathol.*, 17, 506, 1980.

22. Fairchild, S. S., Shannon, K., Kwan, E., and Mishell, R. I., T cell-derived glucosteroid response-modifying factor (GRMF$_T$): a unique lymphokine made by normal T lymphocytes and a T cell hybridoma, *J. Immunol.*, 132, 821, 1984.

23. Schleimer, R. P., Jacques, A., Shin, H. S., Lichtenstein, L. M., and Plaut, M., Inhibition of T cell-mediated cytotoxicity by anti-inflammatory steroids, *J. Immunol.*, 132, 266, 1984.

24. Hirschberg, H., Hirschberg, T., Nousianen, H., Braathen, L. R., and Jaffe, E., The effects of corticosteroids on the antigen presenting properties of human monocytes and endothelial cells, *Clin. Immunol. Immunopathol.*, 23, 577, 1982.

25. Mishell, R. I., Bradley, L. M., Chen, Y. H. U., Grabstein, K. H., Mishell, B. B., Shigi, J. M., and Shigi, S. M., Inhibition of steroid-induced immune suppression by adjuvant stimulated accessory cells, *J. Reticuloendothel. Soc.*, 24, 439, 1978.

26. Mishell, R. I., Lucas, A., and Mishell, B. B., The role of activated accessory cells in preventing immunosuppression by hydrocortisone, *J. Immunol.*, 119, 118, 1977.

27. Mishell, R. I., Shiigi, J. M., Mishell, B. B., Grabstein, K. H., and Shiigi, S. M., Prevention of the immunosuppressive effects of glucocorticosteroids by cell-free factors from adjuvant activated accessory cells, *Immunopharmacology*, 2, 233, 1980.

28. Moore, R. N., Goodrum, K. J., Couch, R., Jr., and Berry, L. J., Factors affecting macrophage function: glucocorticoid antagonizing factor, *J. Reticuloendothel. Soc.*, 23, 321, 1978.

29. Orson, F. M., Grayson, J., Pike, S., De Seau, V., and Blaese, R. M., T cell-replacing factor for glucocorticosteroid-induced immunoglobulin production. A unique steroid-dependent cytokine, *J. Exp. Med.*, 158, 1473, 1983.

30. Stevenson, R. D., Polymorph migration stimulator. A new factor produced by hydrocortisone-treated monocytes, *Clin. Exp. Immunol.*, 17, 603, 1974.

31. Hochman, P. S. and Cudkowicz, G., Suppression of natural cytotoxicity by spleen cells of hydrocortisone-treated mice, *J. Immunol.*, 123, 968, 1979.

32. Holbrook, N. J., Cox, W. I., and Horner, H. C., Direct suppression of natural killer activity in human peripheral blood leukocyte cultures by glucocorticoids and its modulation by interferon, *Cancer Res.*, 43, 4019, 1983.

33. Nair, M. P. N. and Schwartz, S. A., Immunomodulatory effects of corticosteroids on natural killer and antibody-dependent cellular cytotoxic activities of human lymphocytes, *J. Immunol.*, 132, 2876, 1984.

34. Klempner, M. S. and Gallin, J. I., Inhibition of neutrophil Fc receptor function by corticosteroids, *Clin. Exp. Immunol.*, 34, 137, 1978.

35. Hammerschmidt, D. E., White, J. G., Craddock, P. R., and Jacob, H. S., Corticosteroids inhibit complement-induced granulocyte aggregation: possible mechanisms for their efficacy in shock states, *J. Clin. Invest.*, 63, 798, 1979.

36. Skubitz, K. M., Craddock, P. R., Hammerschmidt, D. E., and August, J. T., Corticosteroids block binding of chemotactic peptide to its receptor on granulocytes and cause disaggregation of granulocyte aggregates in vitro, *J. Clin. Invest.*, 68, 13, 1981.

37. Ambrose, C. T., The requirements for hydrocortisone in antibody-forming tissue cultivated in serum-free medium, *J. Exp. Med.*, 119, 1027, 1964.

38. Ambrose, C. T., The essential role of corticosteroids in the induction of the immune response in vitro, in *Hormones and the Immune Response*, CIBA Study Group 36, Wolstenholme, G. E. and Knight, J., Eds., Churchill Livingstone, London, 1970, 100.

39. Cohen, I. R., Stavy, L., and Feldman, M., Glucocorticoids and cellular immunity in vitro. Facilitation of the sensitization phase and inhibition of the effector phase of a lymphocyte anti-fibroblast reaction, *J. Exp. Med.*, 132, 1055, 1970.

40. Stavy, L., Cohen, I. R., and Feldman, M., The effect of hydrocortisone on lymphocyte-mediated cytolysis, *Cell. Immunol.*, 7, 302, 1973.

41. Stavy, L., Cohen, I. R., and Feldman, M., Stimulation of rat lymphocyte proliferation by hydrocortisone during the induction of cell-mediated immunity in vitro, *Transplantation*, 17, 173, 1974.

42. Recant, L., Hume, D. M., Forsham, P. H., and Thorn, G. W., Studies on the effect of epinephrine on the pituitary-adrenocortical system, *J. Clin. Endocrinol. Metab.*, 10, 187, 1950.

43. Chatterton, R. T., Jr., Murray, C. L., and Hellman, L., Endocrine effects on leukocytopoiesis in the rat. I. Evidence for growth hormone secretion as the leukocytopoietic stimulus following acute cortisol-induced lymphopenia, *Endocrinology*, 92, 775, 1973.

44. Comsa, J., Schwarz, J. A., and Neu, H., Interaction between thymic hormone and hypophyseal growth hormone on production of precipitating antibodies in the rat, *Immunol. Commun.*, 3, 11, 1974.

45. Comsa, J., Leonhardt, H., and Schwarz, J. A., Influence of the thymus-corticotropin-growth hormone interaction on the rejection of skin allografts in the rat, *Ann. N. Y. Acad. Sci.,* 249, 387, 1975.

46. Shiu, R. P. C., Elsholtz, H. P., Tanaka, T., Friesen, H. G., Gout, P. W., Beer, C. T., and Noble, R. L., Receptor-mediated mitogenic action of prolactin in rat lymphoma cell line, *Endocrinology,* 113, 159, 1983.

47. Russell, D. H., Matrisian, L., Kibler, R., Larson, D. F., Poulos, B., and Magun, B. E., Prolactin receptors on human lymphocytes and their modulation by cyclosporine, *Biochem. Biophys. Res. Commun.,* 121, 899, 1984.

48. Weisz-Carrington, P., Roux, M. E., McWilliams, M., Phillips-Quagliata, J. M., and Lamm, M. E., Organ and isotype distribution of plasma cells producing specific antibody after oral immunization: evidence for a generalized secretory immune system, *J. Immunol.,* 123, 1705, 1979.

49. Jerne, N. K., Towards a network theory of the immune system, *Ann. Immunol. (Inst. Pasteur),* 125C, 373, 1974.

50. Munster, A. M., Immunologic response of trauma and burns. An overview, *Am. J. Med.,* March 30, 142, 1984.

51. Anderson, J. R., Buchanan, W. W., and Goudie, R. B., *Autoimmunity. Clinical and Experimental,* Charles C. Thomas, Springfield, Ill., 1967.

52. Talal, N., Ed., *Autoimmunity. Genetic, Immunologic, Virologic and Clinical Aspects,* Academic Press, New York, 1977.

53. Milich, D. R. and Gershwin, M. E., Murine autoimmune hemolytic anemia induced via xenogenic erythrocyte immunization. III. Influences of sex, *Clin. Immunol. Immunopathol.,* 18, 1, 1981.

54. Barkley, M. S., Bartke, A., Gross, D. S., and Sinha, Y. N., Prolactin status of hereditary dwarf mice, *Endocrinology,* 110, 2088, 1981.

55. Kaplan, S. L., Grumbach, M. M., Friesen, H. G., and Costom, B. H., Thyrotropin-releasing factor (TRF) effect on secretion of human pituitary prolactin and thyrotropin in children and in idiopathic hypopituitary dwarfism: further evidence for hypophysiotropic hormone deficiencies, *J. Clin. Endocrinol. Metab.,* 35, 825, 1972.

56. Tolis, G., Goldstein, M., and Friesen, H. G., Functional evaluation of prolactin secretion in patients with hypothalamic-pituitary disorders, *J. Clin. Invest.,* 52, 783, 1973.

57. Ramos-Zepeda, R., Kretschmer, R., López-Osuna, M., Parra-Covarrubias, A., and Pérez-Pastén, E., Evaluation of immunological function in human hypopituitarism, *Arch. Invest. Med.,* 4, 197, 1973.

58. Nagy, E., Berczi, I., and Friesen, H. G., Regulation of immunity in rats by lactogenic and growth hormones, *Acta Endocrinol.,* 102, 351, 1983.

59. Ritter, M. A., Embryonic mouse thymocyte development: enhancing effect of corticosterone at physiological levels, *Immunology,* 33, 241, 1977.

60. Barr, R. D., Koekebakker, M., and Milner, R. A., Hydrocortisone — a possible physiological regulator of human granulopoiesis, *Scand. J. Haematol.,* 31, 31, 1983.

61. Kawate, T., Abo, T., Hinuma, S., and Kumagai, K., Studies on the bioperiodicity of the immune response. II. Co-variations of murine T and B cells and a role of corticosteroid, *J. Immunol.,* 126, 1364, 1981.

62. Homo, F., Dardenne, M., and Duval, D., Effect of steroids on concanavalin A-induced blast transformation of mouse lymphoid cells, *Cell. Immunol.,* 56, 381, 1980.

63. Bradley, L. M. and Mishell, R. I., Differential effects of glucocorticoids on the functions of helper and suppressor lymphocytes-T, *Proc. Natl. Acad. Sci. U.S.A. Biol. Sci.,* 78, 3155, 1981.

64. Duncan, M. R., Sadlik, J. R., and Hadden, J. W., Glucocorticoid modulation of lymphokine-induced macrophage proliferation, *Cell. Immunol.,* 67, 23, 1982.

65. Schultz, R. M., Chirigos, M. A., Stoychkov, J. N., and Pavlidis, N. A., Factors affecting macrophage cytotoxic activity with particular emphasis on corticosteroids and acute stress, *J. Reticuloendothel. Soc.,* 26, 83, 1979.

66. Rühl, H., Vogt, W., Rühl, U., Bochert, G., and Schmidt, S., Effects of hydrocortisone treatment and whole body irradiation of mouse lymphocyte stimulation in vitro, *Immunology,* 25, 753, 1973.

67. Thurman, G. B., Rossio, J. L., and Goldstein, A. L., Thymosin-induced recovery of murine T-cell functions following treatment with hydrocortisone acetate, *Transplant. Proc.,* 9, 1201, 1977.

68. Ranelletti, F. O., Musiani, P., Maggiano, N., Lauriola, L., and Piantelli, M., Modulation of glucocorticoid inhibitory action on human lymphocyte mitogenesis: dependence on mitogen concentration and T-cell maturity, *Cell. Immunol.,* 76, 22, 1983.

69. Jokay, I., Kelemenics, K., Karczag, E., and Foldes, I., Interactions of glucocorticoids and heparin on the humoral immune response of mice, *Immunobiology,* 157, 390, 1980.

70. Liddle, G. W., The adrenals, in *Textbook of Endocrinology,* 6th ed., Williams, R. H., Ed., W. B. Saunders, Philadelphia, 1981, 249.

71. Seltzer, A. and Donoso, A. O., Involvement of specific receptors in the histamine stimulation of the pituitary-corticoadrenal system in the rat, *Neuroendocrinol. Lett.,* 4, 299, 1982.

72. Badger, A. M., Griswold, D. E., Dimartino, M. J., and Poste, G., Inhibition of antibody synthesis by histamine in concanavalin A-treated mice: the possible role of glucocorticosteroids, *J. Immunol.,* 129, 1017, 1982.

73. Besedovsky, H. O., del Rey, A., and Sorkin, E., Lymphokine-containing supernatants from Con A-stimulated cells increase corticosterone blood levels, *J. Immunol.,* 126, 385, 1981.

74. Besedovsky, H. O., del Rey, A., Sorkin E., Lotz, W., and Schwulera, U., Lymphoid cells produce an immunoregulatory glucocorticoid increasing factor (GIF) acting through the pituitary gland, *Clin. Exp. Immunol.,* in press.

75. Vahouny, G. V., Kyeyune-Nyombi, E., McGillis, J. P., Tare, N. S., Huang, K.-Y., Tombes, R., Goldstein, A. L., and Hall, N. R., Thymosin peptides and lymphokines do not directly stimulate adrenal corticosteroid production in vitro, *J. Immunol.,* 130, 791, 1983.

76. Healy, D. L., Hodgen, G. D., Schulte, H. M., Chrousos, G. P., Loriaux, D. L., Hall, N. R., and Goldstein, A. L., The thymus-adrenal connection: thymosin has corticotropin-releasing activity in primates, *Science,* 222, 1353, 1983.

77. Daughaday, W. H., The adrenohypophysis, in *Textbook of Endocrinology,* 6th ed., Williams, R. H., Ed., W. B. Saunders, Philadelphia, 1981, 73.

78. Falliers, C. J., Tan, L. S., Szentivanyi, J., Jorgensen, J. R., and Bukantz, S. C., Childhood asthma and steroid therapy as influences on growth, *Am. J. Dis. Child.,* 105, 127, 1963.

79. Ferguson, A. C. and Murray, A. B., Short stature and delayed skeletal maturation in children with allergic disease, *J. Allergy Clin. Immunol.,* 69, 461, 1982.

80. Rebar, R. W., Miyake, A., Low, T. L. K., and Goldstein, A. L., Thymosin stimulates secretion of luteinizing hormone-releasing factor, *Science,* 214, 669, 1981.

Chapter 11

REGULATORY IMMUNE-NEUROENDOCRINE FEEDBACK SIGNALS*

Hugo Besedovsky, Adriana del Rey, and Ernst Sorkin

TABLE OF CONTENTS

* This work was supported by the Swiss National Science Foundation Grant No. 3.399.0.83 SR.

I. INTRODUCTION

The pituitary gland controls directly or indirectly the activity of almost all endocrine glands, and by its connections with the hypothalamus it is associated with sensorial-visceral and autonomic processes. These characteristics make this gland a major integrator of homeostatic mechanisms. The immune response may be considered as a homeostatic response since antigens elicit an immune response not only because of their potential risk for the host (harmless foreign agents can be good immunogens), but also because it leads to a perturbation of the "milieu interieur". The capacity of the immune system to discriminate between self and non-self has its basis in the wide range of specificities expressed by immune cells, a high proportion of which is directed towards recognition of modified or altered self-cells or -molecules. This characteristic of the immune system implies that it can perceive an internal image of body constituents and react to particular distortions of this image. The immune response as a homeostatic response is therefore under physiological conditions contributing to the maintenance of the constancy and integrity of body cells and tissues. This concept also suggests the participation of neuroendocrine mechanisms in immunoregulation and thus, integration at the pituitary level as well.

The better known immunoregulatory mechanisms suggest that the immune system is a self contained, self monitored system. In fact, several autoregulatory mechanisms exist such as antibody feedback, idiotypic-anti-idiotypic network, suppressor/helper cells, and regulatory lymphokines and monokines. The aforementioned regulatory mechanisms confer a degree of autonomy to the immune system that is attested by the fact that immunological cells can also perform in vitro.

However, hormones and neurotransmitters that are present in the microenvironment of immunological cells can restrict this autonomy, probably by their action on receptors for these neuroendocrine agents. Furthermore, we suggested that the activity of hormones and neurotransmitters is interwoven and integrated with intrinsic immunoregulatory processes, thereby leading to common feedback circuits between neuroendocrine structures and the immune system.[1]

In the following text we shall provide a few examples on how manipulation of neuroendocrine mechanisms can limit the autonomy of the immune system. On the basis of our own work we shall then concentrate on the main topic of this contribution: regulatory immune-neuroendocrine feedback signals.

II. NEUROENDOCRINE MECHANISMS LIMIT THE AUTONOMY OF THE IMMUNE SYSTEM

Many experimental data show that, as other body cells, immune cells with their extremely versatile and complex tasks also do not escape neuroendocrine influences. Obvious levels of control by hormones and neurotransmitters concern the general cellular metabolism and cell division. In fact, the immune response is perhaps the only physiological response in which amplification is based on cell proliferation and transformation. These processes require metabolic changes and growth factors that make the immune response particularly dependent on neuroendocrine mechanisms. Even so, we believe that the control of metabolism and proliferation is by no means the only influence which hormones and neurotransmitters exert on immune cells. It suffices to mention that the production of several lymphokines and monokines is known to be affected by certain hormones and neurotransmitters.[2-4] Also the intracellular level of those cyclic nucleotides that participate in the processes of activation or suppression of immune cells can be affected by these agents.[5] Furthermore, it is known that manipulation of brain, autonomic, and endocrine structures as well as psychosocial stimuli result in some cases in subtle influences on the behavior of different subsets of immunological cells.[6]

Two examples of the postulated restriction of autonomy are given in the following. The first derives from manipulation of endocrine mechanisms and the second from disruption of sympathetic connections.

Work over several decades has shown that adrenal cortical hormones can influence immune phenomena. The protein A plaque assay has permitted us to evaluate the effect of reduced endogenous glucocorticoid levels (adrenalectomy) on the total number of immunoglobulin secreting cells (Ig-SC).[7] This parameter is usually taken as an overall expression of B cell and indirectly also of T cell activity. Adrenalectomized and sham operated mice were killed 9 days after surgery, and the total number of splenic immunoglobulin secreting cells were counted. Adrenalectomized animals showed a more than twofold increase in total number of Ig-SC. It is unlikely that the increased number of Ig-SC is caused only by clonal expansion of already activated cells, because of the high degree of cross-reactivity and also because of the polyclonal effects of certain lymphokines and monokines known to be under adrenal control.[4] The most likely interpretation is that the increase of Ig-SC caused by adrenalectomy results in a much higher incidence of immunological cell interactions, for example, within the idiotypic network. The latter is generally considered as a representative expression of immunological autonomy.

The other example showing external restriction imposed on immune mechanisms is given by the exploration of influences of the sympathetic innervation. In the spleen, nerve fibers follow the arterioles and penetrate into the periarteriolar sheath where T cells are located. From there, some fibers spread into the white pulp and form a mesh around lymphoid cells.[8]

We have surgically denervated the spleen, a procedure that resulted in an increased immune response to sheep red blood cells (SRBC). In a related approach we have chemically sympathectomized rats with 6-HO-dopamine. When this procedure was associated with adrenalectomy a clear-cut increase in plaque-forming cells (PFC) against SRBC was again noticed.[9] Other authors have confirmed these results and indeed achieved even more striking results by choosing another type of antigen. The antigens used in these instances elicited T-independent immune responses that were severalfold enhanced by chemical sympathectomy.[10]

The above described experiments showed that hormones and neurotransmitters are not mere innocent bystanders in the microenvironment of immunological cells, but that they can restrain the autonomy of the immune system.

III. IMMUNOREGULATION BASED ON IMMUNE AND NEUROENDOCRINE SIGNALS

The knowledge that hormones and neurotransmitters can influence immune processes, while providing essential information on potential extrinsic immunoregulatory agencies, is in our view not sufficient to prove neuroendocrine immunoregulation. Such evidence must be based on identification of information channels between immunological cells and the neuroendocrine system. Since the immune response is a phasic phenomenon, it is a prerequisite that its extrinsic regulation must necessarily also be reflected in phasic neural and endocrine changes. Such changes should, in turn, be capable of modifying the activity of immunological cells.

Our approach to this obviously complicated problem was basically oriented to:

1. Search for neuroendocrine changes induced by the immune response.
2. Identify and characterize messengers derived from immunological cells that mediate the anticipated neuroendocrine responses.

3.   Evaluate the final effect of the immunologically elicited neuroendocrine responses on immune mechanisms.

The results obtained by applying this methodology, particularly with regard to the adrenal cortex, the sympathetic system, and hypothalamus involvement in immunoregulation are summarized below.

IV. IMMUNOREGULATORY CIRCUIT INTEGRATED AT THE LEVEL OF THE HYPOTHALAMUS-PITUITARY-ADRENAL AXIS

Although glucocorticoid hormones exert well-known multifaceted effects on immunity, it has remained unclear whether these hormones are relevant to immunoregulation under physiological conditions. The following data have provided the primary evidence for this view.

After antigenic challenge with three different antigens — sheep red blood cells (SRBC) or horse red blood cells (HRBC); trinitrophenyl-haemocyanin (TNP-Hae) in two species (rats, mice) — increased glucocorticoid blood levels were noted at about the time of the peak of the immune response.[11] This increase in blood glucocorticoid levels was directly related to the magnitude of the immune response.[29] The reached hormone levels are known to be immunosuppressive,[12] and furthermore we have shown earlier that they are capable of suppressing the response to unrelated antigens. In fact, inhibition of this hormone increase by adrenalectomy can overcome sequential antigenic competition.[13] The increase in corticosterone levels, however, seems not to be a general reaction caused by all types of immune responses, since we have also observed the opposite effect, namely a decrease in the levels of this hormone during skin graft rejection.[14]

How are these changes of glucocorticoid blood levels brought about? Do immunological signals to neuroendocrine structures exist that control blood glucocorticoid levels? If this were so, one might expect that in vitro stimulation of immunological cells would lead to a release of mediators that, when injected into normal recipients, affect the adrenal gland in a manner similar to that observed in immunized animals. Such types of experiments were performed using supernatants obtained from immunological cells stimulated in vitro with concanavalin A (Con A)[15] or allogeneic lymphocytes.[16] These supernatants were not pyrogenic and did not change the blood pressure in the rat. The outcome was unequivocal. A severalfold increase in blood corticosterone levels was obtained that, in its magnitude, was similar to that observed in antigenically stimulated rats. However, as expected the hormone increase occurred within 30 to 60 min after application of preformed mediators instead of after several days. Therefore, injection of mediators derived from immunological cells can mimic the events occurring after antigen injection.

Some of the supernatants used were obtained from cultures of an almost pure population of human peripheral blood lymphocytes containing less than 0.1% monocytes. This fact practically proves the lymphoid cell origin of the factor that increases corticosterone blood levels. We have named this activity glucocorticoid increasing factor (GIF). The existence of GIF has recently been confirmed by other authors.[17,18] The potency of GIF is indicated by the fact that the amount produced by less than 5×10^5 lymphoid cells can increase corticosterone blood level in an adult rat severalfold.

At which level does GIF act? Does it act directly on the adrenal cortex or through the hypothalamus-pituitary axis? Experimental evidence shows that the immunological messenger GIF does not act directly on the adrenal cortex,[19] but that the pituitary gland is involved as is attested by increased ACTH blood levels following GIF injection. Furthermore, blockade of ACTH output by hypophysectomy or by administration of dexamethasone prior to injection of GIF led to the entire ceasing of the glucocortico-steroid output.[16] Experiments showing that intracerebro-ventricular injection of supernatants containing GIF produces increased glucocorticoid blood levels, strongly suggest that at least one pathway of action of this factor is via the hypothalamus, presumably by increasing CRF production.[30]

In summary, these data permit us to postulate the first immunoregulatory circuit linking neuroendocrine structures and the immune system. Stimulation of lymphoid cells induces the release of a factor (GIF) that in turn increases the blood glucocorticoid level via hypothalamus-pituitary axis to a level known to affect the functions of several types of immunological cells.

What could be the regulatory meaning of this circuit? It is known that apart from metabolic effects, glucocorticoids at increased but still physiological concentrations inhibit IL-1 and IL-2 production and/or action.[2-4] In this way, increased glucocorticoid levels can control the clonal expansion of committed cells with high affinity for the antigen. On the other hand, since resting immunological cells are much more sensitive to glucocorticoids than activated cells, we postulate that this circuit may have the function of preventing the excessive expansion of cells with low affinity for the antigen or of those cells which are recruited under the polyclonal influence of lymphokines. It is conceivable that this circuit, by impeding a cumulative excessive expansion of lymphoid and accessory cells, plays a role in preventing autoimmune and lymphoproliferative diseases. It was also shown that under certain conditions lymphocytes can produce an ACTH-like substance. This finding, if confirmed, would suggest the existence of a short loop between lymphoid cells and the adrenal cortex.[20] How this loop may operate under physiological conditions needs further investigation.

V. SYMPATHETIC IMMUNOREGULATION

One of the reasons for studying the role of sympathetic mechanisms in immunoregulation is the existence of interactions between sympathetic adrenocortical hormones. As we mentioned, lymphoid organs are sympathetically innervated[8,21] and disruption of this innervation results in enhanced immune responses.[9,10]

The counterpart of these experiments was the study of the immune response following in vitro and in vivo administration of alpha-agonists, (e.g., methoxamine), which have no central effects. The result was inhibition of the immune response.[9,22] We concluded from these results that sympathetic innervation mediates a mechanism restraining immunological cells in their activity. Interesting as these data are, they do not permit us to decide whether such effects reflect the existence of sympathetic immunoregulation. Therefore we analyzed whether sympathetic nerve activity, as reflected by the noradrenaline (NA) level, changes during the immune response. After antigen challenge (SRBC) we found a marked decrease in NA content in rat spleen on days 3 and 4. The degree and persistence of this NA decrease is inversely related to the magnitude of the response.[23] No change in the NA content of a nonlymphoid organ, the heart, was discerned. Studies on NA turnover rates that reflect the degree of NA synthesis were also performed in the spleen of immunized and control animals. These studies showed a decrease in splenic NA turnover rates in immunized rats.[31]

These findings constitute definitive evidence that a significant change in the sympathetic system, as reflected by a decreased NA content of the spleen, occurs in the environment of immunological cells. Taken with the data described on denervation and effects of alpha-agonists, this decrease in NA can be expected to affect the performance of immunological cells.

Since animals are constantly developing immune responses to environmental antigens, the basal degree of activity of sympathetic nerves may be influenced by the degree of immunological activity. Germ-free (GF) animals, which are subjected to a minimal degree of external antigenic challenge, and specific pathogen-free (SPF) animals, which are constantly exposed to external antigens but protected against pathogens, and which offer an excellent model to study the basal levels of catecholamines in lymphoid organs. According to the above-described results and rationale, the prediction was that the immunologically more engaged SPF rats should have lower NA levels in their lymphoid organs than their germ-free (GF) counterparts. As predicted, lymphoid tissues of SPF rats such as spleen, thymus, and lymph nodes had about half the NA content of GF animals. The NA content of rat stomach and duodenum was similar in SPF and in GF conditions.[24] We explain these results by postulating that antigenic exposure of conventional or SPF animals over their whole lifespan contributes to, or even causes, the described lower NA content in the lymphoid organs. In the same experiments the adrenaline (A) and NA contents of the adrenal gland were also determined. SPF animals had smaller adrenals than GF animals and the total adrenal NA and A content was significantly lower in SPF animals. This fact indicates that the products of immunological cells reach central structures, which directly or indirectly control the function of the adrenal medulla.

In summary, the above data suggest that the sympathetic nervous system participates in immunoregulation. In particular, the phasic decrease of NA levels during the immune response in the spleen, but not in nonlymphoid organs, can be interpreted as the expression of a sympathetic reflex mechanism that frees immunological cells from restraining sympathetic influences. The same process may also favor recirculation of these cells by affecting the blood flow in lymphoid organs. As the decrease in splenic NA content is inversely related to the magnitude of the immune response, this additional evidence seems to favor a relevant role for sympathetic signals in immunoregulation. The mechanisms underlying the NA decrease the nature of the afferent signals, and the type of immunological cells affected by sympathetic signals need to be elucidated.

VI. IMMUNOREGULATION INTEGRATED AT THE HYPOTHALAMIC LEVEL

The hypothalamus controls numerous pituitary and autonomic functions. The above described data about the involvement of the pituitary and the sympathetic nervous system in immunoregulation suggest that the immune response can evoke hypothalamic responses. Our first approach to this problem was a study in the same animal (rat) of both the immune response and the rate of firing of individual hypothalamic neurons at various intervals after injection of SRBC or TNP-Hae.[25] Rat hypothalamic responses (ventromedial nucleus) to TNP-Hae showed increased frequency of neuronal firing during the immune response, the highest activation occurred on day 2, a time close to the peak number of direct PFC. Animals stimulated with SRBC showed on day 1 no PFC and no changes in firing frequency. On day 5, PFC in spleen were maximal, and there was a more than twofold increase in the firing rate of the ventromedial neurons. In several rats that were immunological nonresponders, no increase in firing rates occurred. Furthermore, no changes in firing rates were observed in the anterior hypothalamic nucleus in simultaneous recordings in the immunologically responding rats.

It is well known that aminergic brain pathways modulate the activity of hypothalamic neurons. In order to study whether noradrenergic pathways in the brain are affected by the immune response and its products, we analyzed catecholamine levels in the hypothalamus.[26] In immunologically high responder rats, a marked decrease was noted in hypothalamic NA turnover rate 4 days after antigen administration as compared with saline injected controls.

In order to study whether soluble products derived from immunological cells mediate NA changes in the hypothalamus, we administered such type of material to rats. Two hours after injection of supernatants from rat spleen cells stimulated with Con A, NA concentration in the hypothalamus was reduced when compared with the supernatants obtained from nonstimulated lymphoid cells. The magnitude of the NA reduction observed in the hypothalamus corresponded to about 50% of that obtained by applying alpha-methyl-p-tyrosine, a powerful inhibitor of NA synthesis. We interpret these results as evidence that activation of immunological cells leads to a decrease in the rate of NA synthesis in the hypothalamus, which is possibly mediated by a factor released by immunological cells.

The fact that hypothalamic NA synthesis is inhibited during the immune response permits us now to attempt to integrate the described evidence. First of all, the inhibitor influence of NA on hypothalamic neurons is well-known.[27] Therefore the decrease in NA may explain the increase in the firing rates of hypothalamic neurons during the immune response. Previous experimental evidence from other laboratories has also shown that a NA increase in the hypothalamus leads to a decrease in activity of neurons producing corticotrophin releasing factor.[28] Hence, the hypothalamic NA decrease during the immune response may also mediate the increase in CRF-producing neuron activity and thus, provide a link to the glucocorticoid-associated circuit.

VII. SYNTHESIS

The evidence presented in this chapter proves that the immune response can by itself bring about neuroendocrine responses with immunoregulatory effects. Some of these responses can be attributed to immunological cell-derived soluble messengers. Although these messengers are not yet characterized, we believe that they fulfill requirements that allow us to call them immunological cell-derived hormones. As an example can serve the glucocorticoid increasing factor (GIF), which acts through the hypothalamus-pituitary axis, and therefore is integrated in the network of neuroendocrine homeostatic mechanisms. This situation makes it clear that these immunohormones, aside from their immunological effects, influence other nonimmunological mechanisms.

We have defined the immune response as a homeostatic response. We have provided evidence that it is subject to levels of neuroendocrine regulation as it occurs with other homeostatic mechanisms. This concept implies that afferent information channels exist between immune cells and the brain. In this sense the data could also be considered in a broader context. One of the major functions of the brain is to process information on changes in the external and internal environment detected by receptor organs. The above discussed evidence shows that the brain is informed about the intrusion of antigenic macromolecules and possibly also about modified self-antigens. Immunological cells that express a huge repertoire of specific receptors for antigenic agents may, by way of releasing appropriate but different combinations of immunohormonal messengers, be the ultimate source of this information for the brain. The immune system may thus act as the peripheral receptor organ for this type of external or internal stimuli.

REFERENCES

1. Besedovsky, H. O., del Rey, A., and Sorkin, E., Neuroendocrine immunoregulation, in *Immunoregulation,* Fabris, N., Garaci, E., Hadden, J., and Mitchison, N. A., Eds., Plenum Press, New York, 1983, 315.
2. Gillis, S., Crabtree, G. R., and Smith, K., Glucocorticoid-induced inhibition of T cell growth factor production. I. The effect on mitogen-induced lymphocyte proliferation, *J. Immunol.,* 123, 1624, 1979.
3. Snyder, D. S. and Unanue, E. R., Corticosteroids inhibit murine macrophage Ia expression and interleukin 1 production, *J. Immunol.,* 129, 1803, 1982.
4. Kelso, A. and Munck, A., Glucocorticoid inhibition of lymphokine secretion by alloreactive T lymphocyte clones, *J. Immunol.,* 133, 784, 1984.
5. Hadden, J. W., Cyclic nucleotides and related mechanism in immune regulation — a mini review, in *Immunoregulation,* Fabris, N., Garaci, E., Hadden, J., and Mitchison, N. A., Eds., Plenum Press, New York, 1983, 201.
6. Ader, R., Ed., *Psychoneuroimmunology,* Academic Press, New York, 1981.
7. del Rey, A., Besedovsky, H. O., and Sorkin, E., Endogenous blood levels of corticosterone control the immunologic cell mass and B cell activity in mice, *J. Immunol.,* 133, 572, 1984.
8. Williams, J. M. and Felten, D. L., Sympathetic innervation of murine thymus and spleen: a comparative histofluorescence study, *Anat. Rec.,* 199, 531, 1981.
9. Besedovsky, H. O., del Rey, A., Sorkin E., Da Prada, M., and Keller, H. H., Immunoregulation mediated by the sympathetic nervous system, *Cell. Immunol.,* 48, 346, 1979.
10. Miles, K., Quintans, J., Chelmicka-Schorr, E., and Arnason, B. G., The sympathetic nervous system modulates antibody response to thymus-independent antigens, *J. Neuroimmunol.,* 1, 101, 1981.
11. Besedovsky, H. O., Sorkin, E., Keller, M., and Muller, J., Changes in blood hormone levels during the immune reponse, *Proc. Soc. Exp. Biol. Med.,* 150, 466, 1975.
12. Gisler, R. H. and Schenkel-Hulliger, L., Hormonal regulation of the immune response. II. Influence of pituitary and adrenal activity on immune responsiveness in vitro, *Cell. Immunol.,* 2, 646, 1971.
13. Besedovsky, H. O., del Rey, A., and Sorkin, E., Antigenic competition between horse and sheep red blood cells as a hormone-dependent phenomenon, *Clin. Exp. Immunol.,* 37, 106, 1979.
14. Besedovsky, H. O., Sorkin, E., and Keller, M., Changes in the concentration of corticosterone in the blood during skin-graft rejection in the rat, *J. Endocrinol.,* 76, 175, 1978.
15. Besedovsky, H. O., del Rey, A., and Sorkin, E., Lymphokine containing supernatants from Con A stimulated cells increase corticosterone blood levels, *J. Immunol.,* 126, 385, 1981.
16. Besedovsky, H. O., del Rey, A., Sorkin, E., Lotz, W., and Schwulera, U., Lymphoid cells produce an immunoregulatory glucocorticoid increasing factor (GIF) acting through the pituitary gland, *Clin. Exp. Immunol.,* 59, 622, 1985.
17. Pulley, M. S., Dumonde, D. C., Carter, G., Muller, B., Fleck, A., Southcott, B. M., and den Hollander, F., Hormonal, haematological and acute phase protein responses of advanced cancer patients to the intravenous injection of lymphoid-cell lymphokine (LCL-LK), in *Human Lymphokines,* Kahn, A. and Hill, N. O., Eds., Academic Press, New York, 1982. 651.
18. Bindon, C., Czerniecki, M., Ruell, P., Edwards, A., McCarthy, W. H., Harris, R., and Hersey, P., Clearance rates and systemic effects of intravenously administered interleukin 2 (IL-2) containing preparations in human subjects, *Br. J. Cancer,* 47, 123, 1983.
19. Vahouny, G. V., Kyeyune-Nyombi, E., McGillis, J. P., Tare, N. S., Huang, K.-Y., Tombes, R., Goldstein, A. L., and Hall, N. R., Thymosin peptides and lymphokines do not directly stimulate adrenal corticosteroid production in vitro, *J. Immunol.,* 130, 791, 1983.
20. Smith, E., Meyer, W., and Blalock, J. E., Virus-induced corticosterone in hypophysectomized mice: a possible lymphoid adrenal axis, *Science,* 218, 1311, 1982.
21. Bulloch, K. and Moore, R. Y., Innervation of the thymus gland by brain stem and spinal cord in mouse and rat, *Am. J. Anat.,* 162, 157, 1981.
22. Besedovsky, H. O., Da Prada, M., del Rey, A., and Sorkin, E., Immunoregulation by sympathetic nervous sytem, *Trends Pharmacol. Sci.,* 2, 236, 1981.
23. del Rey, A., Besedovsky, H. O., Sorkin, E., Da Prada, M., and Bondiolotti, G. P., Sympathetic immunoregulation: difference between immunological high and low responder animals, *Am. J. Physiol.,* 242, R30, 1982.
24. del Rey, A., Besedovsky, H. O., Sorkin, E., Da Prada, M., and Arrenbrecht, S., Immunoregulation mediated by the sympathetic nervous system. II, *Cell. Immunol.,* 63, 329, 1981.
25. Besedovsky, H. O., Sorkin, E., Felix, D., and Haas, H., Hypothalamic changes during the immune response, *Eur. J. Immunol.,* 7, 323, 1977.
26. Besedovsky, H. O., del Rey, A., Sorkin, E., Da Prada, M., Burri, R., and Honegger, C., The immune response evokes changes in brain noradrenergic neurons, *Science,* 221, 564, 1983.

27. Nishino, H., Suprachiasmatic nuclei and circadian rhythm. Role of suprachiasmatic nuclei in rhythmic activity of neurons in lateral hypothalamic area, ventromedian nuclei and pineal gland, *Folia Pharmacol. Jpn.,* 72, 941, 1976.

28. Ganong, W. F., The role of catecholamines and acetylcholine in the regulation of endocrine function, *Life Sci.,* 15, 1401, 1974.

29. Besedovsky, H., del Rey, A., and Sorkin, E., unpublished results.

30. Besedovsky, H., del Rey, A., and Sorkin, E., unpublished results.

31. Besedovsky, H., del Rey, A., and Sorkin, E., unpublished results.

Chapter 12

THE CENTRAL NERVOUS SYSTEM AND LEARNING: FEEDFORWARD REGULATION OF IMMUNE RESPONSES

Dana Bovbjerg and Robert Ader

TABLE OF CONTENTS

I. INTRODUCTION

The central nervous system (CNS) regulates bodily systems by means of two basic regulatory strategies — feedback and feedforward.[1] CNS regulation of the immune system is no exception. Other sections of this book have amply demonstrated feedback regulation of the immune system. We will focus instead on the evidence for feedforward regulation of the immune system by the CNS.

Feedback mechanisms require the direct monitoring of some regulated physiologic variable. Deviation from the regulated levels of this product triggers compensatory responses that act to return the levels to normal (the familiar analogy is that of a thermostat controlling room temperature). Feedforward regulation, on the other hand, can come into play before any changes in the regulated variable takes place. Potential disturbances are directly monitored and compensatory changes are made in anticipation of need. For example, major cardiovascular changes occur in anticipation of exertion, prior to any feedback signal to drive them.[1]

II. FEEDFORWARD REGULATION

Clearly, there are advantages to such anticipatory regulation, particularly when a rapid response to a challenge is necessary. The complex tasks of feedforward regulation require a sophisticated controlling system, a system that can monitor sensory inputs, extract the meaningful material, predict impending challenges, and direct appropriate anticipatory responses. Thus, unlike feedback regulation, all known examples of feedforward regulation require a nervous system. The most thoroughly studied instances of feedforward regulation involve classical conditioning, sometimes called Pavlovian conditioning. Pavlov, who systematically studied feedforward regulation of digestion, paired the presentation of two types of stimuli to an animal: an *unconditional stimulus* (for example, food) that elicits a response (salivation) and a *conditional stimulus* (the ringing of a bell) that initially has no effect on that response.[2] After one or more presentations of the conditional stimulus followed by the unconditional stimulus, the animal became responsive to the conditional stimulus presented alone (when the bell rang, the dog salivated), thus demonstrating conditioning.

The elaboration of classical conditioning that has occurred since Pavlov's seminal studies need not concern us here.[3] Suffice it to say that the range of physiologic responses known to be altered by conditioning appears to be limited only by the ingenuity of the investigator and, of course, the existence of appropriate neural pathways. It should be noted that a wide variety of drugs have been used as unconditional stimuli.[4-6]

III. EXPERIMENTAL STUDIES

Feedforward regulation of the immune system by the CNS has been little studied. The first demonstration of classically conditioned modulation of an immune response came over 50 years ago from Russian investigators, the inheritors of the Pavlovian tradition.[7,8] This early Soviet literature, largely ignored in the West, has recently been critically reviewed elsewhere.[9,10]

Our own involvement in conditioned alteration of immune responses began with a serendipitous observation made during the course of an experiment designed to induce an aversion to a novel flavor.[11] Rats were given a saccharin solution to drink and then immediately injected with cyclophosphamide, to cause a transient stomach upset. After this single conditioning trial, subsequent consumption of saccharin was dramatically reduced, as expected. Unexpectedly, these animals began to die during the course of repeated exposures to the saccharin solution alone. Noting that cyclophosphamide is a potent suppressor of immune response, Ader[11] suggested that the pairing of saccharin and cyclophosphamide might have conditioned immunosuppression. Reexposure to saccharin, the conditional stimulus, in the absence of cyclophosphamide, the unconditional stimulus, might thus have rendered these rats susceptible to latent pathogens in the animal colony.

In a subsequent study, conditioned suppression of an immune response was explicitly demonstrated.[12] Rats were conditioned by pairing the presentation of a 0.1% sodium saccharin solution with an injection of 50 mg/kg cyclophosphamide. These animals were reexposed to saccharin three days later and injected with sheep red blood cells, a classic thymus-dependent antigen, to induce an antibody response. Conditioned animals reexposed to the saccharin had significantly reduced antibody responses compared to control animals (Figure 1).

The importance of appropriate control groups should be stressed. Control groups were included to assess the effects of both the conditioning procedure by itself and the reexposure procedure itself (Table 1). Thus, possible nonspecific stresses associated with the experimental manipulations were not confounded with the conditioned suppression.

Some confusion has resulted from the fact that Ader's initial observations were made in an experiment designed to study cyclophosphamide-induced taste aversion.[13,14] The immunosuppression seen after reexposure to the saccharin could have been the result of the rats' aversion per se. This possibility, however, was explicitly tested by the inclusion of a group of rats receiving an injection of LiCl rather than cyclophosphamide. Although these animals showed equal aversion to the saccharin solution, they did not have reduced antibody titers to sheep red blood cells (SRBC).[12] Furthermore, conditioned immunosuppression has also been achieved using different conditional stimuli and with other immunosuppressive agents.[15,16] We conclude that the pairing of the saccharin solution with cyclophosphamide establishes two different responses: taste aversion and a classically conditioned suppression of immune response.[14] Such multiple effects of conditioning have proven to be more the rule than the exception in the conditioning literature.[17,18]

Cyclophosphamide-induced conditioned suppression of the primary antibody response to sheep red blood cells was subsequently confirmed (Figure 1) by two independent laboratories.[19,20]

More recent studies have demonstrated the range of immune responses that can be altered by conditioning. Changing both the species and antigen, we have demonstrated cyclophosphamide-induced conditioned suppression of the primary antibody responses in mice challenged with the hapten, 2,4,6-trinitrophenol coupled to the relatively thymus-independent carrier, lipopolysaccharide.[21] Thus, this conditioned response may (like the unconditioned response) have direct effects on B cell function. It should be noted that there is one report of a failure to condition suppression of the antibody response to another putative thymus-independent antigen, *Brucella abortus*.[20] Whether this reflects differences in response to the two antigens or other methodological differences is not yet clear.

We have also conditioned suppression of a classic cell-mediated response, the popliteal graft-vs.-host reaction.[22,23] The reaction was quantified in F_1 hybrid animals by the increased weight of the popliteal lymph nodes that drain the site of the footpad injection of parental strain lymphocytes.[24] Preliminary experiments showed that a low (10 mg/kg) dose of cyclophosphamide given on the day of the graft and on each of the following 2 days was significantly more suppressive than the same dose given only once, the day after the graft.[25] For the conditioned animals, the day 0 and day +2 injections of drug were replaced by reexposure to the conditional stimulus, which had

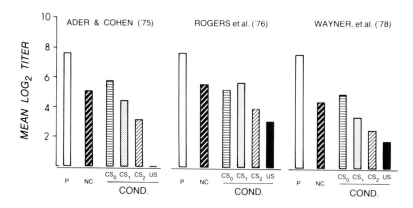

FIGURE 1.   Hemagglutinating antibody titers (mean ± SE) measured 6 days after the injection of sheep red blood cells. NC, nonconditioned rats; CS_0, conditioned animals that were not reexposed to the conditional stimulus; CS_1 and CS_2, conditioned animals reexposed to the conditional stimulus one time or two; US, conditioned animals injected with cyclophosphamide at the time of antigen injection; P, placebo-treated animals. (From Ader, R., in *Advances in Immunopharmacology*, Hadden, J. et al., Eds., Pergamon Press, Oxford, 1981. With permission.)

Table 1
CONDITIONED IMMUNOSUPPRESSION: EXPERIMENTAL GROUPS

Group	Pairing	Reexposure	Expectation
CS (Conditioned: CS reexposure)	SAC + CY	SAC + SAL + AG	Conditioned response
US (Conditioned: US reexposure)	SAC + CY	H_2O + CY + AG	Unconditioned response to CY
CS_0 (Conditioned: No CS reexposure)	SAC + CY	H_2O + AG	Effects of conditioning per se (residual effects of SAC + CY)
NC (Nonconditioned)	H_2O + CY	SAC + AG	Effect of SAC and residual effects of CY
P (Placebo treated)	H_2O + SAL	H_2O + SAL + AG	Effects of handling

Note: Abbreviations: CY = Cyclophosphamide; SAC = sodium saccharin solution; SAL = physiological saline; AG = antigen.

originally been paired with cyclophosphamide *7 weeks* before. As a result, the conditioned animals had significantly reduced graft-vs.-host responses compared to control rats receiving the same amount of drug (Figure 2).

Moreover, conditioned suppression of the response was extinguished by unpaired presentations of saccharin during the 7-week interval between the time of conditioning and induction of the immune response. Loss of a conditioned response after repeated unreinforced presentations of the conditional stimulus is a hallmark of classical conditioning and thus, reaffirms that conditioned immunosuppression is a result of learning processes (Figure 3).

Although the conditioned suppression of specific immune responses has been statistically significant and replicable, the effect has been relatively small in comparison to the immunosuppression achieved with drugs. Such modest effects can, however, have potent biological significance. A dramatic example comes from a recent study[26] in which conditioned immunosuppression delayed the onset of autoimmune disease in mice. Female New Zealand hybrid BW mice — an experimental model of systemic lupus erythematosus — were conditioned by weekly exposure to saccharin over an 8-

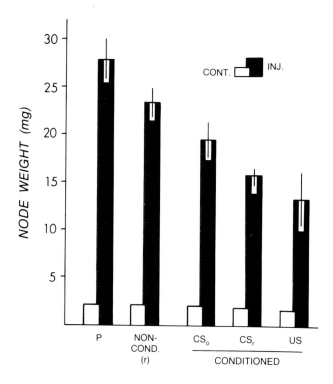

FIGURE 2.   Popliteal lymph node weights (graft-vs.-host response) of Lewis × Brown Norway (F_1) female rats 5 days after foot pad injection of splenic leukocytes from Lewis rat donors. Mean (±SE) weights for stimulated and contralateral unstimulated nodes. P, placebo-treated rats; NCr, nonconditioned animals injected with a single low dose of cyclophosphamide (10 mg/kg) 1 day after the cellular graft (day 1); CS_o, conditioned animals injected with the single low dose of cyclophosphamide but not reexposed to the conditional stimulus; CSr, conditioned animals given the single low dose of cyclophosphamide and also reexposed to the conditional stimulus on days 0, 1, and 2 after the cellular graft; US, conditioned animals injected with the low dose of cyclophosphamide on days 0, 1, and 2. (From Ader, R. and Cohen, N., in *Psychoneuroimmunology,* Ader, R., Ed., Academic Press, New York, 1981. With permission.)

week period, beginning when the mice were 4 months old. Half of these exposures were followed by injection of cyclophosphamide, half by injection of saline. Compared to a nonconditioned group that received the same amount of saccharin and drug, conditioned mice had a slower development of proteinurea and mortality (Figure 4).

As has been discussed at length elsewhere,[27] the explicit inclusion of conditioning procedures may thus, enhance conventional drug treatment protocols and reduce the dose of drug(s) needed for therapeutic effects.

IV. DISCUSSION

The evolutionary value of feedforward regulation of the immune system obviously does not rest on cyclophosphamide-induced conditioned immunosuppression. Rodents would rarely encounter saccharin or cyclophosphamide in the real world (for that matter, they are also unlikely to be exposed to SRBC). Such agents can, however, serve as useful probes for the experimental analysis of the capabilities of the organism. The

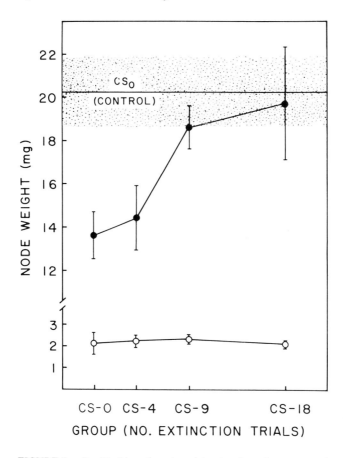

FIGURE 3.   Popliteal lymph node weights (graft-vs.-host response) in conditioned Lewis × Brown Norway (F_1) rats 5 days after foot pad injection of splenic leukocytes from Lewis donors. Mean (±SE) weights of stimulated (●) and contralateral unstimulated (○) nodes. CS_0, conditioned rats never reexposed to the conditional stimulus; CSO, CS4, CS9, CS18, conditioned animals reexposed to the conditional stimulus either 0, 4, 9, or 18 times (unreinforced extinction trials) prior to reexposure to the conditional stimulus at the time of the cellular graft. (From Boubjerg, R., et al., *J. Immunol.*, 1984. With permission.)

potential biological utility of feedforward regulation of immunity is perhaps more obvious when antigenic challenge itself is used as an unconditional stimulus for conditioning alterations in immune response. Examples of this more naturalistic possibility come primarily from the Soviet lierature.[9,10] Although most of these studies are poorly controlled and technically primitive, they are cumulatively persuasive.[10] Also, there has been a recent Western report of conditioned effects of antigenic challenge. Mice, conditioned by the repeated grafting of allogeneic skin, subsequently responded to a sham graft with an increase in cytotoxic T lymphocyte precursor cells characteristic of the allogeneic reaction.[28] In this case, the grafting procedure itself served as the conditional stimulus. Repeated sham grafting resulted in the extinction of this conditioned response.

These demonstrations of classically conditioned effects of antigenic challenge have yet to be confirmed; we mention them here as more obvious examples of the potential survival value of feedforward regulation. An ability to enhance immune responses prior to any actual infection might well provide distinct advantages. Defenses could be

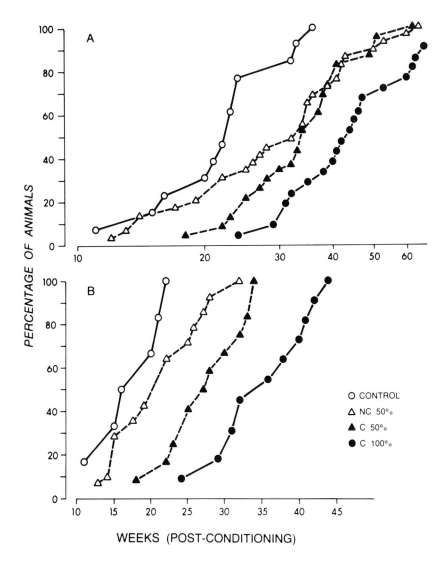

FIGURE 4. (A) Cumulative mortality rate in NZBW (F_1) female mice. Group C 100%, received saccharin followed by an injection of cyclophosphamide weekly; group C 50%, received saccharin weekly followed by cyclophosphamide 50% of the time; group NC 50%, received the same saccharin and drug doses as group C 50% but not temporally paired; control mice, received saccharin weekly but were never injected with cyclophosphamide. (B) Rate of development of unremitting proteinurea in NZBW (F_1) female mice. Groups are the same as above. (From Ader, R., in *Immunoregulation,* Fabris, N., Ed., Plenum Press, New York, 1983. With permission.)

mobilized early and kept to the minimum. Feedforward suppression of immune responses could help to avoid unnecessary concomitant damage to the host and would help husband vital resources. The extent of such capabilities remains speculative. Feedforward regulation may exert only general influences (e.g., enhancement or suppression), or it may be highly specific (e.g., modifying the response to a single antigen). These two possibilities must be carefully distinguished. The reduced immune responses after conditioning may reflect a general suppression of cellular proliferation rather than an effect limited to lymphocytes. Specific neural control is difficult to prove without knowing the steps between cause and effect. For example, lesions in the hypothalamus might alter immune response directly, (e.g., by severing neural links to the spleen) or indirectly, (e.g., by altering body temperature).

We do not yet know the sequence of events that takes place after a conditioned animal is reexposed to the conditional stimulus. In most studies, we have injected animals with antigen immediately after the reexposure and measured the immune response several days later. Thus, the suppression of immune responses that we and others have documented is the interactive net result of the cyclophosphamide-induced conditioned response (for suppression) and the unconditional effects of the antigenic challenge (for elicitation of an immune response). As has been discussed in greater detail elsewhere,[15] this concurrent presentation of conditional and unconditional stimuli with opposing effects may help to explain the modest levels of conditioned suppression. In one recent study, we avoided this confounding effect; conditioned rats were not challenged with antigen until 2 weeks after their last reexposure to the conditional stimulus.[29] Conditioned immunosuppression was still evident and was actually more robust than in previous experiments. This long-lasting effect of reexposure to the conditional stimulus need not be the result of a continuously suppressive neural influence. A short-lived conditioned response might have long lasting consequences on the immune system. Future studies that examine conditioned immunosuppressive effects in vitro should help resolve this issue.

The physiologic means by which the brain can regulate the immune system have been discussed at length in the rest of this volume. As yet, it is not known which (if any) of these might be involved in cyclophosphamide-induced conditioned immunosuppression. Because of their well-known immunosuppressive effects,[30] adrenocorticosteroid hormones might appear to be obvious candidates for the role. Explicit tests of the hypothesis that corticosteroids mediate conditioned immunosuppression, however, failed to confirm this possibility.[12,31] In circumstances where conditioning significantly suppressed serum antibody titers, exogenous or endogenous elevation of corticosteroid levels had no suppressive effects.[31] These results and other corroborative evidence[14] do not foreclose the possibility that increases in corticosteroid levels can be conditioned. Indeed they can[32] and under certain circumstances, such a conditioned response, might be immunosuppressive. Obviously, there may be a number of physiologic mechanisms by which the brain might suppress immune responses. There need not be any single final common path. Moreover, these different physiochemical pathways may each prove to be conditionable, as has been reported for other conditioned effects.[4] The mechanisms responsible for immunosuppression after cyclophosphamide-induced conditioning, for example, may be different from the mechanisms when antilymphocyte serum is used as the unconditional stimulus. Thus, skepticism is warranted for any study proporting to demonstrate "the" mechanism of conditioned modulation of immune response.

Although the mechanisms have yet to be determined, the data are clear — feedforward regulation has a significant impact on the immune system. Classical conditioning procedures can be used to probe the extent of these capabilities and the physiological basis of the interactions between the brain and the immune system.

REFERENCES

1. Houk, J. C., Homeostasis and control principles, in *Medical Physiology,* Mountcastle, V. B., Ed., C. V. Mosby, St. Louis, 1980, 246.
2. Pavlov, I. P., *Lectures on Conditioned Reflexes,* Liveright, New York, 1928.
3. Dickinson, A. and Mackintosh, N. J., Classical conditioning in animals, *Ann. Rev. Psychol.,* 29, 587, 1978.
4. Wikler, A., Conditioning of successive adaptive responses to the initial effects of drugs, *Cond. Ref.,* 8, 193, 1973.

5. Siegel, S., Morphine tolerance acquisition as an associative process, *J. Exp. Psychol. A.,* 3, 1, 1977.

6. Eikelboom, R. and Stewart, J., Conditioning of drug-induced physiological responses, *Psychol. Rev.,* 89, 507, 1982.

7. Metal'nikov, S. and Chorine, V., Role des reflexes conditionnels dans l'immunite, *Ann. Inst. Pasteur,* 40, 893, 1926.

8. Metal'nikov, S. and Chorine, V., Role des reflexes conditionnels dans la formation des anticorps, *C. R. Soc. Biol.,* 102, 133, 1928.

9. Spector, N. H. and Korneva, E. A., Neurophysiology, immunophysiology, and neuroimmunomodulation, in *Psychoneuroimmunology,* Ader, R., Ed., Academic Press, New York, 1981, 449.

10. Ader, R., A historical account of conditioned immunobiologic responses, in *Psychoneuroimmunology,* Ader, R., Ed., Academic Press, New York, 1981, 321.

11. Ader, R., Letter to the editor, *Psychosom. Med.,* 36, 183, 1974.

12. Ader, R. and Cohen, N., Behaviorally conditioned immunosuppression, *Psychosom. Med.,* 37, 333, 1975.

13. Dwyer, D. S., Conditioning immune responses (letter), *Immunol. Today,* 4, 63, 1983.

14. Bovbjerg, D., Cohen, N., and Ader, R., Conditioning immune responses (letter), *Immunol. Today,* 4, 63, 1983.

15. Ader, R. and Cohen, N., Conditioned immunopharmacologic responses, in *Psychoneuroimmunology,* Ader, R., Ed., Academic Press, New York, 1981, 281.

16. Kusnecov, A. W., Sivyer, M., King, M. G., Husband, A. J., Cripps, A. W., and Clancy, R. L., Behaviorally-conditioned suppression of the immune response by antilymphocyte serum, *J. Immunol.,* 130, 2117, 1983.

17. Harris, A. H. and Brady, J. V., Animal learning — visceral and autonomic conditioning, *Ann. Rev. Psychol.,* 25, 107, 1974.

18. Schiff, S. R., Conditioned dopaminergic activity, *Biol. Psychiatr.,* 17, 135, 1982.

19. Rogers, M. P., Reich, P., Strom, T. B., and Carpenter, C. B., Behaviorally conditioned immunosuppression: replication of a recent study, *Psychosom. Med.,* 38, 447,1976.

20. Wayner, E. A., Flannery, G. R., and Singer, G., The effects of taste aversion conditioning on the primary antibody response to sheep red blood cells and *Brucella abortus* in the albino rat, *Physiol. Behav.,* 21, 995, 1978.

21. Cohen, N., Ader, R., Green, N., and Bovbjerg, D., Conditioned suppression of a thymus independent antibody resonse, *Psychosom. Med.,* 41, 487, 1979.

22. Bovbjerg, D., Ader, R., and Cohen, N., Behaviorally conditioned suppression of a graft-versus-host response, *Proc. Natl. Acad. Sci. U.S.A.,* 79, 583, 1982.

23. Bovbjerg, D., Ader, R., and Cohen, N., Acquisition and extinction of conditioned suppression of a graft-vs-host response in the rat, *J. Immunol.,* 132, 111, 1984.

24. Ford, W. L., Burr, W., and Simonsen, M., A lymph-node weight assay for graft versus host activity of rat lymphoid-cells, *Transplantation,* 10, 258, 1970.

25. Bovbjerg, D., Classically Conditioned Alterations in Two Cell-Mediated Immune Responses, Ph.D. thesis, University of Rochester, N. Y., 1983.

26. Ader, R. and Cohen, N., Behaviorally conditioned immunosuppression and murine systemic lupus erythematosus, *Science,* 215, 1534, 1982.

27. Ader, R., Conditioned immunopharmacologic effects in animals: implications for a conditioning model of pharmacotherapy, in *Placebo: Clinical Phenomena and New Insights,* White, L., Jursky, B., and Schwartz, G. E., Eds., Guilford Press, New York, 1985.

28. Gorczynski, R. M., Macrae, S., and Kennedy, M., Conditioned immune response associated with allogeneic skin grafts in mice, *J. Immunol.,* 129, 704, 1982.

29. Ader, R., Cohen, N., and Bovbjerg, D., Conditioned suppression of humoral immunity in the rat, *J. Comp. Physiol. Psychol.,* 96, 517, 1982.

30. Compsa, J., Leonhardt, H., and Wekerle, H., Hormonal coordination of the immune response, *Rev. Physiol. Biochem. Pharmacol.,* 92, 115, 1982.

31. Ader, R., Cohen, N., and Grota, L., Adrenal involvement in conditioned immunosuppression, *Int. J. Immunopharmacol.,* 1, 141, 1979.

32. Ader, R., Conditioned adrenocortical steroid evaluations in the rat, *J. Comp. Physiol. Psychol.,* 90, 1156, 1976.

Chapter 13

ROLE OF HORMONAL IMMUNOREGULATION IN REPRODUCTION

David A. Clark

TABLE OF CONTENTS

I. INTRODUCTION

Successful viviparous reproduction in an outbred population such as man almost invariably generates an intrauterine fetus that bears major histocompatibility antigens (MHC) derived from the father. These antigens elicit an immune response in the mother during the first or second allogeneic pregnancy.[1-5] It had been proposed on the basis of experiments by Simmons and Russell[6,7] that the fetal trophoblast cells that form the maternal-fetal interface lack paternally-derived MHC antigens. Thus, the trophoblast could act as an inert shield or barrier between the antigenic fetal allograft and the immunocompetent mother.[8] However, the fact that the mother does develop sensitized T cells that secrete migration inhibitor factor (MIF) and produces antibodies in response to the antigens of her husband suggests that the trophoblast barrier must be imperfect.[2-6] Furthermore, several independent groups have now demonstrated that in both the mouse and man at least some types of trophoblast cells that contact maternal tissue *in situ* do express paternal Class I MHC antigens.[9-13] The trophoblast also bears two distinct non-MHC antigens, one of which cross-reacts with a lymphocyte surface antigen.[14] Therefore, the concept of an antigenically inert barrier created by the trophoblast can no longer be sustained, and one must search for alternative mechanisms to explain the success of the allogeneic fetus.

It is an intriguing observation that the type of immunity elicited by allogeneic pregnancy does not mediate the rejection of transplanted allografts.[15,16] Indeed, repeated mating to the same husband appears to generate a state of tolerance towards grafts of paternal tissue,[17-19] and this tolerance has been associated with the presence of suppressor T lymphocytes that react specifically with the antigens on paternal cells.[19,20] Therefore, one is tempted to speculate that allogeneic pregnancy succeeds through the generation of suppressor T cells that prevent the generation of cellular immune responses capable of graft rejection. However, Woodruff[21] transplanted the tissue from one of several intrauterine rat fetuses into the thigh muscle of the mother and found that this tissue elicited a normal rejection response.[21] Thus, a female can reject the tissues of her fetus at an extrauterine site while she is pregnant and without any apparent harm to the remaining embryos within the uterus. This finding is entirely consistent with the observation that immunization against paternal MHC antigens has little if any effect on fetal survival.[22] Two conclusions can be drawn from these results. First, it is possible that it is non-MHC antigens that play the key role at the maternal-fetal interface. Thus, immunization of rodents against embryonic and tumor associated antigens, unlike immunity directed against MHC epitopes, can result in infertility, recurrent abortion (resorptions), and post-partum wasting of the newborns.[23-25] The role of the suppressor mechanism during normal reproduction would be to block the generation of effector cells capable of rejecting embryos bearing these non-MHC antigens. Second, it is possible that local intrauterine factors, rather than systemic suppressor mechanisms, block the expression of transplantation immunity against the antigens of the fetus and its associated trophoblast. For example, Smith[26] has recently shown that murine trophoblast cells may be susceptible to cell mediated cytolysis in vitro. What is the mechanism that prevents lysis of trophoblast in vivo?

An important function of placental trophoblast cells in vivo is the production of gestational hormones.[27,28] Some of these hormones, such as progesterone and their synthetic analogs, can suppress immune responses when given in sufficient dose.[29-34] Thus, it is possible that local production of hormones might explain the immunological success of the fetus. This hypothesis is attractive since it explains how the mother can remain competent to deal with infectious agents during pregnancy. I shall discuss briefly the current information bearing on this question.

II. HORMONES AND SUCCESSFUL PREGNANCY

In both mouse and man, the ovarian hormones estrogen and progesterone prepare the uterine lining cells for the implantation of the fertilized ovum.[35,37] Implantation in the mouse requires a surge of estrogen,[35-37] and the development of the trophoblast that will form the early placenta is also estrogen dependent.[38] Continuation of the pregnancy following implantation requires secretion of progesterone. Prior to implantation, in women, ovarian hormone secretion is regulated by the pituitary gland through luteinizing hormone (LH) and prolactin (PRL).[37] Later, chorionic gonadotrophin (HCG), a polypeptide produced by the trophoblast, plays a major regulatory role.[39] In the mouse, where pregnancy lasts only 19 to 21 days, the endocrine situation is different only in that the first half of pregnancy is dependent upon continued production of FSH, LH, and PRL by the pituitary.[37] Pituitary hormone production is triggered by cervical stimulation at the time of mating, and in the absence of fertilization and implantation the mouse becomes pseudopregnant.[40] At 10.5 to 11.5 days of pregnancy, the mouse trophoblast acquires the enzymatic machinery to produce steroid hormones such as progesterone.[27,28] It does not appear that pregnancy in the mouse is of sufficient duration for trophoblast progesterone production to supplant the need for continued hormone production by the ovary. However, as in man, 5 to 7 days following implantation, pituitary hormones that stimulate the ovary to produce estrogen and progesterone are replaced by trophic factors elaborated within the uterus.[41] A PRL-like luteotropic agent is produced by decidua,[42-44] and HCG may also be elaborated from the implantation site.[41]

III. GESTATIONAL HORMONES AND THE SYSTEMIC IMMUNE RESPONSE

Estrogens, at physiologic doses, stimulate the antibody response[45-47] while having little effect on cellular immunity as assessed by delayed hypersensitivity (DTH) and in vitro lymphocyte stimulation assay.[48-50] In contrast, progestational hormones impair cellular immune reactions such as DTH, lymphocyte proliferation, and generation of cytotoxic T cells (CTL).[48-54] Progestational agents, particularly synthetic progestins, can inhibit both humoral and cellular immunity including the rejection of allografts.[31,33,34,55] The human placenta can also produce corticosteroids which, in pharmacologic doses, can suppress both cellular and humoral immunity.[49,55-57]

To decide whether any of these effects mimic the physiological alterations of pregnancy one must first define the changes in the systemic immune response during normal pregnancy, and second, determine if similar changes occur when one gives gestational hormones, (e.g., estrogen plus progesterone). In women, pregnancy was found to have no effect,[58] neither an enhancing[59] nor a suppressive[60] effect on the humoral immune response. Skin graft rejection was only slightly retarded,[61] the mixed lymphocyte (MLC) and mitogen responses were impaired,[62] and DTH, as measured by the tuberculin response in vivo, was impaired in late pregnancy.[63] In the allopregnant mouse, the antibody response was reported to be unaffected,[64,65] enhanced,[66-69] or suppressed.[69-71] Suppression is modest, affects primarily the T cell-dependent IgG response, and is detected only towards the end of pregnancy. The type of antigen used to measure the response and the route of immunization can also affect the result. Furthermore, pregnancy is associated with a significant increase in blood volume and in spleen cellularity, for which corrections should be made, when the response of pregnant animals is compared to nonpregnant controls. In contrast, the controversy concerning the effect of pregnancy on the humoral immune response, cellular immunity as assessed by DTH, and generation of CTL was shown to be suppressed significantly.[50,65,67] It is interesting in this context that combinations of estrogen and progesterone, as administered in the form of an oral contraceptive, either suppress slightly or stimulate the antibody response.[30,72] Administration of HCG to mice, which stimulates estrogen and progesterone production by the ovary, also enhances the antibody response, while inhibiting the DTH and MLC responses.[50,73]

Taken together, one may conclude that the hormonal alterations associated with pregnancy may exert a significant suppressive effect in the cellular arm of the immune system. However, it must be stressed that pregnancy has little effect on the rejection of allografts placed at extrauterine sites in mice and humans.[6,15,16,21,56,62] Furthermore, nonspecific systemic immunosuppression to a degree sufficient to prevent graft rejection would render the pregnant female unduly susceptible to infection. Thus, attention has turned towards the local effects that hormonal agents may have on immune response and graft rejection within the uterus.

IV. LOCAL IMMUNE SUPPRESSION BY GESTATIONAL HORMONES

A. Direct Effects on Cells of the Immune System

In 1977, Siiteri et al.[74] demonstrated that skin allografts could be protected from rejection by implanting a silastic container of progesterone pellets adjacent to the graft. This result was repeated by Beer and Billingham[75] who noted that the progesterone treatment had only a slight suppressive effect on the titer of hemagglutinating antibodies elicited by the graft. It was subsequently reported that progesterone could block lymphocyte responses to mitogens and allogeneic cells in vitro. In man, this was achieved with concentrations of 4 to 10 μg/mℓ,[48,52,76] and in mouse, at 1 to 2 μg/mℓ.[51,65] Two investigators were able to detect the onset of impairment of proliferation of mouse lymphocytes at a concentration of progesterone of 0.1 to 0.5 μg/mℓ,[51,77] and an additional investigation obtained a similar result with human lymphocytes.[52] Taken together, these studies suggest that progesterone might be "Nature's immunosuppressant" that accounts for survival of the fetus.

There are several problems with the interpretation of the preceding data. It was clear from previous studies that suppression of graft rejection required pharmacologic doses of progesterone or their analogs.[31,33,55] Were the concentrations of progesterone found to be effective locally, both in vivo and in vitro, physiologic? In the human placental syncytiotrophoblast membrane, the concentration of progesterone was found to be only 1 to 2 μg/g wet weight by radioimmunoassay[78] — a level below that required for clear-cut suppression of lymphocyte responses in vitro. The circulating level of progesterone in rats bearing skin allografts with local progesterone implants was reported to be ten times the normal physiologic level measured in pregnancy.[75,79] Although circulating progesterone levels in the pregnant mouse can transiently reach 0.1 μg/mℓ in the second half of pregnancy,[80,81] similar to the concentration found to exert some suppressive effects in vitro,[51,77] circulating progesterone in the plasma of pregnant individuals is protein bound with less than 20% free.[82] Thus, the circulating free progesterone level in the mouse is approximately one fifth that required for suppressive effects in vitro. In the mouse and rat, during the first 10 to 12 days of pregnancy, all of the progesterone is produced by the ovary rather than the placenta.[28,37,79,80] Therefore, one would not expect to find a high local progesterone level in fetal tissues for the first 6 to 8 days following implantation. Cytotoxic cells and their progenitors appear in allografts within 5 to 6 days of transplantation and thus, would infiltrate the fetal allograft prior to local production of progesterone by the trophoblast.[27,28,83-85] Furthermore, in the mouse, the component of the trophoblast in direct contact with maternal blood does not have the enzymatic machinery to secrete progesterone.[27,28] It should also be noted that cytotoxic T effector cells are completely resistant to suppression by concentrations of progesterone that inhibit the immune response in vitro.[51] Taken together, these data suggest that although high local concentrations of progesterone can prevent graft rejection, this mechanism is unlikely to account for the physiologic success of the fetal allograft in utero.

B. Indirect Effects on the Immune System

The suppressive effects of progesterone described above appear to arise from a direct suppression of lymphocyte functions, such as thymidine incorporation,[48,86] and may therefore, represent toxic rather than physiologic effects. However, the gestational hormones, estrogen and progesterone, may alter the immune system by indirect mechanisms. For example, estrogen stimulates the production of α_2-macroglobulin (pregnancy zone protein), which has immunosuppressive effects.[87-89] The thymic epithelium contains receptors for estrogen,[90] and estrogen administration induces production of low molecular weight suppressor factors.[91] Morton and co-workers[92,93] have described a factor elaborated early in pregnancy that suppresses the adoptive transfer of delayed hypersensitivity reactions. This material, called early pregnancy factor (EPF), is produced by combination of a molecule elaborated by the oviduct that can directly bind to lymphocytes, and an ovarian factor that is stimulated by a low molecular weight factor from the ovum together with PRL produced by the pituitary.[94-96] EPF appears to account for the immunosuppressive activity that had been associated with impure preparations of HCG.[97] Progesterone has also been reported to induce secretion of small sized immunosuppressive proteins by the uterus in the pig.[98] Thus, hormones can stimulate production of both systemic and local uterine suppressor molecules that may collaborate in inhibiting immune reactivity with the uterus.

Another indirect mechanism by which the immune system may be modified by hormones derives from the fact that the immune system is highly compartmentalized. For example, mucosal surfaces appear to be linked together by preferential migration of sensitized lymphocytes from one mucosal surface to another, — an observation that led to the concept of a common mucosal immune system.[99] A skin ''specific'' system of lymphocyte traffic has also been identified.[100] Wira and Sandoe[101,102] have demonstrated that physiologic elevations in the levels of estrogen and progesterone increase B cell localization and IgA antibody levels in genital secretions.[103] Along similar lines, Tchernitchin and Tchernitchin[104] showed that estrogen stimulates the infiltration of the uterus by eosinophils. While the immune system can be modified by altering the cell traffic of lymphocytes, one must also be aware that alterations in the phagocytic cells that participate in inflammation and immune responses may be produced by hormones. Progesterone, for example, may impair the generation of oxygen radicals that kill parasites in phagosomes.[105]

Although a variety of indirect effects of gestational hormones have been described, the net effect within the context of the pregnancy where levels of several different hormones are changing simultaneously has not been defined. Whether any of these alterations can account for prolonged survival of intrauterine allografts is also unknown.

V. THE ROLE OF THE DECIDUA

The tissue in which the developing ovum implants undergoes a series of cellular alterations known as decidualization,[106] which are dependent upon ovarian estrogen and progesterone, and a stimulus delivered by the implanting ovum that may act in part by increasing the number of progesterone receptors in the adjacent endometrium.[107,108] Decidualization is associated with important endocrine and immunologic effects. The decidualized endometrium can produce hormones such as PRL that stimulate both EPF production and production of progesterone by the ovary.[42,44,109] The decidua also manufactures and secretes α_2-globulin and other proteins that may have immunosuppressive effects in vitro.[110-112]

Several observations suggest that decidua or decidua-associated factors may block certain aspects of graft rejection. Allografts placed on decidua implant and enjoy prolonged survival compared to such grafts transplanted to extrauterine sites.[16,113] Indeed, Moriyama and Sugawa[114] showed a striking enhancement of growth of paternal tumor in the uterus of hamsters given progesterone. Beer and Billingham[16] noted that skin grafts on rodent decidua were promptly rejected if the animal was sensitized, but Dodd et al.[115] found such rejection to be characterized by infiltration of the graft by polymorphonuclear leukocytes rather than lymphocytes. This observation suggested the rejection was mediated by an antibody-dependent cytotoxicity mechanism.[115] Kirby et al.[116] found that allogeneic blastocysts that were rejected when placed under the kidney capsule of immunized recipients implanted and developed normally when placed in the uterus. Taken together, these observations suggest that decidua may protect the fetal allograft from lymphocyte-mediated rejection in early pregnancy.

Some interesting information has been obtained concerning the cellular basis for immunosuppression by decidua. As mentioned before, Kirkwood and Bell[112] have shown that murine decidua elaborates an immunosuppressive factor in vitro. The production of this factor during the initial 72 hr culture period was associated with the presence in the cultures of small round cells bearing Fc receptors.[112] In our laboratory, we have been able to isolate small round lymphoid cells from decidua of allopregnant and isopregnant mice. These cells suppress nonspecifically the generation of cytotoxic T cells in vitro, can prevent the infiltration of sponge-matrix allografts by CTL in vivo, and elaborate a soluble suppressor activity when cultured at 37°C in vitro for 24 to 72 hr.[117,118] The suppressor cells lack T cell markers and are also present in uterine venous blood and the lymph nodes draining the uterus (albeit in lower activity).[53,65,117-119] Cell separation experiments revealed that suppressor activity is associated with small lymphocytic cells that possess cytoplasmic granules.[117] The only markers that have been found on these suppressor cells so far are Fc receptors for IgG.[129] An intriguing observation is the absence of suppressor cell activity in the lymph nodes draining the uterus (DLN) of allopregnant CBA mice resorbing their litters.[53,65] A similar observation was reported by Smith[120] in C57BL/6 mice.

We have recently studied the role of decidual suppressor cells in fetal resorption using a model system in which blastocysts from *Mus caroli* were transferred together with *Mus musculus* blastocysts into the uterus of a pseudopregnant *M. musculus* recipient.[121] The *M. caroli* blastocysts implant and develop normally for 5 days, whereupon they are infiltrated by maternal cytotoxic T lymphoblasts and are resorbed, whereas the *M. musculus* embryos remain healthy.[121] The presence of xenoantigens on *M. caroli* trophoblast does not explain the apparent immunological attack on the fetus.[122] Rather, there is a deficiency of suppressor cell activity in the decidua bearing the xenoembryo at the time when infiltration by maternal lymphoblast is evident.[121,123] This correlation between absence of maternal suppressor cells and resorption of xenoembryos suggests, but does not prove, that localized intrauterine suppressor cells may prevent the immunologic rejection of the fetus.

The mechanisms of localization of non-T suppressor cells in the decidua remains speculative. In experiments using chimeric *M. musculus-M. caroli* embryos, healthy *M. caroli* fetuses can be gestated within the uterus of *M. musculus* recipients by creating blastocyst injection chimeras where the trophoblast is entirely of the *M. musculus* genotype.[124,125] If one reverses the situation and envelops *M. musculus* embryos in a *M. caroli* trophoblast, resorption occurs.[124,125] Thus, it appears that trophoblast-decidua interaction may be crucial for the local recruitment of adequate levels of suppression. The molecular and cellular basis for this recruitment has not yet been elucidated. Currently under investigation are three possible mechanisms. First, the xenotrophoblast may fail to interact with *M. musculus* decidual cells in the normal manner, thereby leading to a primary and nonimmunological failure of the function of trophoblast in early embryo-decidua interaction. Second, there may be a failure to acquire and produce low levels of steroid hormones such as progesterone[28] or the luteotrophic chorionic gonadotropin[41] at the correct time, or to stimulate the decidua to produce hormones such as PRL that may be required for tissue infiltration by lymphoid cells in DTH-type reactions.[126] A DTH-like cellular infiltrate has been seen at early implantation sites,[127] and Beer and Billingham[16] have shown that localized hypersensitivity reaction in one horn of a rodent's uterus enhances fertility in that horn. Furthermore, even though DTH reactivity of sensitized T lymphocytes may be blocked in the peripheral circulation during pregnancy,[5,50,67] detection of MIF in the circulation of pregnant rats suggests an ongoing DTH reaction may be occurring.[3] That the DLN are required for both optimal fecundity and serum MIF production suggests that this pregnancy-associated DTH-type reaction may be localized to the genital tract. Third, Bernard et al.[128] have described uptake of antibody by the early embryo and trophoblast, and thus it is possible that the Fc component of antibody may localize or activate suppressor cells through their Fc receptors. Further experiments will be needed to determine if any of these possible models for localization of non-T suppressor cells in the decidua are correct.

VI. SUMMARY

Both steroid and peptide hormones play a crucial role in successful gestation. Although these hormones may have some effects on systemic immunity, the immunocompetence of the mother to resist infection is preserved and local impairment of intrauterine immunity by hormone-dependent mechanisms seems to explain protection of the antigenic fetal graft from attack by the maternal cytotoxic cells. Endocrine factors do not, however, appear to act to directly suppress the immune system, but rather by promoting decidualization and by maintaining the function of the trophoblast. The interaction between trophoblast and decidua seems to play a key role in recruitment of a population of non-T suppressor cells. Absence of these suppressor cells correlates with resorption and invasion of the resorbing mouse fetus by maternal cytotoxic cells.

REFERENCES

1. Johnson, L. V. and Calarco, P. G., Mammalian preimplantation development: the cell surface, *Anat. Rec.*, 196, 201, 1980.
2. Youtananukorn, V., Matangkasombut, P., and Osathanondh, V., Onset of human cell-mediated immune reaction to placental antigens during first pregnancy, *Clin. Exp. Immunol.*, 16, 593, 1974.
3. Tofoski, J. G. and Gill, T. J., III, The production of migration inhibitory factor and reproductive capacity in allogeneic pregnancy, *Am. J. Pathol.*, 88, 333, 1977.
4. Bell, S. C. and Billington, W. D., Humoral immune responses in murine pregnancy. I. Anti-paternal alloantibody levels in maternal serum, *J. Reprod. Immunol.*, 3, 3, 1981.
5. Rocklin, R. E., Kitzmiller, J. L., Carpenter, C. B., Garovoy, M. R., and David, J. R., Maternal-fetal relation: absence of an immunologic blocking factor from the serum of women with chronic abortion, *N. Engl. J. Med.*, 295, 1209, 1976.
6. Simmons, R. L. and Russell, P. S., The antigenicity of mouse trophoblast, *Ann. N.Y. Acad. Sci.*, 99, 717, 1962.
7. Simmons, R. L. and Russell, P. S., The histocompatibility antigens of fertilized mouse eggs and trophoblast, *Ann. N.Y. Acad. Sci.*, 129, 35, 1966.

8. Beer, A. E. and Billingham, R. E., *The Immunobiology of Mammalian Reproduction,* Prentice-Hall, Englewood Cliffs, N. J., 1976.
9. Chatterjee-Hasrouni, S. and Lala, P. K., Localization of paternal H-2K antigens on murine trophoblast cells in vivo, *J. Exp. Med.,* 155, 1679, 1982.
10. Jenkinson, E. J. and Owen, V., Ontogeny and distribution of major histocompatibility complex (MHC) antigens on mouse placental trophoblast, *J. Reprod. Immunol.,* 2, 173, 1980.
11. Wegmann, T. G., The presence of class I MHC antigens at the maternal-fetal interface and hypotheses concerning survival of the fetal allograft, *J. Reprod. Immunol.,* 3, 267, 1981.
12. Sunderland, C. A., Redman, C. W., and Stirrat, G. M., HLA A,B,C antigens are expressed on nonvillous trophoblast of the early human placenta, *J. Immunol.,* 127, 2614, 1981.
13. Sunderland, C. A., Naiem, M., Mason, D. Y., Redman, C. W., and Stirrat, G. M., The expression of major histocompatibility antigens by human chorionic villi, *J. Reprod. Immunol.,* 3, 323, 1981.
14. Faulk, W. P., Yeager, C., McIntyre, J. A., and Ueda, M., Oncofoetal antigens of human trophoblast, *Proc. R. Soc. London Ser. B,* 206, 163, 1979.
15. Wegmann, T. G., Waters, C. A., Drell, D. W., and Carlson, G. A., Pregnant mice are not primed but can be primed to fetal alloantigens, *Proc. Natl. Acad. Sci. U.S.A.,* 76, 2410, 1979.
16. Beer, A. E. and Billingham, R. E., Host responses to intra-uterine tissue, cellular, and fetal allografts, *J. Reprod. Fertil.,* Suppl. 21, 59, 1974.
17. Breyere, E. J. and Barrett, M. K., Tolerance induced by parity in mice incompatible at the H-2 locus, *J. Natl. Cancer Inst.,* 27, 409, 1961.
18. Prehn, R. T., Specific homograft tolerance induced by successive matings and implications concerning choriocarcinoma, *J. Natl. Cancer Inst.,* 25, 883, 1960.
19. Smith, R. N. and Powell, A. E., The adoptive transfer of pregnancy-induced unresponsiveness to male skin grafts with thymus-dependent cells, *J. Exp. Med.,* 146, 899, 1977.
20. Chaouat, G., Voisin, G. A., Escalier, D., and Robert, P., Facilitation reactin (enhancing antibodies and suppressor cells) and rejection reaction (sensitized cells) from the mother to the paternal antigens of the conceptus, *Clin. Exp. Immunol.,* 35, 13, 1979.
21. Woodruff, M. F. A., Transplantation immunity and the immunological problem of pregnancy, *Proc. R. Soc. London Ser. B,* 148, 68, 1958.
22. Mitchison, N. A., The effect on offspring of maternal immunization in mice. *J. Genet.,* 51, 406, 1953.
23. Parmiani, G. and Della Porta, G., Effects of antitumor immunity on pregnancy in the mouse, *Nature (London) New Biol.,* 241, 26, 1973.
24. Milgrom, E., Comini-Andrada, E., Chaudhry, A. P., Fetal and neonatal fatality in rat hybrids from mothers stimulated with paternal skin, *Transplant. Proc.,* 9, 1409, 1977.
25. Hamilton, M. S., Beer, A. E., May, R. D., and Vitetta, E. S., The influence of immunization of female mice with F9 teratocarcinoma cells on their reproductive performance, *Transplant. Proc.,* 11, 1069, 1979.
26. Smith, G., In vitro susceptibility of mouse placental trophoblast to cytotoxic effector cells, *J. Reprod. Immunol.,* 5, 39, 1983.
27. Deane, H. W., Rubin, B. L., Driks, E. C., Lobel, B. L., and Leipsner, G., Trophoblastic giant cells in the placentas of rats and mice and their probable role in steroid-hormone production, *Endocrinology,* 70, 407, 1962.
28. Chew, N. J. and Sherman, M. I., Biochemistry of differentiation of mouse trophoblast: Δ^5, 3_β hydroxysteroid dehydrogenase, *Biol. Reprod.,* 12, 351, 1975.
29. Munroe, J. S., Progesteroids as immunosuppressive agents, *J. Reticuloendothel. Soc.,* 9, 361, 1971.
30. Joshi, U. M., Rao, S., Kora, S. J., Dikshit, S. S., and Virkar, K. D., Effect of steroidal contraceptives on antibody formation in the human female, *Contraception,* 3, 327, 1971.
31. Hulka, J. F., Mohr, K., and Lieberman, M. W., Effect of synthetic progestational agents on allograft rejection and circulating antibody production, *Endocrinology,* 77, 897, 1965.
32. Baker, D. A., Phillips, C. A., Roessner, K., Albertini, R. J., and Mann, L. I., Suppression by progesterone of nonspecific in vitro lymphocyte stimulation in mice as a mechanism for the enhancement of herpes simplex virus type 2 vaginal infection, *Am. J. Obstet. Gynecol.,* 136, 440, 1980.
33. Turcotte, J. G., Haines, R. F., Brody, G. L., Meyer, T. J., and Schwartz, S. A., Immunosuppression with medroxyprogesterone acetate, *Transplantation,* 6, 248, 1968.
34. Enein, A. -A., Sakai, A., and Kountz, S. L., The synergistic effect of melengestrol acetate and antilymphocyte serum on heart allograft survival in rats, *Transplantation,* 23, 453, 1977.
35. Nalbandov, A. V., Endocrine control of implantation, in *Biology of the Blastocyst,* Blandau, R. J., Ed., University of Chicago Press, Chicago, Ill., 1971, 383.
36. Dickmann, Z., Systemic versus local hormonal requirements for blastocyst implantation: a hypothesis, *Perspect. Biol. Med.,* 22, 390, 1979.
37. Gidley-Baird, A. A. and Emmens, G. W., Pituitary hormone control of implantation in the mouse, *Aust. J. Biol. Sci.,* 31, 657, 1978.

38. Roy, S. K., Sengupta, J., Paria, B. C., and Manchanda, S. K., In vitro inhibition of trophoblast maturation and expansion of early rat blastocysts by an oestrogen antagonist, *Acta Endocrinol.*, 99, 129, 1982.

39. Saxena, B. B., Hasan, S. H., Haour, F., and Schmidt-Gollwitzer, M., Radioreceptor assay of human chorionic gonadotropin: detection of early pregnancy, *Science*, 184, 793, 1974.

40. Gunnet, J. W. and Freeman, M. E., The mating-induced release of prolactin: a unique neuroendocrine response, *Endocrine Rev.*, 4, 44, 1983.

41. Wide, L. and Wide, M., Chorionic gonadotropin in the mouse from implantation to term, *J. Reprod. Fertil.*, 57, 5, 1979.

42. Basuray, R. and Gibori, G., Luteotropic action of the decidual tissue of the pregnant rat, *Biol. Reprod.*, 23, 507, 1980.

43. Soares, M. J. and Talamantes, F., Gestational effects on placental and serum androgen, progesterone and prolactin-like activity in the mouse, *J. Endocrinol.*, 95, 29, 1982.

44. Golander, A., Barrett, J., Hurley, T., Barry, S., and Handwerger, S., Failure of bromocriptine, dopamine and thyrotropin-releasing hormone to affect prolactin secretion by human decidual tissue *in vitro*, *J. Clin. Endocrinol. Metab.*, 49, 787, 1979.

45. Kenny, J. F., Pangburn, P. C., and Trail, G., Effect of estradiol on immune competence: in vivo and in vitro studies, *Infect. Immunity*, 13, 448, 1976.

46. Eidinger, D. and Garrett, T. J., Studies on the regulatory effects of the sex hormones on antibody formation and stem cell differentiation, *J. Exp. Med.*, 136, 1098, 1972.

47. Terres, G., Morrison, S. L., and Habicht, G. S., A quantitative difference in the immune response between male and female mice, *Proc. Soc. Exp. Biol. Med.*, 127, 664, 1968.

48. Clemens, L. E., Siiteri, P. K., and Stites, D. P., Mechanism of immunosuppression of progesterone on maternal lymphocyte activation during pregnancy, *J. Immunol.*, 122, 1978, 1979.

49. Skinnider, L. F. and Laxdal, V., The effect of progesterone, oestrogens and hydrocortisone on the mitogenic response of lymphocytes to phytohaemagglutinin in pregnant and non-pregnant women, *Br. J. Obstet. Gynecol.*, 88, 1110, 1981.

50. Carter, J., The effect of progesterone, oestradiol, and HC6 on cell-mediated immunity in pregnant mice, *J. Reprod. Fertil.*, 46, 211, 1976.

51. Pavia, C., Siiteri, P. K., Perlman, J. D., and Stites, D. P., Suppression of murine allogeneic cell interactions by sex hormones, *J. Reprod. Immunol.*, 1, 33, 1979.

52. Mori, T., Kobayashi, H., Nishimura, T., and Mori, T., Possible role of progesterone in immunoregulation during pregnancy, in *Immunological Influences on Human Fertility*, Boettcher, B., Ed., Academic Press, New York, 1978, 175.

53. Clark, D. A. and McDermott, M. R., Active suppression of host-vs-graft reaction in pregnant mice. III. Developmental kinetics, properties, and mechanism of induction of suppressor cells during first pregnancy, *J. Immunol.*, 127, 1267, 1981.

54. Gehrz, R. C., Christianson, W. R., Linner, K. M., Conroy, M. M., McCue, S. A., and Balfour, H. H., Jr., Cytomegalovirus-specific humoral and cellular immune response in human pregnancy, *J. Infect. Dis.*, 143, 391, 1981.

55. Kountz, S. L. and Wechter, W. J., Immunosuppression with melengestrol, *Transplant. Proc.*, 9, 1447, 1977.

56. Medawar, P. B. and Sparrow, E. M., The effects of adrenocortical hormones, adrenocorticotrophic hormone, and pregnancy on skin transplantation immunity in mice, *J. Endocrinol.*, 14, 240, 1956.

57. Barlow, S. M., Morrison, P. J., and Sullivan, F. M., Plasma corticosterone levels during pregnancy in the mouse: the relative contributions of the adrenal glands and foeto-placental units, *J. Endocrinol.*, 60, 473, 1974.

58. Murray, D. L., Imagawa, D. T., Okada, D. M., and St. Geme, J. W., Jr., Antibody response to monovalent A/New Jersey/8/76 influenza vaccine in pregnant women, *J. Clin. Microbiol.*, 10, 184, 1979.

59. Mitchell, G. W., Jr., McRipley, R. J., Selvaraj, R. J., and Sbarra, A. J., The role of the phagocyte in host-parasite interactions. IV. The phagocytic activity of leukocytes in pregnancy and its relationship to urinary tract infections, *Am. J. Obstet. Gynecol.*, 96, 687, 1966.

60. Rangnekar, K. N., Rao, S. S., Joshi, U. M., Virkar, K. D., Kora, S. J., and Dikshit, S. S., Humoral antibody formation during pregnancy, *J. Reprod. Fertil.*, 38, 237, 1974.

61. Billingham, R. E., Transplantation immunity and the maternal-fetal relation, *N. Engl. J. Med.*, 270, 667, 1964.

62. Thong, Y. H., Steele, R. W., Vincent, M. M., Hensen, S. A., and Bellanti, J. A., Impaired in vitro cell-mediated immunity to rubella virus during pregnancy, *N. Engl. J. Med.*, 289, 604, 1973.

63. Covelli, H. D. and Wilson, R. T., Immunologic and medical considerations in tuberculin-sensitized pregnant patients, *Am. J. Obstet. Gynecol.*, 132, 256, 1978.

64. Merritt, K. and Galton, M., Antibody formation during pregnancy, *Transplantation*, 7, 562, 1969.

65. Clark, D. A., McDermott, M. R., and Szewczuk, M. R., Impairment of host-versus-graft reaction in pregnant mice. II. Selective suppression of cytotoxic T-cell generation correlates with soluble suppressor activity and with successful allogeneic pregnancy, *Cell. Immunol.,* 52, 106, 1980.

66. Kenny, J. F. and Diamond, M., Immunological responsiveness to *Escherichia coli* during pregnancy, *Infect. Immunity,* 16, 174, 1977.

67. Fabris, N., Immunological reactivity during pregnancy in the mouse, *Experientia,* 29, 610, 1973.

68. Woodrow, J. C., Elson, C. J., and Donohoe, W. T. A., Effect of pregnancy on the isoantibody response in rabbits, *Nature (London),* 233, 62, 1971.

69. Baines, M. G., Pross, H. F., and Millar, K. G., Effects of pregnancy on the maternal lymphoid system in mice, *Obstet. Gynecol.,* 50, 457, 1977.

70. Baines, M. G. and Pross, H. F., Impairment of the thymus-dependent humoral immune response by syngeneic or allogeneic pregnancy, *J. Reprod. Immunol.,* 4, 337, 1982.

71. Sasaki, K. and Ishida, N., Diminished immune response in pregnant mice, *Tohoku J. Exp. Med.,* 116, 391, 1975.

72. Rojo, J. M., Portoles, M. P., and Portoles, A., Immune-responses and lymphocyte mitogenic activation in mice under oral-contraceptive treatment, *J. Reprod. Immunol.,* 2, 29, 1980.

73. Fabris, N., Piantanelli, L., and Muzzioli, M., Differential effect of pregnancy or gestagens on humoral and cell-mediated immunity, *Clin. Exp. Immunol.,* 28, 306, 1977.

74. Siiteri, P. K., Febres, F., Clemens, L. E., Chang, R. J., Gondos, B., and Stites, D. P., Progesterone and the maintenance of pregnancy: is progesterone nature's immunosuppressant, *Ann. N.Y. Acad. Sci.,* 286, 384, 1977.

75. Beer, A. E. and Billingham, R. E., Maternal immunological recognition mechanisms during pregnancy, in *Maternal Recognition of Pregnancy,* Ciba Foundation Symposium 64 (new series), Whelan, J., Ed., Excerpta Medica, Amsterdam, 1979, 293.

76. Schiff, R. I., Mercier, D., and Buckley, R. H., Inability of gestational hormones to account for the inhibitory effects of pregnancy plasmas on lymphocyte responses *in vitro, Cell. Immunol.,* 20, 69, 1975.

77. Hirokawa, K., Okayasu, I., and Hatakeyana, S., Effect of pregnancy and its related hormones on the in vitro proliferation activity of mouse spleen cells, *Acta Pathol. Jpn.,* 29, 837, 1979.

78. Smith, N. C. and Brush, M. G., Prepraation and characterization of human syncytiotrophoblast plasma membranes, *Med. Biol.,* 56, 272, 1978.

79. Sanyal, M. K., Secretion of progesterone during gestation in the rat, *J. Endocrinol.,* 79, 179, 1978.

80. Holinka, C. F., Tseng, Y.-C., and Finch, C. E., Reproductive aging in C57BL/6J mice: plasma progesterone, viable embryos and resorption frequency throughout pregnancy, *Biol. Reprod.,* 20, 1201, 1979.

81. Murr, S. M., Stabenfeldt, G. H., Bradford, G. E., and Gechwind, I. I., Plasma progesterone during pregnancy in the mouse, *Endocrinology,* 94, 1209, 1974.

82. Batra, S., The regulation of oestradiol and progesterone concentrations in the female reproductive tissues, *Acta Obstet. Gynecol. Scand.,* Suppl. 82, 1, 1979.

83. Botte, V., Tramontana, S., and Chieffi, G., Histochemical distribution of some hydroxysteroid dehydrogenases in the placenta, foetal membranes and uterine mucosa of the mouse, *J. Endocrinol.,* 40, 189, 1968.

84. Hayry, P., von Willebrand, E., and Soots, A., In situ effector mechanisms in rat kidney allograft rejection. III. Kinetics of the inflammatory response and generation of donor-directed killer cells, *Scand. J. Immunol.,* 10, 95, 1979.

85. Ascher, N. L., Chen, S., Hoffman, R., and Simmons, R. L., Maturation of cytotoxic effector cells at the site of allograft rejection, *Transplant. Proc.,* 13, 1105, 1981.

86. Mendelsohn, J., Multe, M. M., and Bernheim, J. L., Inhibition of human lymphocyte stimulation by steroid hormones: cytokinetic mechanisms, *Clin. Exp. Immunol.,* 27, 127, 1977.

87. Horne, C. H. W., Thomson, A. W., Hunter, C. B. J., van Heyningen, V., Deane, D. L., and Steel, C. M., Association between pregnancy-associated α_2-glycoprotein (α_2-PAG) and mixed leucocyte reaction determinants on the leucocyte surface, *Experientia,* 35, 411, 1979.

88. Stimson, W. H., Studies on the immunosuppressive properties of a pregnancy-associated α-macroglobulin, *Clin. Exp. Immunol.,* 25, 199, 1976.

89. Stimson, W. H., Are pregnancy-associated serum proteins responsible for the inhibition of lymphocyte transformation by pregnancy serum, *Clin. Exp. Immunol.,* 40, 157, 1980.

90. Thompson, E. A., Jr., The effects of estradiol upon the thymus of the sexually immature female mouse, *J. Steroid Biochem.,* 14, 167, 1981.

91. Stimson, W. H. and Hunter, I. C., Oestrogen-induced immunoregulation mediated through the thymus, *J. Clin. Lab. Immunol.,* 4, 27, 1980.

92. Morton, H., Rolfe, B., Clunie, G. J. A., Anderson, J. J., and Morrison, J., An early pregnancy factor detected in human serum by the rosette inhibition test, *Lancet,* 1, 394, 1977.

93. Noonan, F. P., Halliday, W. J., Morton, H., and Clunie, G. J. A., Early pregnancy factor is immunosuppressive, *Nature (London)*, 278, 649, 1979.
94. Morton, H., Rolfe, B. E., McNeill, L., Clarke, P., Clarke, F. M., and Clunie, G. J. A., Early pregnancy factor-tissues involved in its production in the mouse, *J. Reprod. Immunol.*, 2, 73, 1980.
95. Clarke, F. M., Morton, H., Rolfe, B. E., and Clunie, G. J. A., Partial characterization of early pregnancy factor in the sheep, *J. Reprod. Immunol.*, 2, 151, 1980.
96. Cavanagh, A. C., Morton, H., Rolfe, B. E., and Gidley-Baird, A. A., Ovum factor: a first signal of pregnancy, *Am. J. Reprod. Immunol.*, 2, 97, 1982.
97. Rolfe, B. E., Morton, H., and Clarke, F. M., Early pregnancy factor is an immunosuppressive contaminant of commercial preparations of human chorionic gonadotrophin, *Clin. Exp. Immunol.*, 51, 45, 1983.
98. Murray, F. A., Segerson, E. C., and Brown, F. T., Suppression of lymphocytes in vitro by porcine uterine secretory protein, *Biol. Reprod.*, 19, 15, 1978.
99. McDermott, M. R. and Bienenstock, J., Evidence for a common mucosal immunologic system. I. Migration of B immunoblasts into intestinal, respiratory, and genital tissues, *J. Immunol.*, 122, 1892, 1979.
100. Streilein, J. W., Lymphocyte traffic, T-cell malignancies and the skin, *J. Invest. Dermatol.*, 71, 167, 1978.
101. Wira, C. R. and Sandoe, C. P., Hormonal regulation of immunoglobulins: influence of estradiol on immunoglobulin A and G in the rat uterus, *Endocrinology*, 106, 1020, 1980.
102. Wira, C. R., Hyde, E., Sandoe, C. P., Sullivan, D., and Spencer, S., Cellular aspects of the rat uterine IgA response to estradiol and progesterone, *J. Steroid Biochem.*, 12, 451, 1980.
103. McDermott, M. R., Clark, D. A., and Bienenstock, J., Evidence for a common mucosal immunologic system. II. Influence of the estrous cycle on B immunoblast migration into genital and intestinal tissues, *J. Immunol.*, 124, 2536, 1980.
104. Tchernitchin, A. and Tchernitchin, X., Characterization of the estrogen receptors in the uterine and blood eosinophil leukocytes, *Experientia*, 32, 1240, 1976.
105. Siiteri, P. K. and Stites, D. P., Immunologic and endocrine interrelationships in pregnancy, *Biol. Reprod.*, 26, 1, 1982.
106. Bell, S. C., Decidualization: regional differentiation and associated function, in *Oxford Reviews of Reproductive Biology*, Vol. 5, Oxford University Press, New York, 1983, 220.
107. Puri, R. K. and Roy, S. K., The binding of progesterone in different parts of the rabbit uterus during implantation, *J. Biosci.*, 2, 349, 1980.
108. Logeat, F., Sartor, P., Hai, M. T. V., and Milgrom, E., Local effect of the blastocyst on estrogen and progesterone receptors in the rat endometrium, *Science*, 207, 1083, 1980.
109. Rothchild, I. and Gibori, G., The luteotrophic action of decidual tissue: the stimulating effect of decidualization on the serum progesterone level in pseudopregnant rats, *Endocrinology*, 97, 838, 1975.
110. Denari, J. H., Germino, N. I., and Rosner, J. M., Early synthesis of uterine proteins after a decidual stimulus in the pseudopregnant rat, *Biol. Reprod.*, 15, 1, 1976.
111. Bell, S. C., Immunochemical identity of "decidualization-associated protein" and alpha 2 acute-phase macroglobulin in the pregnant rat, *J. Reprod. Immunol.*, 1, 193, 1979.
112. Kirkwood, K. J. and Bell, S. C., Inhibitory activity of supernatants from murine decidual cell cultures on the mixed lymphocyte reaction, *J. Reprod. Immunol.*, 3, 243, 1981.
113. Watnick, A. S. and Russo, R. A., Survival of skin homografts in uteri of pregnant and progesterone-estrogen treated rats, *Proc. Soc. Exp. Biol. Med.*, 128, 1, 1968.
114. Moriyama, I. and Sugawa, T., Progesterone facilitates implantation of xenogenic cultured cells in hamster uterus, *Nature (London) New Biol.*, 236, 150, 1972.
115. Dodd, M., Andrew, T. A., and Cotes, J. S., Functional behavior of skin allografts transplanted to rabbit deciduomata, *J. Anat.*, 130, 381, 1980.
116. Kirby, D. R. S., Billington, W. D., and James, D. A., Transplantation of eggs to the kidney and uterus of immunised mice, *Transplantation*, 4, 713, 1966.
117. Slapsys, R. M. and Clark, D. A., Active suppression of host-vs-graft reaction in pregnant mice. IV. Local suppressor cells in decidua and uterine blood, *J. Reprod. Immunol.*, 4, 355, 1982.
118. Slapsys, R. and Clark, D. A., Active suppression of host-versus-graft reaction in pregnant mice. V. Kinetics, specificity, and in vivo activity on non-T suppressor cells localized to the genital tract of mice during first pregnancy, *Am. J. Reprod. Immunol.*, 3, 65, 1983.
119. Clark, D. A., Slapsys, R. M., Croy, B. A., Rossant, J., and McDermott, M. R., Regulation of cytotoxic T cells in pregnant mice, in *Immunology of Reproduction*, Gill, T. and Wegmann, T., Eds., Oxford University Press, New York, 1983, 343.
120. Smith, G., Maternal regulator cells during pregnancy, *Clin. Exp. Immunol.*, 44, 90, 1981.
121. Croy, B. A., Rossant, J., and Clark, D. A., Histological and immunological studies of post implantation death of *Mus caroli* embryos in the *Mus musculus* uterus, *J. Reprod. Immunol.*, 4, 277, 1982.

122. Croy, B. A., Rossant, J., and Clark, D. A., Ectopic grafts of xenogeneic but not allogeneic tropho-blast recruit cytotoxic cells, *Transplantation,* 37, 84, 1984.
123. Clark, D. A., Slapsys, R. M., Croy, B. A., and Rossant, J., Suppressor cell activity in uterine decidua correlates with success or failure of murine pregnancies, *J. Immunol.,* 131, 540, 1983.
124. Rossant, J., Croy, B. A., Clark, D. A., and Chapman, V. M., Interspecific hybrids and chimeras in mice, *J. Exp. Zool.,* 228, 223, 1983.
125. Rossant, J., Mauro, V. M., and Croy, B. A., Importance of trophoblast genotype for survival of interspecific murine chimaeras, *J. Embryol. Exp. Morphol.,* 69, 141, 1982.
126. Nagy, E. and Berczi, I., Prolactin and contact sensitivity, *Allergy,* 36, 429, 1981.
127. Johnson, M. H., Fertilization and implantation, in *Immunology of Human Reproduction,* Scott, J. S. and Jones, W. R., Eds., Grune & Stratton, New York, 1976, 50.
128. Bernard, O., Ripoche, M. A., and Bennett, D., Distribution of maternal immunoglobulins in the mouse uterus and embryo in the days after implantation, *J. Exp. Med.,* 145, 58, 1977.
129. Slapsys, R. M. and Clark, D. A., unpublished data.

Chapter 14

THE INFLUENCE OF HORMONES ON INFECTIOUS AND PARASITIC DISEASE

I. Berczi

TABLE OF CONTENTS

I. INTRODUCTION

Historians frequently recorded that wars and natural disasters were associated with sweeping epidemics of infectious disease. In veterinary epidemiology certain weakening conditions, such as transportation and translocation, deficiencies in care and feeding, or even climatic changes, are often cited as factors that influence the susceptibility of animals to infectious disease. Man-made or natural disasters usually create severe deficiencies in nutrition, housing, and sanitary conditions that can explain satisfactorily the occurrence of epidemics. However, such conditions also elicit, both in man and animals, profound neurohormonal responses, which were first described by Selye[1] in 1936 and became known as stress. The essence of the stress reaction is a neurohormonal imbalance. This can be caused by a variety of external and internal stimuli that either upset, or have the potential to upset the normal functioning, or even the survival, of the animal/human being. Many stress situations have a diverse effect on the organism and for this reason, it is difficult, if not impossible, to separate the effects mediated by the neurohormonal system from other effects, some of which may influence directly the immune system. There is a voluminous literature on the effect of stress on various immune reactions and resistance to infectious disease, which cannot be discussed here. Instead the interested reader is referred to reviews on this subject.[2-7] However, it is interesting to note in this context, that all the pituitary hormones that have major influences on the immune system, namely ACTH, growth hormone (GH), and prolactin (PRL), have been classified as stress hormones.[8-12] In this chapter, some recent work on the endocrine response to infection and the possible role of some hormones in host resistance to infectious agents will be surveyed briefly. For an exhaustive treatment of this subject the reader is referred to earlier publications.[13,14]

II. ENDOCRINE RESPONSE TO INFECTION

Fever has been recognized as a sign of infectious disease from at least the time of Hippocrates. The recognition of the potential significance of fever, however, did not occur until recently. The first indication for the biological significance of fever was the observation of Kluger et al.[15] that lizards seek warmer environments to raise their body temperature to febrile levels when infected. This behavioral modification of body temperature has survival value. Other poikilotherms, including fish, behave similarly. In mammals, fever is induced by an endogenous pyrogenic substance produced by monocyte/macrophage-type cells. This pyrogen appears to be identical with interleukin 1, which is a lymphocyte activating factor, playing a fundamental role in the initiation of most, if not all, immune reactions.[16,17] Several in vitro functions of mammalian lymphoid cells, such as lectin induced mitogenesis of thymocytes, lymphokine production, interleukin 1 induced T cell proliferation, and antibody production are elevated significantly at febrile temperature ($39°C$).[18-20]

Pyrogens are potent stimulators of ACTH release, and the injection of pyrogen is accepted in medicine as a test of the ACTH reserve in patients.[21] Both ACTH and a related peptide, α-MSH, were shown to reduce fever in rabbits.[22-24] This may represent an important regulatory mechanism, also activated by pyrogens. One of the most potent exogenous pyrogenic material is the lipopolysaccharide component (LPS), or endotoxin, derived from the cell walls of gram-negative bacteria. In rats, endotoxin caused a biphasic temperature response, manifesting in hypothermia for 1 hr, which was followed by hyperthermia for 5 to 8 hr after injection. The normal pulsatile GH release, which could be observed on the 1st day, was abolished on the 2nd day after endotoxin treatment. On the 3rd day, GH secretion was greater than the initial level prior to treatment. The release of thyroid stimulating hormone (TSH) was suppressed also by endotoxin, and a rebound release was observed on the subsequent day. The suppression of GH secretion by endotoxin could be reversed by treatment with an antiserum to somatostatin, suggesting that hypothalamic somatostatin mediates adenohypophyseal hormone release.[25] Treatment of sows with endotoxin caused a marked increase in plasma glucocorticoids, and inhibited the release of PRL. This inhibition was not related to the elevated levels of glucocorticoids. Endotoxin induced hypoprolactinemia was suggested as the pathomechanism for agalactia, which occurs frequently in sows with mastitis caused by gram-negative bacteria. The mechanism of LPS induced inhibition of PRL secretion is unknown.[26]

Acute bacterial and viral infections of moderate severity in patients were characterized by elevated levels of plasma glucose, insulin, GH, and cortisol, whereas plasma glucagon, epinephrine, and norepinephrine levels were normal. Such patients exhibited insulin resistance, but monocyte insulin receptors were found to be normal, suggesting that post-receptor impairment was responsible for the resistant state. The diurnal variation of cortisol was abolished also, which led to elevated levels, particularly during the afternoon-evening hours.[27,28]

Before discussing the endocrine response to infections any further, one must emphasize that infections lead to diverse and complex changes in host metabolism,[29] which, in conjunction with secondary factors, such as fever, endotoxin, and nutritional state, could lead to a great variety of hormonal changes. There is little doubt, however, that at least part of the endocrine response to each infection is designed to strengthen host resistance. Other changes may be less specific, or could even be the result of manipulation of the endocrine system by pathogens, in order to avoid host resistance. Yet some other infection induced endocrine alterations may be purely coincidental, due to the affinity of the virus for particular endocrine glands. Virus induced diabetes and polyendocrinopathy are examples of the latter.[30,31] An intriguing action of cholera and pertussis toxins is their interference with the regulatory effect of dopamine on PRL secretion, and of somatostatin on GH secretion.[32-34]

III. THE INFLUENCE OF HORMONES ON HOST RESISTANCE TO INFECTIONS

A. Glucocorticoids

In patients treated with glucocorticoids, gram-negative bacterial and staphylococcal infections, tuberculosis, diphtheria, certain types of fungal, viral, and protozoal infections are frequently encountered.[35] The efficacy of glucocorticoids in chronic active hepatitis, positive for B surface antigen, was studied in 51 pair-randomized patients. Initially, 15 to 20 mg of prednisolone were given per day, and after remission, the maintenance dose was 10 mg/day. The patients were followed for up to $3^{1}/_{2}$ years. Prednisolone decreased significantly serum bilirubin and globulin at 3 months, delayed other biochemical indicators of remission, and accelerated relapse, as well as it increased the frequency of complications and the death rate. Thus, prednisolone had an overall harmful effect in patients with type B viral hepatitis.[36] Hydrocortisone and methylprednisolone inhibited the response of T lymphocytes to stimulation by autologous monocytes, preincubated with viral, or bacterial soluble antigens. Methylprednisolone, but not hydrocortisone, had an inhibitory effect on the stimulatory capacity of antigen pulsed monocytes at relatively high doses (10 $\mu g/m\ell$) and also inhibited the stimulatory properties of antigen pulsed umbilical vein endothelial cells.[37]

Cortisone treatment of guinea pigs inhibited the development of skin reactivity and of antibody formation, after infection with *Mycobacterium tuberculosis*. Cortisone also hastened the progress of the disease in the initial stages, but its effect was not obvious in later stages. The adverse effect of cortisone on the progress of tuberculosis was more marked, throughout the period of study, in prevaccinated animals.[38]

Cortisone acetate, administered to separate groups of rabbits during the 1st, 2nd, or 4th week after intratesticular injection of *Treponema pallidum* altered significantly the kinetics of the immune response, the nature of cellular infiltration, bacterial clearance, and healing. In rabbits, treated with cortisone during the 1st week of infection, a delayed appearance of specific humoral and cellular immunity was observed. After cessation of cortisone treatment, specific immunity appeared rapidly. Cellular infiltration and bacterial clearance were also delayed, but proceeded thereafter, normally. In animals given cortisone during the 2nd week of infection, only slight and temporary reductions were observed in antibody titers and in specific antigen-induced blastogenic lymphocyte responses in vitro. However, the steroid-treated animals had a decreased capacity to eliminate effectively the treponema organisms from the site of infection. In the infected lesions of such animals, macrophages phagocytosed the organisms, but were unable to digest the bacteria, as indicated by the large amounts of treponema antigen present in these phagocytic cells. Cortisone therapy during healing (4th week) reversed temporarily the fibrotic process, and the treponemas reappeared at the primary site. Thus, the course of experimental syphilis infection is determined largely by host immunity, which can be inhibited in the inductive, effector, and healing phases by cortisone treatment.[39]

Short-term treatment with cortisone acetate prevented the expulsion of *Trichuris muris,* and allowed the establishment and survival of an adult worm population in mice for at least 70 days. Serum taken from tolerant mice transferred passive immunity to naive mice, but cells transferred from such donors were ineffective. Cells from immune mice caused a significant reduction in worm numbers, when given on the same day as a secondary infection. It was suggested that corticosteroid treatment deleted an accessory cell population, which led to tolerization of immunocompetent T cells.[40]

Treatment of sheep with dexamethasone decreased the number of established worms after infection with *Haemonchus contortus.* This was not due to direct action of dexamethasone on the nematodes. Sheep, continuously treated with dexamethasone, harbored similar numbers of worms as controls, whereas animals given dexamethasone around the time of infection, had 32 to 36% of the burden of untreated animals. The inhibition of suppressor lymphocytes by dexamethasone was suggested as the mechanism of increased resistance to infection.[41]

B. Diabetes

The presence of oral yeasts and precipitating antibodies to *Candida* was estimated in 204 unselected, diabetic patients. Yeasts, mostly *Candida albicans,* were isolated from 41% of outpatients (out of 172 total), and antibodies were found in 17.5%, although none of these patients had clinically evident disease. The extent of oral yeast colonization and the incidence of antibodies was not related to treatment, or to the duration of the disease, but rather, it correlated directly with blood and urinary glucose levels.[42] The course of *Staphylococcus aureus* bacteremia in 27 diabetic patients (18 insulin dependent) was compared with that in 34 nondiabetic patients matched for age, preexisting cardiac valvular disease, community acquired bacteremia, fever, and leukocytosis. Diabetics with staphylococcal bacteremia were more likely to develop endocarditis than nondiabetics, in the presence of a primary focus. There was no mortality difference between those with and without endocarditis.[43]

C. Sex Hormones
1. Sex-Related Difference in Resistance to Infections
a. Mouse

Male mice exhibited a stronger cell mediated immune response to *Coxsackievirus B-3* infection, as measured by cytotoxicity on day 3 after inoculation. Male cytotoxicity

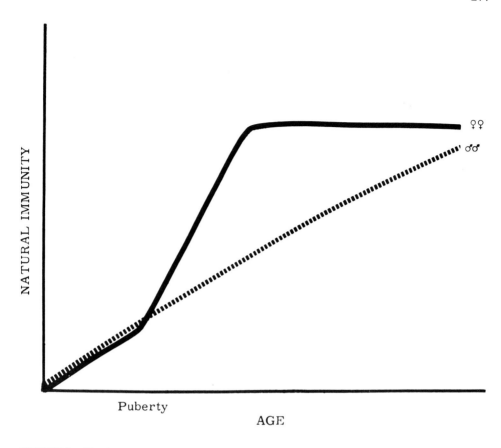

FIGURE 1.   The development of age immunity to direct-infection nematodes in male and female hosts.[52]

was nonspecific on day 3 and peaked on day 7, with a virus specific response. Day 7 female immune cells caused little or no target cell lysis, but significant levels of cytotoxicity were observed earlier on days 3 and 6. A second wave of reactivity was observed in some animals between the 10th and 17th day. Female cytotoxicity was not virus specific at any time and uninfected target cells were lysed as well as, or better, than viral infected cells. In males, both the specific and nonspecific cytotoxicity was mediated by T cells. Whereas in females, a mixture of different effector populations participated with T cells being responsible for only a portion of the activity. These sex-related differences were not observed with *Vaccinia virus*.[44] A cardiotropic strain of Coxsackie B-3 virus induced more cytotoxicity to uninfected myofibers than a noncardiotropic strain. Cytotoxicity was stronger in female than in male animals and was mediated by natural killer (NK) cells. Later killer T lymphocytes occurred in male animals, whereas the cytolytic cells in females maintained the characteristics of NK cells.[45]

The 129 strain of mice have circulating C-type viral glycoproteins (G_{IX}-gp70) in their serum. Males had a significantly higher level, which was reduced by castration to the level of females and was fully restored to male levels by testosterone treatment.[46] Female mice exhibited a higher immune reactivity to both viable, or heat-killed *Paracoccidioides brasiliensis* yeast cells than did males, as measured by delayed hypersensitivity response in vivo, or by the migration inhibition assay.[47]

b. Man

Carriers of *Hepatitis-B virus* are more prevalent among males than females. Chronic liver disease, including active hepatitis, postnecrotic sclerosis, and primary hepatocellular carcinoma, which are associated with hepatitis B infection, show a marked male predominance. Hepatitis B virus-related cancer of the liver is four to nine times more common in males than in females.[48-50] A survey conducted in Ghana, West Africa, showed that individuals in rural areas responded earlier to *Epstein Barr virus* than those in urban areas, and that antibody levels were consistently higher in females than in males in every age group.[51]

c. Other Species

Observations with regard to sex-related differences in resistance to nematode infections showed, in several species, that males and females are not different until puberty, when a sudden increase of immunity occurs in females. In the male, immunity develops gradually, from shortly after birth to adulthood (Figure 1).[52]

2. Gonadectomy

Mortality and necrosis in the heart was greater in male mice than in females, after infection with a heart adapted strain of *Coxsackie B-3 virus*. Castration of the males prior to infection reduced mortality and the development of autoimmune T lymphocytes. This could be reversed by testosterone and antagonized by estrone treatment.[53] Male Swiss mice are more susceptible to infection with *Ancylostoma caninum* than are females. Orchidectomy decreased the survival of filariform larvae in males, whereas ovariectomy increased larval survival in females significantly.[54]

Castration enhanced the resistance of rats to infection with the larvae of *Taenia taeniaeformis, Cysticercus crassicollis,* in males and diminished resistance in females.[55] Alteration of the sex hormonal environment in both sexes of guinea pigs affected significantly their immunity to *Toxoplasma gondii.* Gonadectomy enhanced delayed hypersensitivity, which led to greater prominence of lesions in the nonlymphoid organs of both sexes.[56]

3. The Effect of Estrous Cycle on Genital Tract Infections

Rats were infected intravaginally with *Pasteurella pneumotropica* and the vaginal microflora was analyzed in relation to the estrus cycle. *P. pneumatropica* was the dominant organism and the bacterial count was significantly increased at estrus, which correlated with an increase in cornified nonnucleated cells, with large numbers of adherent gram-negative coccobacilli.[57] *Escherichia coli* was inoculated into the uterine lumen of rats and rabbits at different stages of the estrus cycle. In rats, a large number of *E. coli* were retained in the ligated uterine horns, independent of the estrus stage. *E. coli,* inoculated at diestrus, induced purulent endometritis, but the organisms caused asymptomatic infection when inoculated at proestrus-estrus. Large numbers of *E. coli* were retained in the nonligated horn at proestrus, due to the *physiological* constriction of the cervix. In rabbits, the inoculation of *E. coli* into ligated uterine horns caused purulent inflammation, regardless of ovarian status.[58] Estradiol treatment of intact, or ovariectomized, rats caused accumulation of a significant amount of fluid in the uterine horns, which also facilitated the movement of vaginal bacteria into the uterine lumen. Ligation of the uterine body above the cervix, or treatment with antibiotics, did not suppress such infections.[59]

4. The Influence of Estrogens on Immunity to Infectious Agents
a. Mouse

A single dose of 2.5 μg of estradiol given to male mice before and up to 3.5 days after the administration of 3×10^5 heat-killed *E. coli* increased significantly the numbers of antibody producing cells in the spleen, 4 days after immunization. Estrogen had no effect, when given 2 days before the antigen, or 2 hr before sacrifice. The number of antibody producing cells was significantly increased in the spleen from male animals immunized with *E. coli* 3 days earlier and exposed in vitro to estradiol at 500 to 5000 pg/ml concentrations, whereas at higher concentrations (20 ng/ml) some decrease was observed. Furthermore, uptake of tritiated thymidine was increased in thymic and spleen cells incubated for 24 hr with 500 pg/ml of estradiol, whereas 20 ng/ml was slightly, but significantly, inhibitory. Therefore, estradiol in concentrations that approximate physiological serum levels enhances the proliferation of immunocompetent cells.[60] Treatment with estrone increased the resistance of mice to a laboratory strain of type I *Pneumococcus*.[61]

Treatment of ovariectomized NIH Swiss mice with estrogens elevated the level of circulating *Murine leukemia virus* group specific antigen and the activity of RNA-directed DNA polymerase in the uterus.[62] The susceptibility of Swiss mice to infection with MM virus was increased markedly by estrone treatment. The titers of circulating interferon, induced by the virus, was lower in estrone pretreated animals, when compared with controls.[63]

b. Rat

Significantly higher bacterial counts, with lower proportions of antibody coated bacteria, were found in estradiol treated rats (0.5 mg/kg/wk), than in controls, 4 weeks after intravesical infection with *E. coli*.[64] Treatment of intact or ovariectomized rats with estradiol decreased their susceptibility to uterine infections that originated from the movement of vaginal bacteria into the uterus.[59] Estrogen treatment of orchidectomized male rats increased their resistance to infection with larvae of *Taenia taeniaeformis*.[55]

c. Man

A higher incidence of bacteriurea and of genitourinary infections with *Candida albicans* and erosion (possibly due to Trichomonadosis) was found in users of oral contraceptives. Bacteriurea was associated with oral contraceptives containing ethynyl estradiol, or those with higher estrogen doses.[65,66] However, other investigators found no relations between genitourinary infections and the use of oral contraceptives.[67]

d. Other Species

Chronic treatment of guinea pigs with hexoestrol led to overwhelming disease in animals infected with *Toxoplasma gondii*.[56] Female guinea pigs were treated for 14 days i.m. with 1 mg of beta-estradiol-3-benzoate and then inoculated intravaginally with the chlamydial agent of guinea pig inclusion conjunctivitis. Estradiol treated animals manifested infections of greater intensity and longer duration than did controls. Moreover, ascending infections were observed, resulting in endometritis, cystic salpingitis, and cystitis. Humoral and cell mediated immune responses of estradiol treated and untreated animals were similar to the chlamydial agent.[68]

Hamsters of both sexes, treated with estrone, exhibited delayed tumor development after s.c. inoculation with *Simian virus 40*.[69]

5. Androgens

Treatment of male and female mice with testosterone protected them against pneumococcus infection, but to a lesser degree than did estrogens.[61] In male mice castration reduced Coxsackie B-3 virus induced necrotic lesions and T cell mediated cytotoxicity, which would be reversed by testosterone treatment.[53] The administration of androgen to ovariectomized female rats lowered their resistance to infection with larvae of *Taenia taeniaeformis*.[55] *Simian virus 40* oncogenesis in adult male hamsters was accelerated by testosterone treatment.[69] Purulent oophoritis and metritis occurred in female rats injected with 250 μg of testosterone propionate at 3 days of age. This infectious disease was caused by mycoplasma organisms.[70]

6. Progesterone

Progesterone had no effect on pneumococcus infection in mice.[61] However, progesterone treatment of monkeys made them susceptible to the Carr-Zibler strain of Rous chicken sarcoma virus. Eight juvenile monkeys (five *M. mulatta,* four *M. speciosa,* and one *C. aethipos)* and two adults were conditioned with 5 mg/kg progesterone injections daily, given i.m. All animals developed tumors (fibrosarcomas) at the site of inoculation in 8 to 15 days. Virus was demonstrated in all these tumors by back passage to chickens.[71] Further investigations revealed that 5-day-old nontreated monkeys were also susceptible to tumor induction by this virus. Physiological doses of progesterone rendered 30 otherwise resistant juvenile and adult monkeys susceptible to the oncogenic effect of chicken sarcoma virus.[72]

REFERENCES

1. Selye, H., A syndrome produced by diverse nocuous agents, *Nature (London),* 138, 32, 1936.
2. Rasmussen, A. F., Jr., Emotions and immunity, *Ann. N.Y. Acad. Sci.,* 164, 458, 1969.
3. Solomon, G. F., Amkraut, A. A., and Kasper, P., Immunity, emotions and stress with special reference to the mechanisms of stress effects on the immune system, *Ann. Clin. Res.,* 6, 313, 1974.
4. Walton, B., Anaesthesia, surgery and immunology, *Anaesthesia,* 33, 322, 1978.
5. Furst, J. B., Emotional stress reactions to surgery; review of some therapeutic implications, *N.Y. State J. Med.,* 78, 1083, 1978.
6. Cheville, N. F., Environmental factors affecting the immune response of birds — a review, *Avian Dis.,* 23, 308, 1979.
7. Brocker, E. B. and Macher, E., The effect of anaesthesia and surgery on immune function — a review, *Klin. Wochenschr.,* 59, 1297, 1981.
8. Selye, H., The general adaptation syndrome and the diseases of adaptation, *J. Clin. Endocrinol.,* 6, 117, 1946.
9. Volpé, A., Mazza, V., and Direnzo, G. C., Prolactin and certain obstetric stress conditions, *Int. J. Biol. Res. Preg.,* 3, 161, 1982.
10. Johansson, G. G., Karonen, S.-L., and Laakso, M.-L., Reversal of an elevated plasma level of prolactin during prolonged psychological stress, *Acta Physiol. Scand.,* 119, 463, 1983.
11. Kant, G. J., Mougey, E. H., Pennington, L. L., and Mayerhoff, J. L., Graded footshock stress elevates pituitary cyclic AMP and plasma β-endorphin, β-LPH, corticosterone and prolactin, *Life Sci.,* 33, 2657, 1983.
12. Kosten, T. R., Jacobs, S., Mason, J., Wahby, V., and Atkins, S., Psychological correlates of growth hormone response to stress, *Psychosom. Med.,* 46, 49, 1984.
13. Jackson, G. J., Herman, R., and Singer, I., Eds., *Immunity to Parasitic Animals,* Vol. 2, Appleton-Century-Crofts, New York, 1970.
14. Selye, H., *Hormones and Resistance,* Vols. 1, 2, Springer-Verlag, Basel, 1971.
15. Kluger, M. J., Ringler, D. H., and Anver, M. R., Fever and survival, *Science,* 188, 166, 1984.
16. Rosenwasser, L. J., Dinarello, C. A., and Rosenthal, A. S., Adherent cell function in murine T-lymphocyte antigen recognition. IV. Enhancement of murine T-cell antigen recognition by human leukocytic pyrogen, *J. Exp. Med.,* 150, 707, 1979.
17. Murphy, P. A., Simon, P. L., and Willoughby, W. F., Endogenous pyrogens made by rabbit peritoneal exudate cells are identical with lymphocyte activating factors made by rabbit alveolar macrophages, *J. Immunol.,* 124, 2498, 1980.
18. Roberts, N. J., Jr., Temperature and host defense, *Microbiol. Rev.,* 42, 241, 1979.
19. Duff, G. W. and Durum, S. K., Fever and immunoregulation: hyperthermia, interleukins 1 and 2, and T cell proliferation, *Yale J. Biol. Med.,* 55, 437, 1982.
20. Jampel, H. D., Duff, G. D., Gershon, R. K., Atkins, E., and Durum, S. K., Fever and immunoregulation. III. Hyperthermia augments the primary in vitro humoral immune response, *J. Exp. Med.,* 157, 1229, 1983.

21. Liddle, G. W., The adrenals, in *Textbook of Endocrinology,* 6th ed., Williams, R. H., Ed., W. B. Saunders, Philadelphia, 1981, 249.
22. Zimmer, J. A. and Lipton, J. M., Central and peripheral injections of ACTH (1-24) reduce fever in adrenalectomized rabbits, *Peptides,* 2, 413, 1981.
23. Murphy, M. T., Richards, D. B., and Lipton, J. M., Antipyretic potency of centrally administered α-melanocyte stimulating hormone, *Science,* 221, 192, 1983.
24. Glyn-Ballinger, J. R., Bernardini, G. L., and Lipton, J. M., α-MSH injected into the septal region reduces fever in rabbits, *Peptides,* 4, 199, 1983.
25. Kasting, N. W. and Martin, J. B., Altered release of growth hormone and thyrotropin induced by endotoxin in the rat, *Am. J. Physiol.,* 243, E332, 1982.
26. Smith, B. B. and Wagner, W. C., Suppression of prolactin in pigs by *Escherichia coli* endotoxin, *Science,* 224, 605, 1974.
27. Beisel, W. R., Bruton, J., Anderson, K. D., and Sawyer, W. D., Adrenocortical responses during tularemia in human subjects, *J. Clin. Endocrinol. Metab.,* 27, 61, 1967.
28. Drobny, E. C., Abramson, E. C., and Baumann, G., Insulin receptors in acute infection: a study of factors conferring insulin resistance, *J. Clin. Endocrinol. Metab.,* 58, 710, 1984.
29. Beisel, W. R., Metabolic response to infection, *Ann. Rev. Med.,* 26, 9, 1975.
30. Onodera, T., Ray, U. R., Melez, K. A., Suzuki, H., Toniolo, A., and Notkins, A. L., Virus-induced diabetes mellitus: autoimmunity and polyendocrine disease prevented by immunosuppression, *Nature (London),* 297, 66, 1982.
31. Oldstone, M. B. A., Rodriguez, M., Daughaday, W. H., and Lampert, P. W., Viral perturbation of endocrine function: disordered cell function leads to disturbed homeostasis and disease, *Nature (London),* 307, 278, 1984.
32. Cronin, M. J., Myers, G. A., MacLeod, R. M., and Hewlett, E. L., Pertussis toxin actions on the pituitary-derived 235-1 clone: effects of PGE$_1$, cholera toxin, and forskolin on cyclic AMP metabolism and prolactin release, *J. Cyclic Nucl. Prot. Phosph. Res.,* 9, 245, 1983.
33. Cronin, M. J., Rogol, A. D., Myers, G. A., and Hewlett, E. L., Pertussis toxin blocks the somatostatin-induced inhibition of growth hormone release and adenosine 3′,5′-monophosphate accumulation, *Endocrinology,* 113, 209, 1983.
34. Cronin, M. J., Myers, G. A., MacLeod, R. M., and Hewlett, E. L., Pertussis toxin uncouples dopamine agonist inhibition of prolactin release, *Am. J. Physiol.,* 244, E499, 1983.
35. Fauci, A. S., Dale, D. C., and Balow, J. E., Glucocorticoid therapy: mechanisms of action and clinical considerations, *Ann. Intern. Med.,* 84, 304, 1976.
36. Lam, K. C., Lai, C. L., Ng, R. P., Trepo, C., and Wu, P. C., Deleterious effect of prednisolone in HBsAg-positive chronic active hepatitis, *N. Engl. J. Med.,* 304, 380, 1981.
37. Hirschberg, H., Hirschberg, T., Nousianen, H., Braathen, L. R., and Jaffe, E., The effects of corticosteroids on the antigen presenting properties of human monocytes and endothelial cells, *Clin. Immunol. Immunopathol.,* 23, 577, 1982.
38. Venkataraman, M., Kumar, R., Bhuyan, U. N., Shriniwas, Malaviya, A. N., and Mohapatra, L. N., Immune responses in experimental tuberculosis: effect of cortisone treatment, *Indian J. Med. Res.,* 64, 1592, 1976.
39. Lukehart, S. A., Baker-Zander, S. A., Lloyd, R. M. C., and Sell, S., Effect of cortisone administration on host-parasite relationships in early experimental syphilis, *J. Immunol.,* 127, 1361, 1981.
40. Lee, T. D. G. and Wakelin, D., Cortisone-induced immunotolerance to nematode infection in CBA/Ca mice. I. Investigation of the defect in the protective response, *Immunology,* 47, 227, 1982.
41. Adams, D. B. and Davies, H. I., Enhanced resistance to infection with *Haemonchus contortus* in sheep treated with a corticosteroid, *Int. J. Parasitol.,* 12, 523, 1982.
42. Odds, F. C., Evans, E. G. V., Taylor, M. A. R., and Wales, J. K., Prevalence of pathogenic yeasts and humoral antibodies to *Candida* in diabetic patients, *J. Clin. Pathol.,* 31, 840, 1978.
43. Cooper, G. and Platt, R., *Staphylococcus aureus* bacteremia in diabetic patients: endocarditis and mortality, *Am. J. Med.,* 73, 658, 1982.
44. Wong, C. Y., Woodruff, J. J., and Woodruff, J. F., Generation of cytotoxic T lymphocytes during Coxsackievirus B-3 infection. III. Role of sex, *J. Immunol.,* 119, 591, 1977.
45. Huber, S. A., Job, L. P., Auld, K. R., and Woodruff, J. F., Sex-related differences in the rapid production of cytotoxic spleen cells active against uninfected myofibers during Coxsackie virus B-3 infection, *J. Immunol.,* 126, 1336, 1981.
46. Obata, Y., Stockert, E., Yamaguchi, M., and Boyse, E. A., Source and hormone-dependence of G$_{ix}$-gp70 in mouse serum, *J. Exp. Med.,* 148, 793, 1978.
47. Montoya, F. and Garcia-Moreno, L. F., Effect of sex on delayed hypersensitivity responses in experimental mouse paracoccidioidomycosis, *J. Reticuloendothel. Soc.,* 26, 467, 1979.
48. Curtis, J. L., Samper, L., Rodriquez, L. A., and Garrett, M. G., Sex difference in hepatitis-associated (Australia) antigen carrier state one year after hepatitis outbreak, *Pediatrics,* 52, 441, 1973.

49. Blumberg, B. S., Sex differences in response to hepatitis-B virus. I. History. II. Parental responses to HBV infection and the secondary sex ratio of the offspring, *Arthritis Rheum.*, 22, 1261, 1979.

50. London, W. T., Sex differences in response to hepatitis-B virus: introduction, *Arthritis Rheum.*, 22, 1258, 1979.

51. Biggar, R. J., Gardiner, C., Lennett, E., Collins, W. E., Nkrumah, F. K., and Henle, W., Malaria, sex, and place of residence as factors in antibody response to Epstein-Barr virus in Ghana, West Africa, *Lancet,* II, 115, 1981.

52. Thorson, R. E., Direct infection nematodes, in *Immunity to Parasitic Animals,* Vol. 2, Jackson, G. J., Herman, R., and Singer, I., Eds., Appleton-Century-Crofts, New York, 1970, 913.

53. Huber, S. A., Job, L. P., and Auld, K. R., Influence of sex hormones on Coxsackie B-3 virus infection in Balb/c mice, *Cell. Immunol.,* 67, 173, 1982.

54. Bhai, I. and Pandey, A. K., Gonadectomy and survival and *Ancylostomacaninum* (Nematoda) filariform larvae in mice, *Experientia,* 38, 278, 1982.

55. Campbell, D. H. and Melcher, L. R., Relationship of sex factors to resistance against *Cysticercus crassicollis* in rats, *J. Infect. Dis.,* 66, 184, 1940.

56. Kittas, C. and Henry, L., Effect of sex hormones on the immune system of guinea pigs and on the development of toxoplasmic lesions in non-lymphoid organs, *Clin. Exp. Immunol.,* 36, 16, 1979.

57. Yamada, S., Baba, E., and Arakawa, A., Proliferation of *Pasteurella pneumotropica* at oestrus in the vagina of rats, *Lab. Anim.,* 17, 261, 1983.

58. Nishikawa, Y., Baba, T., and Imori, T., Effect of the extrous cycle on uterine infection induced by *Escherichia coli, Infect. Immunity,* 43, 678, 1984.

59. Leland, F. E., Kohn, D. F., and Sirbasku, D. A., Effect of estrogen-promoted bacterial infections of the rat uterus on bioassay of mammalian cell growth factor activities in uterine luminal fluid, *Biol. Reprod.,* 28, 1243, 1983.

60. Kenny, J. F., Pangburn, P. C., and Trail, G., Effects of estradiol on immune competence: in vivo and in vitro studies, *Infect. Immunity,* 13, 448, 1976.

61. Von Hamm, E. and Rosenfeld, I., The effect of various sex hormones upon experimental penumococcus infections in mice, *J. Infect. Dis.,* 70, 243, 1942.

62. Fowler, A. K., Kouttab, N. M., Kind, P. D., Strickland, J. E., and Hellman, A., Oncornaviral protein modulation in mouse uterine tissue by estrogen, *Proc. Soc. Exp. Biol. Med.,* 148, 14, 1975.

63. Giron, D. F., Allen, P. J., Pindak, F. F., and Schmidt, J. P., Inhibition by estrone of the antiviral protection and interferon elicited by interferon inducers in mice, *Infect. Immunity,* 3, 318, 1971.

64. Riedasch, G., Setzis, K., Bersch, W., and Ritz, E., Estrogens influence antibody coating in experimental urinary tract infection, *Klin. Wochenschr.,* 61, 529, 1983.

65. Kålund Jensen, H., Hansen, P. Å., and Blom, J., Incidence of *Candida albicans* in women using oral contraceptives, *Acta Obstet. Gynecol. Scand.,* 49, 293, 1970.

66. Takahashi, M. and Loveland, D. B., Bacteriuria and oral contraceptives, *JAMA,* 227, 762, 1974.

67. Kunin, C. M. and McCormack, R. C., An epidemiologic study of bacteriuria and blood pressure among nuns and working women, *N. Engl. J. Med.,* 278, 635, 1968.

68. Rank, R. G., White, H. J., Hough, A. J., Jr., Pasley, J. N., and Barron, A. L., Effect of estradiol on chlamydial genital infection of female guinea pigs, *Infect. Immunity,* 38, 699, 1982.

69. Ohtaki, S., Suppressive effects on *Simian virus 40*-induced oncogenesis of several immunosuppressive agents and hormonal modifications applied during the latent period, *Cancer Res.,* 38, 4698, 1978.

70. Leader, R. W., Leader, I., and Witschi, E., Genital mycoplasmosis in rats treated with testosterone propionate to produce constant estrus, *J. Am. Vet. Med. Assoc.,* 157, 1923, 1970.

71. Munroe, J. S. and Windle, W. F., Tumors induced by chicken sarcoma in monkeys conditioned with progesterone, *Nature (London),* 216, 811, 1967.

72. Munroe, J. S., Progesteroids as immunosuppressive agents, *J. Reticuloendothel. Soc.,* 9, 361, 1971.

Chapter 15

SEX HORMONES IN AUTOIMMUNITY

Elizabeth S. Raveche and Alfred D. Steinberg

TABLE OF CONTENTS

I. INTRODUCTION

In humans, females are more susceptible to several autoimmune diseases such as systemic lupus erythematosus (SLE),[1] myasthenia gravis,[2] and idiopathic thrombocytopenic purpura. In SLE, the female-male ratio is 10:1 for women in their menstruating years. However, in prepubertal or postmenopausal women this ratio is lower,[3] indicating that sex hormones are involved in the increased prevalence of autoimmunity in females of reproductive age. In addition, reports of an association of lupus and abnormalities of estrogen metabolism in males with Klinefelter's syndrome suggest that persistent estrogen stimulation may be responsible for the development of SLE in this condition.[4] Further evidence for the role of sex hormones in lupus comes from a study of monozygotic twins discordant for SLE, where the unaffected twin was surgically castrated at 15 years of age, prior to the onset of SLE.[5] Symptoms of lupus are exacerbated during pregnancy or after delivery,[6] with the ingestion of oral contraceptives,[7] and at a particular stage of the menstrual cycle.[8] In addition, abnormalities in sex hormone biosynthesis and metabolism have been described. Before discussing the possible mechanism of action of sex hormones in immunity in general and in autoimmunity, in particular, a brief review of the biosynthesis and metabolism of sex hormones might be helpful.

II. OVERVIEW OF SEX HORMONE PHYSIOLOGY

Most of the sex hormones are produced by the gonads and are derived from cholesterol. The conversion of cholesterol to sex hormones is activated by luteinizing hormone (LH). LH, a pituitary hormone, is secreted by anterior pituitary basophilic cells in response to the hypothalamic LH releasing factor (LHRH). The release of LHRH and in turn LH is episodic with estrogen, progesterone, and testosterone altering the amount of LH produced. The significant interrelationship between the pituitary and the gonads has become established since the discovery that the anterior pituitary is essential for the function of the gonads.[9]

In man, the naturally occurring estrogenic hormones are estradiol and estrone. Estrone is less active than estradiol and estriol, (which is a breakdown product) is a very weak estrogenic hormone. The major naturally occurring compounds that possess androgenic activity are testosterone, 5 α-dihydrotestosterone (DHT), and androstenedione. LH accelerates the conversion of cholesterol to pregnenolone, which is a common pathway for the formation of both androgens and estrogens (Figure 1). The androgenic steroids, testosterone and androstenedione, are the immediate precursors of estradiol and estrone, respectively.

The ovaries in females are the main source for estrogens. The testes in males may account for as much as 30% of the estrogen. Peripheral conversion of androgens to estrogens is also very important in the production of estrogen. A significant fraction of androstenedione is converted to estrone. The androstenedione in premenopausal females is derived about equally from the ovaries and the adrenal glands. Following menopause, the ovarian production of androstenedione falls off, but the adrenal gland secretion continues. The conversion of androstenedione to estrone is approximately 1% in lean premenopausal women and rises to 2 to 3% in postmenopausal women. A number of conditions increase the production of estrone from circulating androstenedione, such as aging and obesity. Several studies have suggested that most extraglandular estrogen formation occurs in adipose tissue.

Testosterone is the major androgen produced by the testes and is secreted into the blood. DHT is also secreted, but in very small amounts. Androstenedione, a testosterone precursor, is also secreted by the testes but then it becomes a plasma precursor for estrogens. Testosterone can be metabolized to estradiol or reduced to DHT. In females

SIMPLIFIED BIOSYNTHESIS OF SEX HORMONES:

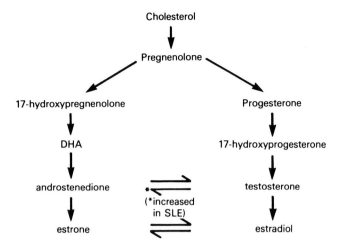

FIGURE 1. Biosynthesis of sex hormones. Abnormalities observed in human SLE are indicated by asterisk. Female lupus patients may have increased oxidation of testosterone to androstenedione that may account for their lower plasma testosterone levels.[13,14]

OUTLINE OF METABOLISM OF ESTROGENS:

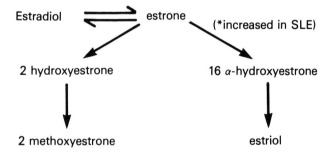

FIGURE 2. Outline of metabolism of estrogen. Abnormalities observed in human SLE are indicated by asterisk. Some patients with SLE manifest increased 16-hydroxylation of estrone.[16] The net outcome may be an increase in estrogenic activity.

about one fourth of the circulating testosterone arises from ovarian secretion and the remainder from the adrenal glands.

A simplified scheme for the metabolism of estrogens is presented in Figure 2. Estriol is the most abundant estrogen in the urine and is the product of the metabolism of estrone and estradiol. Estradiol secretion is increased in obesity.[10] Estriol has been shown to act as an antiestrogen, perhaps because of its short-term occupancy of estrogen receptor.[11] However, if given continuously, it acts as a strong estrogen since the estriol-receptor complexes are continuously translocated to the nucleus where it specifically binds to nonhistone proteins of chromatin eventually leading to messenger RNA production and finally protein formation. 2-Hydroxyestrone, which has a high affinity for the estrogen receptor, behaves as an antiestrogen and is not uterotropic.[12] Testostrone and androstenedione are metabolized to 17-ketosteroids, mainly androsterone and eticholanolone.

III. ABNORMALITIES OF SEX HORMONE METABOLISM IN PATIENTS WITH AUTOIMMUNITY

Abnormalities in steroid biosynthesis have been reported in patients with the autoimmune disorder systemic lupus erythematosus (SLE). Lahita et al.[13] has found that female SLE patients had increased oxidation of testosterone to androstenedione (see Figure 1). In addition, female patients, who were not receiving prednisone, had lower plasma testosterone levels than did normal females.[14] Although conversion of testosterone to androstenedione is a reversible reaction, experiments indicate that these two pathways are frequently dissociated and controlled by distinct enzymes.[15] The increased conversion of testosterone to androstenedione may increase the conversion of androstenedione to estrogens. Thus, both the low plasma levels of testosterone and the increased oxidation of testosterone may play a role in the increased development of autoimmunity in females. Estrogens in turn affect the immune system and promote the development of autoimmunity as it will be discussed in detail later in this chapter.

In addition, patients with SLE were also found to have alterations in the metabolism of estrogens (see Figure 2),[16] namely increased 16-hydroxylation of estrone. The 16-hydroxylated metabolites of estradiol retain substantial peripheral estrogenic activity. Furthermore, 16-hydroxyestrone can form stable covalent adducts with proteins both in vitro and in vivo, which may be recognized in patients with SLE as foreign antigens and trigger autoimmune responses. Pregnancy and phasic estrogen secretion during the menstrual cycle increase the levels of 16-hydroxylated metabolites.[17] Thus, further increases in 16-hydroxyestrone may cause a worsening of the disease either because of the formation of antigenic 16-hydroxyestrone-protein adducts or by modulation of the immune response because of the increase in estrogenic activity. 16-Hydroxyestrone is highly estrogenic in vivo and possesses a low binding affinity for the estrogen receptor.[18] This suggests that abnormal estrogen metabolism may lead to increased estrogenic activity and secondary abnormalities.

IV. GENERALIZED EFFECTS OF SEX HORMONES ON THE IMMUNE SYSTEM

Females have higher immunoglobulin levels and increased resistance to infection in most mammalian species.[19] Female animals made higher antibody responses to specific antigens.[20] Castration of male mice greatly enhanced the specific antibody response, particularly to T-dependent antigens. Female mice rejected allografts earlier than males and castration of males obliterated this difference; whereas, testicular grafts in oophorectomized females decreased the graft rejection rate.[21] In addition, gonadectomy of experimental animals of both sexes increased thymic size. Splenic lymphocytes from female mice made higher responses to both T and B cell mitogens. This increased immunological reactivity in female mice was dependent on the estrous cycle of the female mice. Peak increases in proliferation to mitogens occurred at proestrus when estrogen is elevated.[22] Thus, the gonads and the hormones produced by these organs are intimately involved in the native regulation of the intensity of the immune response. However, sex hormones are not produced and do not function in a vacuum; a complex network of interactions of the various endocrine glands regulates the action of sex hormones.

The literature is replete with the studies of the action of sex hormones on the immune system. The effects of the various sex hormones on the immune system is variable depending on the dose employed and the method of administration. A generalized overview of the effects of sex hormones on the immune system will follow. At low doses, estrogens augment and androgens suppress immunological reactivity. Low doses of estrogens potentiate the antibody response in vivo.[23,24] At high doses, estrogens have a detrimental effect on the immune system and can result in severe wasting and death.[25,26] Progesterone behaves in a similar fashion; low doses cause augmentation and higher doses reduction of immune responses.

Thus, circulating levels of sex hormones influence immunological reactivity. However, a crucial factor in determining the immunological outcome of sex hormone activity is the ability of the hormone to act on the target. A correlation exists between high sensitivity to androgens and low immunological performance.[27] In mice, end organ responses to male hormones were correlated with decreased immunological reactivity in males. High responder strain males, which showed a larger seminal vesicle increase after the injection of testosterone propionate, had lower immunoglobulin levels, and lower specific antibody responses than females of the stain.

V. SEX HORMONE RECEPTORS IN THE IMMUNE SYSTEM

Sex hormones have been found to regulate the magnitude of immune responses. Cells that differentiate in the thymus are involved in immune regulation and have been found to possess receptors for sex hormones. Thymus androgen receptors have been described in the rat[28] and also in the mouse.[29] The mouse was found to have high-affinity DHT binding in the thymus that was indistinguishable from seminal vesicle cytosol binding, which is a known androgen target tissue. Tissue from testicular feminized male mice (TFM) that are known to have no androgen receptors[30] were also negative in our assay. There was no substantial difference in the dissociation constants and maximal binding capacities (Bmax) between male and female mice of the C57BL 6 strain. The presence of thymic androgen receptors allows for the possibility that sex differences in the immune response could be mediated by the action of testosterone or dihydrotestosterone on the thymus via specific androgen receptors. In addition, the murine thymus was found to possess estrogen receptors with maximal binding capacities similar to the uterus, a known estrogen target tissue (Figure 3). Attempts in our laboratory to determine the cell types in the thymus that possess receptors for sex hormones have been inconclusive. In the rat both lymphocytes and thymic epithelial cells have been shown to interact with androgens with a greater percentage of cortical thymic lymphocytes incorporating labeled testosterone than medullary thymic lymphocytes. Thus, specific receptors for sex hormones in the thymus might mediate the effects of sex hormones on immune processes.[31]

VI. SEX HORMONE ALTERATIONS OF LYMPHOCYTE SUBPOPULATIONS

In order to determine if thymocyte subclasses were altered by sex hormones, subpopulations of thymocytes were analyzed using flow cytometric techniques. Thymocytes vary in their expression of different cell surface markers. Peanut agglutinin (PNA), a plant lectin, preferentially binds to immature thymocytes and suppressor cell precursors.[32,33] Lyt surface antigens distinguish other subpopulations of T cells. The helper T-cell phenotype is Lyt $1^+ 2^-$ whereas cytotoxic and suppressor T cells are Lyt $1^+ 2^+$.[34]

ESTRADIOL BINDING IN C57Bl/6 MICE

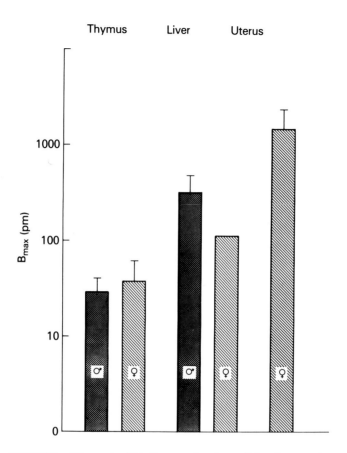

FIGURE 3.   The maximal binding capacity of estradiol to the cytosol of thymus, liver and uterus of 3-month-old male and female CS7BL/ 6 mice is shown in the vertical column. Bars represent SE of the means for three separate experiments.

Another surface antigen, Thy 1, appears in high concentrations on immature T cells and in low concentrations on more mature T Cells.[35] Estradiol treatment of mice resulted in a decrease, both in percentage and absolute numbers of PNA bright, Thy 1 bright, and Lyt 1^+2^+ cells.[36] This decrease in immature thymocytes and suppressor cell precursors following estradiol treatment was observed in both male and female mice, but was more pronounced in females (Figure 4). The ability of estradiol to cause a relative increase in helper T cells and decrease in suppressor thymocytes is consistent with the functional evidence that females have a more reactive immune system than males. In conclusion, the observed effect of sex hormones on subpopulations of thymocytes may, in part, be due to regulation of differentiation and activation via specific sex hormone receptors on cells involved in the immune response.

VII. THYMUS AND SEX HORMONES

The thymus behaves much like an endocrine organ in its regulation of peripheral T cells. Epithelial cells of the thymus produce thymic hormones and T cells regulate the magnitude of immune responses by feedback control mechanisms. In addition, there

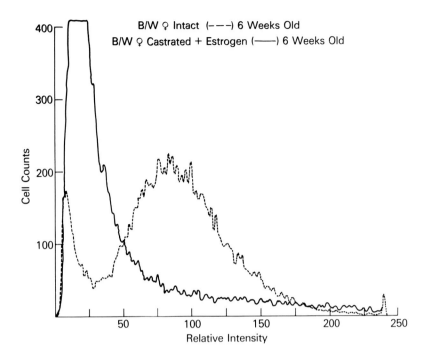

FIGURE 4. Fluorescence profiles obtained after the staining of murine thymocytes with fluorescein-conjugated peanut agglutinin (PNA). The dashed line is the profile obtained from 6-week-old (NZBXNZW)F₁ females. The solid line is the profile obtained after staining thymocytes from 6-week-old (NZBXNZW)F₁ females that had been castrated at 2 weeks and given an implant containing 17-β-estradiol. Estradiol administration resulted in decreased PNA bright cells.

are numerous interactions between the immune and endocrine systems, including a role for hormone receptors on lymphocytes. For example, the number of insulin receptors on lymphocytes increases dramatically following activation.[37]

The thymus has been shown to be affected by the administration of sex hormones. Gonadectomy in experimental animals of both sexes increases the size of the thymus,[38] and exogenous administration of estrogens or testosterone decreases thymus size.[39] The sex hormones may be acting on

1. Thymocytes directly
2. Thymic epithelial cells which produce factors affecting thymocyte differentiation
3. Other organs such as the bone marrow, from which precursor T cells are derived
4. Other endocrine organs causing a stimulation of secretion, e.g., corticosteroid hormones by the adrenal glands, which can then cause thymic involution

Sex steroids may act on the thymus through the action of specific sex hormone receptors. We demonstrated that the thymus of both autoimmune NZB and normal strains of mice possess specific cytoplasmic sex hormone receptors. These may be localized to epithelial cells.[40,41] Sex steroids may act via specific receptors on thymic epithelial cells to release factors that then act on thymocytes. Indeed, thymic epithelial cultures have been shown to release both stimulatory and inhibitory factors when sex steroids are present.[42] Other studies of organ cultured thymocytes showed no effect of either testosterone or estradiol.[43] Organ cultures of 14-day-old fetuses exposed to sex hormones had no effect on the maturation of small Thy 1⁺ cells. In contrast, the glucocorticoid, dexamethasone, inhibited the development of Thy 1⁺ cells. It is possible that sex hormones that are thymolytic act via other organs like the bone marrow, or that fetal thymuses have not developed sex hormone receptors.

The enzyme 20 alpha hydroxysteroid dehydrogenase (20αSDH), a marker of T lymphocytes and bone marrow pre-T cells, is influenced by sex hormones. Castration of male mice decreased both 20αSDH activity as well as the number of large marrow cells. Implantation of testosterone capsules into castrated males increased 20αSDH activity. Castration decreased and testosterone treatment increased the activity of splenic suppressor cells.[44] These studies suggest that testosterone is acting at the bone marrow stem cell as well as in the thymus.

In summary, the thymus, which is where immunoregulatory cells differentiate, has been shown to be a target organ for sex hormones. The thymus appears to be one of the major sites for sex hormone dependent regulation of the immune system.

VIII. MURINE MODELS OF AUTOIMMUNITY

Of the experimental models of lupus, not all display sex-related differences in disease expression. NZB male and female mice have similar survival with average age at death of 17 and 15 months, respectively. NZW mice do not develop a full-blown autoimmune disease, but rather, they exhibit a membranous and proliferative glomerulonephritis associated with deposition of immune complexes in the kidneys. This was more pronounced in females.[45]

F_1 hybrids produced by crossing NZB and NZW mice, neither of which showed a tremendous sex difference in the expression of autoimmune traits, resulted in an F_1 model with a much more severe autoimmune disease in females. Female (NZBXNZW)F_1 (referred to as B/W from here on) live on the average 10 months, whereas males die at 17 months.[45]

Asplenic B/W mice had sex-related differences in longevity. Male asplenic B/W mice lived longer than female asplenic mice.[46] Athymic B/W females also had accelerated disease.[47] These abnormal mice indicate that sex hormones may act at the bone marrow stem cell stage.

Another murine model of lupus MRL/1pr also demonstrates differences in disease patterns between male and female mice. MRL/1pr develop massive lymph node enlargement, glomerulonephritis, and coronary arteritis. Subcutaneous implants of testosterone retarded lymphadenopathy in both male and female MRL/1pr mice.[48]

BXSB mice show a sex difference in disease expression, but this is not hormonal. Autoimmune disease is accelerated in males who develop hypergammaglobulinemia, hemolytic anemia, and glomerulonephritis. Accelerated disease in males is linked to the Y chromosome; castration and hormone treatment did not alter disease expression.[49,50]

Palmerston North mice, which develop renal disease and produce anti-DNA autoantibodies, also display differences in disease expression between males and females. Mean survival was 12 months in females and 16 months in males.[51]

Thus, sex hormones affect the development of autoimmunity in most murine models with females having increased disease expression.

IX. SEX HORMONES AND THE EXPRESSION OF AUTOIMMUNITY

Many laboratories have studied the effects of sex hormones in the B/W model of murine autoimmunity.[52-58] It was noted 15 years ago, that in B/W mice there was not only an age-dependent appearance of anti-DNA antibodies but also a sex-dependence (Figure 5). Even at older ages, males did not develop as high an incidence of anti-DNA antibodies as that observed in female B/W mice.[59] Very early it was found that castra-

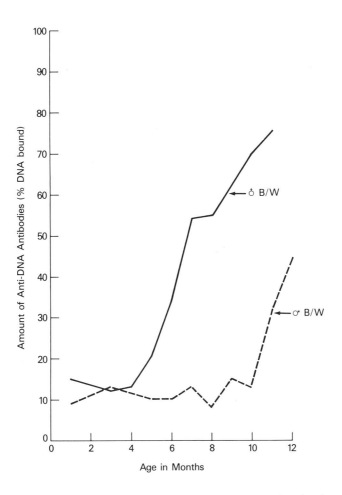

FIGURE 5. The effect of both age and sex on the formation of anti-DNA autoantibodies in B/W mice.

tion of male B/W mice greatly accelerated their disease, and from these studies it was concluded that male sex hormones offer protection against autoimmunity. In female B/W mice younger than 6 months, IgG and IgM anti-DNA antibodies are found. However, after 6 months, the class of antibody produced is almost exclusively IgG in females. Males show this same increase in IgG anti-DNA antibodies, but 3 months later. Prepubertal castration of B/W females alone did not increase survival but prepubertal castration and administration of testosterone prolonged life. In male B/W, prepubertal castration caused early death and an earlier appearance of autoimmune disease. A combination of prepubertal castration of males and the administration of β-estradiol induced disease indistinguishable from that observed in females. In addition administration of testosterone reduced disease in females and males even in postpubertal mice.[58] However, danazol, a synthetic androgen, had very little effect on female B/W disease even though testosterone reduced disease in female B/W (Table 1). Thus, it seems that prepubertal treatment of B/W mice with sex hormones has the more profound effects on their autoimmune disease. Nevertheless, postpubertal androgen treatment of female B/W mice retards their autoimmune disease (Table 2).[60] Progesterone treatment did not reduce autoantibody titers.[45] Estrogen inhibitors were found to retard disease in B/W females,[54] suggesting that estrogens accelerate disease.

Investigations have revealed a sex hormone regulated clearance of immune com-

Table 1

ANTI-ssDNA ANTIBODIES IN FEMALE
(NZB x NZW) F₁ MICE TREATED WITH
ANDROGENS FROM 5 OR 7 MONTHS OF
AGE AND STUDIED 2 MONTHS LATER

| Sex | Treatment | Dose (mg) | Mean % ssDNA binding ± SEM | |
			5 Month group	7 Month group
Female	Control		51 ± 7	58 ± 6
Male	Control		17 ± 4	15 ± 3
Female	Testosterone	8	10 ± 4[a]	57 ± 8
	Danazol	4	60 ± 5	67 ± 7
	Danazol	16	63 ± 3	68 ± 6

[a]   Significantly different from female controls, but not male controls. These same mice had a significant, but incomplete reduction in anti-nDNA (45 ± 4 vs. 65 ± 6 in control females and 21 ± 9 in control males).

Table 2

EFFECT OF PRE- AND POSTPUBERTAL TREATMENT ON
ANTI-DNA AUTOANTIBODIES

| | Amount of anti-DNA autoantibodies | |
	Prepubertal treatment	Postpubertal treatment
B/W ♀	69.7 ± 5.4	62.9 ± 5.3
B/W castrated ♀	51.2 ± 5.2	50.4 ± 3.2
B/W castrated + testosterone ♀	19.6 ± 6.5[a]	43.8 ± 4.1[a]

[a]   Significantly less labeled DNA bound than in control group.

plexes in B/W mice. Young male and female B/W mice cleared IgG-sensitized mouse erythrocytes more rapidly than older B/W mice. Castrated female B/W mice treated with androgen implants from 3 weeks of age showed improved clearance of IgG sensitized erythrocytes at 7 months, whereas estrogen-treated male mice showed delayed clearance.[61] It is possible that androgens act to influence the number or activity of macrophages involved in immune complex clearance.

Many studies in our laboratory have concentrated on the inbred NZB strain. In depth genetic analyses of the mechanism operative in this strain has been performed.[62] NZB mice have been crossed with several nonautoimmune strains, and both spontaneous and induced autoantibodies have been studied. Prior to 9 months of age, (NZBXDBA/2)F₁ mice produce very little autoantibodies. However, they can be in duced to produce anti-single stranded DNA (ssDNA) by the injection of ssDNA complexed to methylated bovine serum albumin (MBSA). Male (NZBXDBA/2)F₁ mice of both reciprocal crosses produced significantly lower amounts of anti-ssDNA antibodies than did their sisters.[63] However, castration plus estrogen implants significantly increased the amount of antibody produced (Figure 6). Testosterone implants were immunosuppressive in both male and female mice. Backcross studies suggested that the ability to respond to ssDNA is inherited as an autosomal dominant trait that is further regulated by sex hormones.

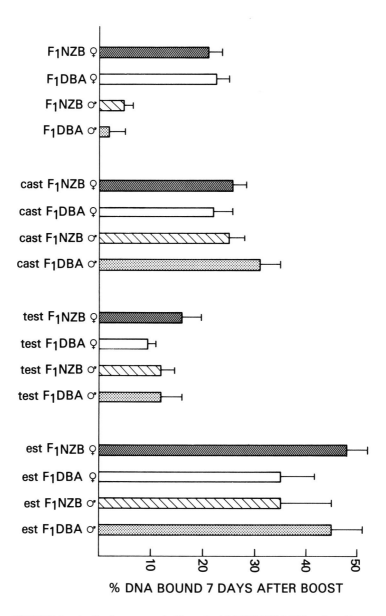

FIGURE 6.   Antibody response in 12-week-old (NZBXDBA/2)F₁ referred to as F₁ NZB and (DBA/2XNZB)F₁ referred to as F₁ DBA, where the first parent in the cross is the mother. Mice were injected on day 0 with 91 μg ssDNA complexed to MBSA in Freund's adjuvant with a boost on day 21 with 91 μg ssDNA complexed to MBSA. The columns represent the mean percent of labeled ssDNA bound by sera measured by a Farr assay. Animals were castrated (cast) at 2 weeks of age and some mice received silastic implants containing either 2.5 mg testosterone (test) or 2.0 mg estradiol (est).

In addition to studying the effects of sex hormones on induced autoantibody production in NZB mice, and their hybrids, spontaneous autoantibody was analyzed. (NZBXDBA/2)F₁ mice produce autoantibodies directed against T cells (NTA). It was found that female F₁ hybrids of NZB and nonautoimmune DBA/2 mice produce much more NTA than do male F₁ littermates (Figure 7). The inhibition of NTA production in the intact F₁ males was eliminated by castration, but not by vasectomy. Furthermore

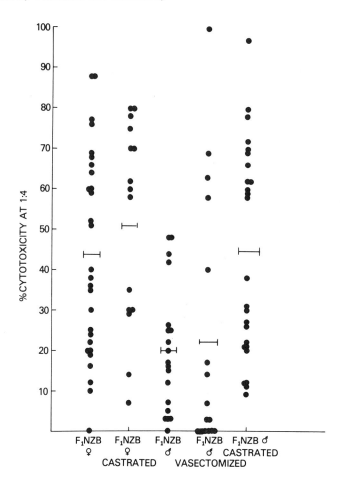

FIGURE 7. Naturally occurring thymocytotoxic autoantibodies
were measured by a cytotoxicity assay involving chromium labeled
target thymocytes. Each dot represents the percent cytotoxicity of sera
from individual year old (NZBXDBA/2)F$_1$ mice. Mice were castrated
or vasectomized at 2 weeks of age.

testosterone administration reduced NTA levels in both female and male mice. Further
study indicated that NZB mice are resistant to the suppressive effects of androgens on
NTA production.[64] Similar to the B/W hybrids, F$_1$ mice of crosses with NZB and
nonautoimmune mice such as the DBA/2 show a marked regulation by sex hormones
of the amount of particular autoantibodies, which is not observed in the autoimmune
NZB parent. The magnitude of autoantibody production may be more sensitive to sex
hormone modulation when all loci involved in the autoantibody production are not
derived from the autoimmune NZB as is the case in the F$_1$ heterozygote. In contrast,
NZB female mice showed a reduction in anti-ssDNA and anti-erythrocyte autoantibodies following androgen treatment.[65] Thus, androgens decrease the production of some
autoantibodies in NZB mice, but have no effect on the levels of other autoantibodies.
Either the pathways or cells involved in the production of the various autoantibodies
are different or regulatory genes that are affected by sex hormones are operative in the
control of some but not all autoantibodies.

We found that many, but not all, of the inherited autoimmune traits of NZB mice
were suppressed by male hormones. Thus, any interpretation of the modes of inherit-

ance operative in autoimmune strains must take into account the lower expression of the trait in males.[62]

NZB and B/W mice have an inability to become tolerant to heterologous serum proteins such as deaggregated bovine γ-globulin (BGG).[66] To test the cellular basis for the NZB tolerance defect, neonatally thymectomized (NZB X DBA/2)F₁ mice were lethally irradiated at 3 months of age and reconstituted with either nonautoimmune DBA/2 or autoimmune NZB T-depleted marrow cells and DBA/2 or NZB thymocytes.[67] The development of tolerance was determined both by the strain of the donor cells and by the sex of the recipient mice. Androgens protected against the tolerance defect imposed by NZB thymocytes and increased the development of tolerance in the presence of normal marrow (Figure 8). These studies further indicate a role of sex hormones in murine autoimmunity.

In addition to studying NZB autoimmune mice, studies have been performed using a congeneic line that is all NZB with the exception of an X-linked immune defect gene (xid), which results in a lack of a subpopulation of B cells.[68] NZB mice with the xid defect have reduced autoantibody production and increased survival.[69] These mice spontaneously produce very little antierythrocyte autoantibodies and thus, have very low Coombs titers. However, stimulation with the polyclonal B cell activator poly rI·rC increased the amount of antierythrocyte autoantibodies for at least 3 months after the cessation of the administration of the polyclonal B cell activator. In contrast, male NZB xid congeneic mice had very low Coombs titers (Figure 9). Thus, female sex hormones prolong the effects of polyclonal B cell activators on cells involved in autoantibody production.[70]

Another murine model of autoimmunity, MRL/1pr has been studied in our laboratory to determine the effects of sex hormones on disease activity. Chronic administration of α-DHT by in vivo silastic implants containing this androgen markedly reduced anti-DNA and proteinuria and prolonged survival (Figure 10).[48] Surprisingly, this did not prevent the massive lymphadenopathy characteristic of this strain. Thus, in MRL/1pr, androgens seem to be selectively depressing those cells involved in autoantibody production.

X. SEX HORMONE MODULATION IN HUMAN LUPUS

The experimental work in murine models of human lupus have suggested that many of the traits of autoimmunity are inherited traits with sex hormones modulating the expression of these autoimmune phenotypes. In addition, these studies have indicated that autoimmunity is a multifactorial disease with independent expression of many traits. Sex hormones have an effect on the expression of only some traits and seem to have a greater effect on levels of expression rather than on the appearance of the trait itself. Hormone modulation of the course of human lupus has also demonstrated that, as in the mouse, differential hormone modulation of the disease is probable.

Danazol has been used to treat human lupus. This attenuated androgen derivative of ethynyltestosterone is an anabolic steroid with mild androgenic side effects.[71] Danazol has been found to be effective in the management of cystic disease of the breast, hereditary angioedema,[72] and hemophilia.[73] The drug binds to sex steroid receptors for androgen and progesterone but not estradiol. At higher concentrations of danazol, estradiol binding can occur. In addition, danazol acts by direct enzymatic inhibition of sex steroid synthesis, but does not seem to alter FSH or LH levels. Danazol has been used to treat several autoimmune diseases. Positive clinical effects were seen in mildly active SLE in a prospective study comparing the drug with placebo. In some instances, thrombocytopenia was dramatically improved and decreased titers of anti-DNA antibodies were observed.[74,75] However, others have reported exacerbations in lupus fol-

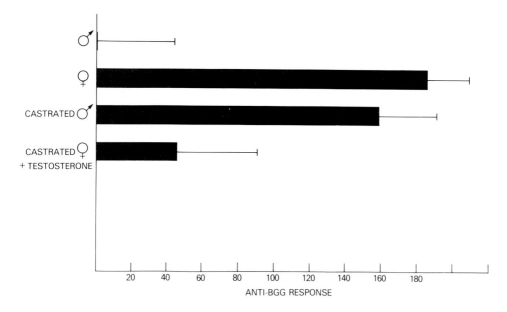

FIGURE 8.   Effect of androgens on the anti-BGG response of neonatally thymectomized (NZBXDBA/2)F₁ mice reconstituted with DBA/2 T-depleted marrow cells and NZB thymus. A solid phase immunoradiometric assay was used to measure anti-BGG antibodies as previously described. Mice were tolerized with 10 mg of deaggregated BGG and challenged 10 days later with 0.5 mg BGG emulsified in Freund's adjuvant and bled 10 days after challenge and assayed for anti-BGG antibodies.

lowing danazol.[76] In addition to the limited effect on the production of autoantibodies against DNA in SLE, danazol has been found to be effective in the treatment of idiopathic thrombocytopenic purpura (ITP).[77] ITP is an autoimmune disorder with a female preponderance in which platelets react with an autoantibody and are destroyed by macrophages. After treatment, circulating anti-platelet antibody titers decreased in most instances.

The variability of the success of danazol modulation of human lupus may reflect differences in the genetic and hormonal component of individual patients. It is possible that in the genetic control of gene expression, those individuals that are heterozygous for a trait may show a greater degree of sex hormone modulation of antibody titer than the homozygous situation. Thus, nonfamilial lupus patients might benefit more from sex hormone therapy. In addition, patients who have been shown to have decreased plasma testosterone levels, increased oxidation of testosterone, or increased hydroxylation of estriol, might also benefit from sex hormone therapy. Thus, not all components of the immunological disorders observed in human autoimmunity are affected by sex hormones, and any possible treatment of human patients must reflect this variability.

XI. SUMMARY

Many experiments indicate that hormones from all the endocrine glands influence lymphatic organs and immunological reactions. A simplified scheme of possible sites of male sex hormone regulation of the immune system is presented in Figure 11. Although both androgens and estrogens exert a profound effect on the immune system, only the effects of androgens are stressed in this figure both for clarity and because the effects of exogenous administration of estradiol are varied. Ovarian and testicular hormones exert a modulating effect on thymic epithelium via specific sex hormone cytoplasmic receptors. This effect secondarily influences the behavior of thymocytes that

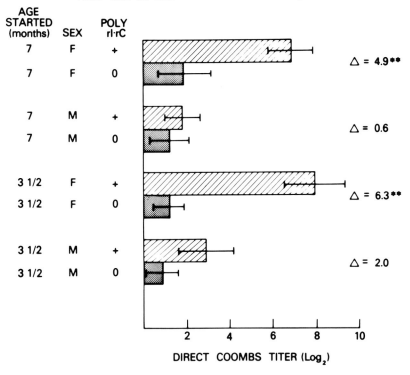

ERYTHROCYTE AUTO ANTIBODIES 3 MONTHS AFTER STOPPING
POLY rI·rC IN NZB *xid/xid* AND NZB *xid*/y MICE

FIGURE 9.   Anti-erythrocyte autoantibodies in female and male NZB mice which possess
the xid defect. NZB xid/xid female and NZB xid/Y congeneic mice were injected daily with
polyrI·rC. One group was injected when the mice were 7 months old and one group when
the mice were $3^1/_2$ months old. The mice were injected for 3 months and then analyzed 3
months later for the presence of anti-erythrocyte autoantibodies by a direct Coombs assay.

in turn regulate the immune response. In addition, other cells involved in the immune
system, such as B lymphocytes or macrophages, may be directly or indirectly affected
by sex hormones. Sex hormones may have a more generalized effect on the immunological system as well by regulating the pathway of differentiation of uncommitted
pluripotent stem cells. Because autoimmunity involves abnormalities of immunoregulation, an understanding of the action of sex hormones on the immune system is vital.

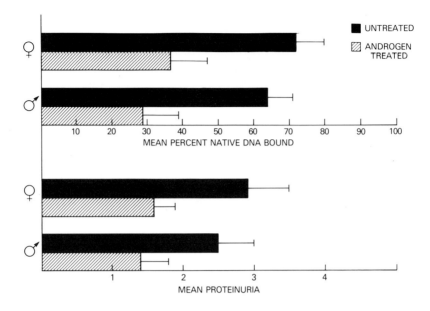

FIGURE 10.   MRL/1pr mice were studied at 4 months of age. Androgen treated mice received silastic implants containing either testosterone or α-dihydrotestosterone at 2 months of age. At least ten mice were studied per group. Antibodies to native DNA were measured by the Farr technique. Results are expressed as mean percent DNA bound ±SEM. Proteinuria was estimated on a 0 to 4 scale by the dip-stick method using tetrabromophenol paper. Bars represent mean proteinuria ±SEM.

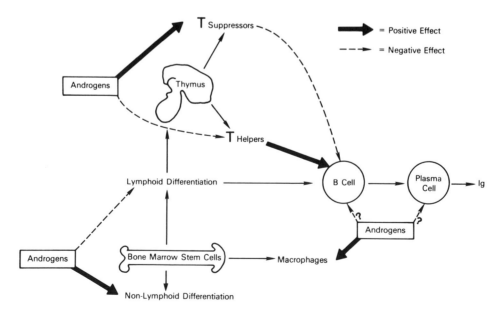

FIGURE 11.   Summary of the effects of androgens on the immune system. Androgens can act at the bone marrow stem cell level and result in decreased lymphoid stem cell differentiation. Androgens can also act at the thymic level and cause an increase in the proportion of suppressor T cells. Androgens may also act to increase macrophage activity and decrease the total amount of immunoglobulin produced.

299

REFERENCES

1. Dubois, E. L., The clinical picture of systemic lupus erythematosus, in *Lupus Erythematosus*, 2nd ed., Dubois, E. L., Ed., University of California Press, Los Angeles, 1974, 232.
2. Osserman, K. E. and Genkins, S. G., Studies in myasthenia gravis: review of twenty years experience in over 1200 patients, *Mt. Sinai J. Med.*, 38, 497, 1971.
3. Kornreich, H., Systemic lupus erythematosus in childhood, *Clin. Rheumatol. Dis.*, 2, 249, 1976.
4. Stern, R., Fishman, J., Brusman, H., and Kunkel, H. G., Systemic lupus erythematosus associated with Klinefelter's syndrome, *Arthritis Rheum.*, 20, 18, 1977.
5. Yocum, M. W., Grossman, J., Waterhouse, C., Abraham, G. N., May, A. G., and Condem, J. J., Monozygotic twins discordant for systemic lupus erythematosus: comparison of immune response, autoantibodies, viral antibody titers, gamma globulin and light chain metabolism, *Arthritis Rheum.*, 18, 193, 1975.
6. Mund, A. and Simson, R. N., Effect of pregnancy on course of SLE, *JAMA*, 183, 917, 1963.
7. Garovich, M., Agudelo, C., and Pisko, E., Oral contraceptives and systemic lupus erythematosus, *Arthritis Rheum.*, 23, 1396, 1980.
8. Rose, E. and Pillsbury, D. M., Lupus erythematosus and ovarian function: observation on possible relationship and report of six cases, *Ann. Intern. Med.*, 21, 1022, 1944.
9. Salomon, Y., Receptors for the glycoprotein hormones: CH, FSH, hCG and TSH, in *Cellular Receptors for Hormones and Neurotransmitters*, Schulster, D. and Levitzki, A., Eds., John Wiley & Sons, New York, 1980, 149.
10. Brown, J. B. and Matthew, G. D., The application of urinary estrogen methods to problems in gynecology, *Recent Prog. Horm. Res.*, 18, 337, 1962.
11. Anderson, J. N., Peck, E. J., and Clark, J. H., Estrogen-induced uterine responses and growth: relationship to receptor estrogen binding by uterine nuclei, *Endocrinology*, 96, 160, 1975.
12. Martucci, C. and Fishman, J., Uterine estrogen receptor binding of catecholstrogens and of estetrol (1,3,5(10)-Estratriene-3,15α,16α,17β-tetrol), *Steroids*, 27, 325, 1976.
13. Lahita, R. G., Kunkel, H. G., and Bradlow, H. L., Increased oxidation of testosterone in systemic lupus erythematosus, *Arthritis Rheum.*, 26, 39, 1983.
14. Jungers, P., Khalil, N., Pellisier, C., Dougados, M., Tron, F., and Bach, J. F., Low plasma androgens in women with active or quiescent SLE, *Arthritis Rheum.*, 25, 454, 1982.
15. Bogovich, F., and Payne, A. H., Purification of rat testicular microsomal 17 ketosteroid reductase, *J. Biol. Chem.*, 255, 5552, 1980.
16. Lahita, R. G., Bradlow, H. L., Kunkel, H. G., and Fishman, J., Alterations of estrogen metabolism in systemic lupus erythematosus, *Arthritis Rheum.*, 22, 1195, 1979.
17. Bucala, R., Fishman, J., and Cerami, A., Formation of covalent adducts between cortisol and 16-α hydroxyestrone and protein: possible role in the pathogenesis of cortisol toxicity and systemic lupus erythematosus, *Proc. Natl. Acad. Sci. U.S.A.*, 79, 3320, 1982.
18. Lipsett, M. B., *Steroid Hormones in Reproductive Endocrinology*, Yen, S. and Jaffe, R. B., Eds., W. B. Saunders, Philadelphia, 1978, 80.
19. Butterworth, M., McClellan, B., and Allansmith, M., Influence of sex on immunoglobulin levels, *Nature (London)*, 214, 1224, 1967.
20. Fujii, H., Nawa, Y., Tsuchiya, H., Matsuno, K., Fukumoto, T., Fukuda, S., and Kotani, M., Effect of a single administration of testosterone on the immune response and lymphoid tissue in mice, *Cell. Immunol.*, 20, 315, 1975.
21. Ahlquist, J., in *Endocrine Influence on Lymphatic Organs, Immune Responses, Inflammation and Autoimmunity*, Acta Endocrinol., Suppl. 206, 3, 1976.
22. Krzych, U., Strausser, H. R., Bressler, J. P., and Goldstein, A. R., Effects of sex hormones on some T and B cell functions as evidenced by differential immune expression between male and female mice and cyclic pattern of immune responsiveness during the estrous cycle, in *Reproductive Immunology*, Ian R. Liss, New York, 1981, 145.
23. Kenny, J. F., Pangburn, P. C., and Trail, G., Effect of estradiol on immune competence: *in vivo* and *in vitro* studies, *Infect. Immunol.*, 13, 448, 1976.
24. Raveche, E. S., Tjio, J. H., Bogel, W., and Steinberg, A. D., Studies of the effects of sex hormones on autosomal and x-linked genetic control of induced and spontaneous antibody production, *Arthritis Rheum.*, 22, 1177, 1979.
25. Roubinian, J., Talal, N., Siiteri, P. K., and Sadakian, J. A., Sex hormone modulation of autoimmunity in NZB/NZW mice, *Arthritis Rheum.*, 22, 1162, 1979.
26. Thompson, J. S., Cranford, M. K., Reilly, R. W., and Severson, C. D., The effect of estrogenic hormones on immune responses in normal and irradiated mice, *J. Immunol.*, 98, 331, 1967.
27. Cohn, D. A., High sensitivity to androgen as a contributing factor in sex differences in the immune response, *Arthritis Rheum.*, 22, 1218, 1979.

28. Grossman, C. J., Nathan, P., Taylor, B. B., and Sholiton, L. J., Rat thymic dihydrotestosterone receptor: preparation, location and physicochemical properties, *Steroids,* 34, 539, 1979.

29. Raveche, E. S., Vigersky, R. A., Rice, M. K., and Steinberg, J. H., Murine thymic androgen receptors, *J. Immunopharmacol.,* 2, 425, 1980.

30. Byron, J. W., Analysis of receptor mechanisms involved in the hemopoietic effects of androgens: use of the Tfm mutant, *Exp. Hematol.,* 5, 429, 1977.

31. Siiteri, P. K., Sex hormone production and action, *Arthritis Rheum.,* 22, 1984, 1979.

32. Reisner, Y., Linker-Israeli, M., and Sharon, N., Separation of mouse thymocytes into two subpopulations by the use of peanut agglutinin, *Cell. Immunol.,* 25, 129, 1976.

33. Rabinovich, H., Umiel, T., Reisner, Y., Sharon, N., and Globerson, A., Characterization of embryonic liver suppressor cells by PNA, *Cell Immunol.,* 47, 347, 1979.

34. Jandinski, J., Cantor, H., Tadakuma, T., Peavy, D. L., and Pierce, C., Separation of helper T cells from suppressor T cells expressing different Ly components. I. Polyclonal activation:suppressor and helper activities are inherent properties of distinct T-cell subclasses, *J. Exp. Med.,* 143, 1382, 1976.

35. Fathman, C. G., Small, M., Herzenberg, L. A., and Weissman, I. L., Thymus cell maturation. II. Differentiation of three "mature" subclasses *in vivo, Cell. Immunol.,* 15, 109, 1975.

36. Novotny, E. A., Raveche, E. S., Sharrow, S., Ottinger, M., and Steinberg, A. D., Analysis of thymocyte subpopulations following treatment with sex hormones, *Clin. Immunol. Immunopathol.,* 28, 205, 1983.

37. Helderman, J. H. and Strom, T. B., Specific insulin binding site on T and B lymphocytes as a marker of cell activation, *Nature (London),* 274, 62, 1978.

38. Eidinger, D. and Garrett, T. J., Studies of the regulatory effects of sex hormones on antibody formation and stem cell differentiation, *J. Exp. Med.,* 136, 1098, 1972.

39. Barr, I. G., Pyke, K. W., Pearce, P., Toh, B., and Funder, J. W., Thymic sensitivity to sex hormones develops post-natally: on *in vivo* and *in vitro* study, *J. Immunol.,* 132, 1095, 1984.

40. Grossman, C. J., Sholiton, L. J., and Roselle, G. A., Estradiol regulation of thymic lymphocyte function in the rat: mediation by serum thymic factors, *J. Steroid Biochem.,* 16, 683, 1982.

41. Pearce, P., Khalid, B. A. K., and Funder, J. W., Androgens and the thymus, *Endocrinology,* 109, 1073, 1981.

42. Stimson, W. H. and Hunter, I. C., Estrogen induced immunoregulation mediated through the thymus, *J. Clin. Lab. Immunol.,* 4, 27, 1980.

43. Barr, I. G., Khalid, B. A. K., Pearce, P., Toh, B.-H., Bartlett, P. F., Scollay, R. G., and Funder, J. W., Dihydrotestosterone and estradiol deplete corticosensitive thymocytes lacking in receptors for these hormones, *J. Immunol.,* 128, 2825, 1982.

44. Weinstein, Y. and Berkovich, Z., Testosterone effect on bone marrow, thymus and suppressor T cells in the (NZBXNZW)F1 mice: its relevance to autoimmunity, *J. Immunol.,* 126, 998, 1981.

45. Roubinian, J. R., Talal, N., Greenspan, J. S., Goodman, J. R., and Siiteri, P. K., Effect of castration and sex hormone treatment on survival, antinucleic acid antibodies and glomerulonephritis in NZB/NZW F mice, *J. Exp. Med.,* 147, 1568, 1978.

46. Gershwin, M. E., Erickson, K., Castles, J. J., Ahmed, A., and Ikeda, R. M., Immunologic characteristics of hereditarily asplenic (Dhl+) New Zealand black and white F₁ mice, *Dev. Comp. Immunol.,* 4, 529, 1980.

47. Gershwin, M. E., Ohsugi, Y., Ahmed, A., Castles, J. J., Scibienski, R., and Ikeda, R. M., Studies of congenitally immunologically mutant New Zealand mice. IV. Development of autoimmunity in congenitally athymic (nude) New Zealand Black X White F₁ hybrid mice, *J. Immunol.,* 125, 1189, 1980.

48. Steinberg, A. D., Roths, J. B., Murphy, E. D., Steinberg, R. T., and Raveche, E. S., Effects of thymectomy or androgen administration upon the autoimmune disease of MRL/1pr mice, *J. Immunol.,* 125, 871, 1980.

49. Eisenberg, R. A., and Dixon, F. J., Effect of castration on male determined acceleration of autoimmune disease in BXSB mice, *J. Immunol.,* 125, 1959, 1980.

50. Eisenberg, R. A., Izui, S., McConahey, P. J., Peters, C. J., Theofilopoulos, A. N., and Dixon, F. J., Male determined accelerated autoimmune disease in BXSB mice: transfer of bone marrow and spleen cells, *J. Immunol.,* 125, 1032, 1980.

51. Walker, S. E., Gray, R. H., Fulton, M., Wigley, R. D., and Schnitzer, B., Palmerston North mice, a new animal model for systemic lupus erythematosus, *J. Lab. Clin. Med.,* 92, 932, 1978.

52. Cooke, A., and Hutchings, P., Sex differences in the regulation of experimentally induced autoantibodies in B/W mice, *Immunology,* 41, 819, 1980.

53. Walker, S. E. and Bole, G. G., Jr., Influence of natural and synthetic estrogens on the course of autoimmune disease in the NZB/NZW mouse, *Arthritis Rheum.,* 16, 231, 1973.

54. Steinberg, A. D., Melez, K. A., Raveche, E. S., Reeves, J. P., Boegel, W. A., Smathers, P. A., Taurog, J. D., Weinlein, L., and Duvic, M., Approach to the study of the role of sex hormones in autoimmunity, *Arthritis Rheum.,* 22, 1170, 1979.

55. Roubinian, J., Talal, N., Greenspan, J. S., Goodman, J. R., and Nussenzweig, V., Danazol's failure to suppress autoimmunity in NZB/NZW F1 mice, *Arthritis Rheum.*, 22, 1399, 1979.

56. Morton, J., Weyant, D. A., Siegel, B. V., and Golding, B., Androgen sensitivity and autoimmune disease, *Immunology*, 44, 661, 1981.

57. Michalski, J., McCombs, C. C., Roubinian, J. R., and Talal, N., Effect of androgen therapy on survival and suppressor activity in aged NZB/NZW F₁ hybrid mice, *Clin. Exp. Immunol.*, 52, 229, 1983.

58. Melez, K. A., Boegel, W. A., and Steinberg, A. D., Therapeutic studies in New Zealand mice. VII. Successful androgen treatment of NZB/NZW F₁ females of different ages, *Arthritis Rheum.*, 23, 41, 1980.

59. Steinberg, A. D., Pincus, T., and Talal, N., DNA-Binding assay for detection of anti-DNA antibodies in NZB/NZW F₁ mice, *J. Immunol.*, 102, 788, 1969.

60. Melez, K. A., Reeves, J. P., and Steinberg, A. D., Regulation of the expression of autoimmunity in NZB X NZW F₁ mice by sex hormones, *J. Immunopharmacol.*, 1, 27, 1978.

61. Shear, H., Roubinian, J. R., Gil, P., and Talal, N., Clearance of sensitized erythrocytes in NZB/NZW mice, effects of castration and sex hormone treatment, *Eur. J. Immunol.*, 11, 776, 1981.

62. Raveche, E. S., Steinberg, A. D., Klassen, L. W., and Tjio, J. H., Genetic studies in NZB mice. I. Spontaneous autoantibody production, *J. Exp. Med.*, 147, 1487, 1978.

63. Raveche, E. S., Tjio, J. H., and Steinberg, A. D., Genetic studies in NZB mice. III. Induced antinucleic acid antibody production, *J. Immunol.*, 122, 1454, 1979.

64. Raveche, E. S., Tjio, J. H., and Steinberg, A. D., Genetic studies in NZB mice. IV. The effect of sex hormones on the spontaneous production of anti-T cell autoantibodies, *Arthritis Rheum.*, 23, 48, 1980.

65. Steinberg, A. D., Smathers, P. A., and Bogel, W. B., Effects of sex hormones on autoantibody production by NZB mice and modification by environmental factors, *Clin. Immunol. Immunopathol.*, 17, 562, 1980.

66. Staples, P. J., Steinberg, A. D., and Talal, N., Induction of immunologic tolerance in older New Zealand mice repopulated with young spleen, bone marrow or thymus, *J. Exp. Med.*, 131, 1223, 1970.

67. Laskin, C. A., Taurog, J. D., Smathers, P. A., and Steinberg, A. D., Studies of defective tolerance in murine lupus, *J. Immunol.*, 127, 1743, 1981.

68. Amsbaugh, D. F., Hansen, C. T., Prescott, B., Stashak, P. W., Barthold, D. R., and Baker, P. J., Genetic control of the antibody response to type III pneumococcal polysaccharide in mice. I. Evidence that an X-linked gene plays a decisive role in determining responsiveness, *J. Exp. Med.*, 136, 931, 1972.

69. Taurog, J. D., Raveche, E. S., Smathers, P. A., Glimcher, L. H., Huston, D. P., Alling, D., and Steinberg, A. D., T cell abnormalities in NZB mice occur independently of autoantibody production, *J. Exp. Med.*, 153, 221, 1981.

70. Smathers, P. A., Steinberg, B. J., Reeves, J. P., and Steinberg, A. D., Effects of polyclonal immune stimulation upon NZB·xid congenic mice, *J. Immunol.*, 128, 1414, 1982.

71. Sherins, R. J., Gandy, H. M., Thorslund, T. W., Paulsen, C. A., Pituitary and testicular function studies. I. Experience with a new gonadal inhibitor 17-α-Pregn-4-en-20-yno-(2,3-d)isoxasol-17-ol (Danazol), *J. Clin. Endocrinol. Metab.*, 32, 522, 1971.

72. Gelfand, J. A., Sherins, R. J., Alling, D. W., and Frank, M. M., Treatment of hereditary angioedema with danazol: reversal of clinical and biochemical abnormalities, *N. Engl. J. Med.*, 295, 1444, 1976.

73. Gralnick, H. R., and Rick, M. E., Danazol increases factor VIII and factor IX in classic hemophilia and Christmas Disease, *N. Engl. J. Med.*, 308, 1393, 1983.

74. Pariser, K., Gell, J., Gelfand, J., Turksay, N., and Agnello, V., Pilot studies in the use of danazol in treatment of patients with systemic lupus erythematosus, *Proc. 15th Int. Congr. Rheumatol.*, (Abstr.), 483, 1981.

75. Morley, K. D., Parke, A., and Hughes, G. R., Systemic lupus erythematosus: two patients treated with danazol, *Br. Med. J.*, 284, 1431, 1982.

76. Fretwell, M. and Altmat, L. C., Exacerbation of lupus erythematosus-like syndrome during treatment of non-Cl-esterase-inhibitor dependent angioedema with danazol, *J. Allergy Clin. Immunol.*, 69, 306, 1982.

77. Ahn, Y. S., Harrington, W., Simon, S., Mylvaganam, R., Pall, L., and So, A., Danazol for the treatment of idiopathic thrombocytopenic purpura, *N. Engl. J. Med.*, 308, 1396, 1983.

Chapter 16

PITUITARY-NEUROHORMONAL IMMUNOREGULATION IN CANCER

Benjamin H. Newberry and Thomas J. Gerstenberger

TABLE OF CONTENTS

I. INTRODUCTION

Pituitary hormones can, both directly and indirectly, alter immune function. Evidence for those relationships is the major topic of this volume and has figured prominently in discussions of psychoneuroimmunology.[1-3] The immune system can influence cancer.[4-6] Our major purpose in this chapter is to present some of the evidence relevant to hypophyseal modulation of neoplastic processes via immune function from the perspective of the empirical requirements for unequivocal demonstration of such effects. We shall also summarize briefly the status of research on psychological responsiveness of cancer, since that question has been considered closely related to pituitary-immune-cancer relationships.[7-10] In keeping with the fact that our interest in this topic stems from an interest in cancer etiology rather than in medical oncology, we shall not discuss hormones as cancer therapeutic agents.

II. RELATIONSHIPS INVOLVING PITUITARY FUNCTION, IMMUNE FUNCTION, AND NEOPLASTIC DISEASE

Relevant effects of pituitary hormones may be direct or indirect. In the direct case, pituitary hormones, themselves influenced by hypothalamic releasing and release-inhibiting factors, would affect some aspect of tumor immunity, most likely through mature effector cells or their precursors. Indirect effects would be those in which other organs or functions stand between pituitary output and the effect on the immune system. In either case, variations in pituitary function could be said to cause variations in neoplastic processes via the immune system.

The most obvious candidates for intermediaries between pituitary hormones and the immune system are the peripheral endocrine organs and their hormones. However, there may be other possibilities as well. One possibility involves loops that include the brain. Hypophyseal hormones influence the brain, as do hypothalamic and peripheral hormones,[11,12] and there is evidence for innervation of immune organs, particularly the thymus.[13-16]

In evaluating the proposition that pituitary function influences cancer through immunomodulation, it is necessary to consider the range of things that might produce covariation between pituitary hormone levels and neoplastic outcomes. Factors other than pituitary effects on immune function might be responsible for such covariation and must be ruled out empirically in order to conclude in favor of a pituitary-immune-cancer causal sequence.

In the first place, it is at least possible for associations between pituitary function and cancer outcomes to occur when there is no causal link, immunologic or otherwise, from pituitary to neoplastic processes. There is, for example, catecholamine involvement in regulation of the immune system[17,18] and reason to suspect more direct catecholamine effects on tumors, given the sensitivity of some tumor cells to cyclic nucleotides.[19,20] Cardiovascular system effects on tumor may also occur.[21,22] One would expect some covariation between such functions and hypophyseal hormones across environmental conditions and perhaps across individual differences, making it possible for pituitary function to covary with neoplastic processes without having produced any effect upon them.

There is a similar problem with exogenous agents having the capability to influence neoplasia. If psychoneural processes that are reflected in pituitary function alter exposure to exogenous agents, or if exogenous agent exposure has independent effects on pituitary output and neoplastic processes, then noncausal associations between pituitary function and neoplasia would appear. Infectious agents,[23-25] even nonobvious drugs,[26,27] and dietary factors[28] present such possibilities.

Yet another possibility is that associations between pituitary function and neoplasia reflect the effects of the disease on the host rather than vice versa. Cancer can exert multiple and strong effects upon hosts.[29] Among the most obvious sources of endocrine alterations in neoplasia are ectopic hormones, which can both mimic and change pituitary function.[30,31]

When variations in pituitary output do produce variations in neoplasia, it is not necessary for them to do so via immunomodulation. Effects on neoplastic processes of pituitary hormones and/or hormones under pituitary influence have long been known.[30-32] A large number of those effects involve tumors of traditional endocrine or endocrine target tissues and the hormones that have the most obvious effects on those tissues. A common effect is for hormones which influence a nonneoplastic tissue to affect the development of tumors derived from that tissue in a similar way.

In a number of cases, it appears possible for endocrine changes to have a tumor-inducing effect — that is, to produce tumors without the known involvement of such usual oncogens as radiation, viruses, or nonendocrine chemical carcinogens. The best studied of such tumors are experimental; they are usually produced by endocrine changes of great magnitude and duration. Examples include tumors of the pituitary, thyroid, testes, ovaries, kidneys,[30] and mammary glands.[30,32,33] Hormones are also capable of modifying the effects of other oncogens[30,34-38] and directly affecting the function of neoplastic cells.[31,39-42] These effects are not limited to the most obvious combinations of hormones and tumor histogenesis.[40,41,43,44]

Evaluating the possibility that pituitary function can affect neoplastic disease via the immune system requires considering another issue, namely immunologic control of cancer. While immune function can affect tumor, it is not clear how general those effects are or whether they operate predominantly in one direction. Many tumors are antigenic.[4-6,45,46] However, several things argue against concluding from this that immunologic control of cancer is a general and strong phenomenon. Tumors are not always effectively immunogenic.[47-49] There are instances in which immune responses protect the tumor rather than the host.[49-52] Immunosuppression does not at present seem to produce a strong, general increase in human susceptibility to cancer, the adequately documented effects being largely confined to the damaged lymphoreticular system itself.[50,53]

Since the pituitary can influence cancer by nonimmunologic means and since immunologic effects on cancer are varied and imperfectly understood, the fact of pituitary influence on the immune system does not by itself imply resulting effects on cancer. Alternative explanations must be eliminated. This is more difficult to do with human than animal cancers because relevant human data must often be correlational and because humans may vary greatly in exposure to relevant exogenous agents.

III. SOME RELEVANT FINDINGS

Endocrine modulation of tumor immunity has not been a major emphasis in work on the hormonal responsiveness of cancers. We are aware of few studies simultaneously involving pituitary-responsive hormones, immune function, and neoplastic processes. The sample of relatively recent studies we describe appears to be representative of the methods that have been used.

Pavelić and Vuk-Pavlović[54] reported inhibition of several types of transplanted tumors by exogenous insulin and/or glucagon. In animals with mammary carcinoma and fibrosarcoma, these hormones increased the number of splenic plaque-forming cells in response to sheep erythrocytes (SRBC) and increased phagocytosis of SRBC. Also increased by these hormones was in vitro cytotoxicity of host lymphocytes against their own fibrosarcoma cells. The authors noted the possibility of direct hormonal effects on tumor cells, but argued that the inconsistency between insulin and glucagon effects in other studies supports an immunologic interpretation of their findings. This report is interesting because it contains an effect on disease development in vivo, a parallel in vitro cytotoxicity effect, and a demonstration of alterations in nontumor immunity as well. From our present perspective, however, it needs to be noted that pituitary effects on pancreatic hormones are not well characterized and may be complex.[55-58]

A report of sex differences in immunity and tumor development implicates the pituitary-gonadal axis.[59] The H-4-II-E hepatoma progressed and disseminated uniformly in male ACI rats, but either failed to take or regressed in females. In females, tumors were infiltrated by lymphocytes and there was considerable inflammation around the tumors. In males, this evidence of immune reaction to tumor was not observed. In addition, labeled lymphocytes injected into tumor-bearing males showed significantly less migration to lymphoid organs than in either tumor-free males or tumor-bearing females. The difference in tumor development was not affected by gonadectomy 2 days prior to tumor inoculation, but that finding does not rule out effects of residual hormones or endocrine effects on the immune system earlier in the animals' development.

Riley and colleagues[60] found that fluocinolone acetonide and dexamethasone enhanced development of 6C3HED lymphosarcoma in C3H/He mice but not in C3H/Bi. The former animals were considered partially histoincompatible with the tumor. The results are difficult to interpret because of the likelihood that the tumor effect was due to histocompatibility antigens rather than tumor-specific antigens and the possibility of substrain differences in factors other than tumor syngeneity.

There have been negative findings. Medroxyprogesterone antagonized 7,12-dimethylbenz(a)anthracene-induced rat mammary tumors, but did not affect splenocyte response to SRBC, concanavalin A, or lipopolysaccharide. Neither did it affect response to L1210 leukemia in mice preimmunized against that tumor.[61] In another study that might be regarded as negative,[62] cortisol enhanced the effects of cyclophosphamide on transplanted sarcomas in mice and reduced the inflammatory response to the tumor. However, neither tumor regrowth nor lifespan were affected by adding cortisol to the cyclophosphamide treatment. The authors suggested that the effect of cortisol resulted from decreased vascular permeability and a consequent reduction of nutrients to tumor cells damaged by cyclophosphamide.

Natural immunity is strongly associated with the study of neoplastic processes.[4,5] The activity of activated macrophages and natural killer (NK) cells is often assessed by tumor cytotoxicity. There is consequently more research on natural than specific immunity that is relevant to our topic. However, since that research is likely to be covered by other contributions to this volume, we will mention only a sample of findings.

Kalland and Forsberg[63] gave the nonsteroid estrogen diethylstilbestrol (DES) to neonatal mice (NMRI and AKR/J) and studied NK activity at 6 to 7 weeks of age. Spleen cells from DES AKR/Js showed reduced activity in vitro against I-522 and YAC-1 lymphoma cells, but not against the NK-resistant I-51 cell line. Corresponding results were obtained in vivo when labeled tumor cells were injected into DES and control mice and when transplanted I-522 and I-51 were allowed to develop. There was some evidence for DES effects on MC-induced sarcoma. DES animals had higher tumor incidence at low MC doses and a lower incidence at high MC doses.

Mathews et al.[64] found that β-endorphin and met-enkephalin enhanced human NK activity against K562 cells by several in vitro measures, including number of tumor-effector cell conjugates, overall NK cytotoxic capacity, and the fraction of NK cells among total mononuclear leukocytes. The enhancement of cytotoxic activity was blocked by naloxone.

Consistent with findings on other aspects of immune function, there is evidence for corticosteroid inhibition of natural immunity. Oehler and Herberman[65] studied the effects of cortisol and polyinosinic-polycytidylic acid (poly I:C) on spleen cell cytotoxicity against cultured W/Fu Gl lymphoma. The cytotoxicity of W/Fu rats given 125 mg/kg cortisol was considerably reduced at 12 hr postcortisol. A second experiment indicated that this suppression had disappeared within 48 hr. The enhancement of cytotoxicity by poly I:C was not impaired by cortisol; the authors suggested that poly I:C acts by activating corticosteroid-resistant NK precursors. Parillo and Fauci[66] found that dexamethasone inhibited the natural cytotoxicity of human blood mononuclear cells whether given in vivo or added to the cytotoxicity cultures. However, their target cells were not tumor cells.

Greenberg et al.[67] have reported hormonal influences on initial host resistance to NK-sensitive SL2-5 lymphoma in DBA/2 mice. Resistance to SL2-5 inocula, presumably mediated by variations in NK activity, was reduced by injections of 1.0 mg cortisol sodium succinate, but enhanced by ACTH. It was also found that the stress of tail shock inhibited host resistance and that resistance was higher in shocked animals given naltrexone.

At least one study implicates pituitary function in the antitumor activity of macrophages.[68] Interferon was given i.p. either alone or with 10 mg/kg cortisol, prednisone, or dexamethasone. Peritoneal macrophages harvested from steroid-treated mice 24 hr later showed reduced cytotoxicity against MBL-2 leukemia cells. Dexamethasone was considerably more potent than the other compounds; it essentially eliminated the effect of interferon activation.

IV. PSYCHOLOGICAL VARIABLES AND NEOPLASTIC PROCESSES

There has been much speculation and data on the possibility that psychological status or psychologically relevant environmental conditions can modulate tumor development by altering endogenous components of host resistance. Discussions of the area are available.[7,8,10,69-72] There have been discussions of using psychotherapy to affect endogenous host resistance,[73-75] though psychotherapy for that purpose is quite premature.[44]

We cannot deal in depth with psychological effects here, but the issue is sufficiently closely related to our topic that some discussion is useful. It seems to be widely believed that immunologic concomitants of psychosocial factors are the major mechanisms of their effects on neoplasia.[9,73-81] Pituitary-adrenocortical activation with consequent immunosuppression and tumor enhancement is frequently suggested. However, there are numerous problems with the empirical support for these ideas. We can only summarize them here and refer the reader to critical discussions[44,70,71,82,83] for more extensive information.

There is little evidence for endogenously mediated psychosocial effects on human cancer. Most research on this question must be correlational, making it difficult to rule out confoundings with exogenous agent exposure, the effects of neoplastic processes on psychosocial variables, and nonneoplastic medical problems. Also, most of the research that has been done has avoidable flaws, including absent control groups, inadequate statistical analyses, and confoundings with patient knowledge of diagnosis, effects of cancer therapy, and researcher expectations.[44,70,71,82] No solid data exist that implicate particular biologic mediators in endogenously mediated psychosocial effects on human cancer.

Research on animal models has shown that psychosocial factors, particularly stress, can influence tumor,[9,44,72,83] but serious questions remain. Stress can both enhance and inhibit tumor development. No generalizations offered have adequately accounted for the pattern of enhancement and inhibition (though in some cases controllability seems able to mitigate the tumor-enhancing effects of stress[81,84] and chronic stress to inhibit tumors enhanced by acute stress[67]). No generalization has been suggested that incorporates the differences among cancers in a useful way.[44] No physiologic mediator has been firmly established, though evidence for immunologic mediation may soon be adequate for some situations. Many studies have been overinterpreted, considering their methodologic inadequacies.

Thus, although there is reason to suspect that endogenously mediated psychosocial effects on cancers can occur, the exploration of these possibilities is in its infancy.

V. DISCUSSION

The data are, as a whole, consistent with the possibility that pituitary function can alter neoplastic processes by means of alterations in tumor immunity. However, we view them as less than conclusive, at least as regards normal variations in pituitary and immune function.

There are three things about the available data that lead us to this reservation. First, in vitro methods, used in many studies,[54,63,64] suffer from the defects of their virtues, namely their inability to deal with the complex interactions that accompany endocrine, immunologic, and neoplastic processes. Hormonal effects on antitumor immunity in vitro do not preclude the occurrence of countervailing effects during normal variations in endocrine activity. For example, while some hormones whose concentrations usually rise under threatening or demanding circumstances are often immunosuppressive, others, such as somatotropin, prolactin, and thyroid hormones,[85] can be immunoenhancing.[86-88]

A second problem is the use of hormonal manipulations that produce, even in vivo, effects unlike those which occur naturally. The temporal patterns of effect of exogenous hormones are unlikely to correspond to naturally occurring patterns. Synthetic hormones,[60,61,63,68] hormones of greater potency than those of the species under study,[62,67,68] or large doses[60,65] may produce effects that could not normally occur. The reduction of resistance to tumor by cortisol under conditions in which ACTH enhances resistance[67] illustrates this problem.

Finally, there is the difficulty of noncausal covariation. Since hormones may influence neoplastic processes in nonimmunologic ways, clear demonstrations of a pituitary-immune-cancer sequence require evidence such as the failure of an endocrine effect when the mediating immunologic processes are blocked. Such steps have rarely been taken, perhaps because simple blockades of immune processes are often not available. Without such confirmation of putative mediating processes, however, causal sequences must remain in doubt.

If evidence for hypophyseal effects on tumor via immunomodulation is incomplete, evidence that psychosocial factors can operate on neoplastic processes via a pituitary-immune sequence is nearly nonexistent. The generality and mechanisms of endogenously mediated psychosocial effects on cancer are still much in doubt. However, as with the more basic question of naturally occurring pituitary-immune-cancer effects, the available evidence suggests that useful generalizations will be discovered.

REFERENCES

1. Ader, R., Ed., *Psychoneuroimmunology,* Academic Press, New York, 1981.
2. Lloyd, R., Mechanisms of psychoneuroimmunological response, in *Impact of Psychoendocrine Systems in Cancer and Immunity,* Fox, B. H. and Newberry, B. H., Eds., C. J. Hogrefe, Toronto, 1983, 1.
3. Solomon, G. F., Amkraut, A. A., and Rubin, R. T., Stress and psychoimmunological response, in *Mind and Cancer Prognosis,* Stoll, B. A., Ed., John Wiley & Sons, New York, 1979, 73.

4. Chirigos, M. A., Mitchell, M., Mastrangelo, M. J., and Krim, M., Eds., *Mediation of Cellular Immunity in Cancer by Immune Modifiers,* Raven Press, New York, 1981.

5. Herberman, R. B. and Ortaldo, J. R., Natural killer cells: their role in defenses against disease, *Science,* 214, 24, 1981.

6. Penn, I., Depressed immunity and the development of cancer, *Clin. Exp. Immunol.,* 46, 459, 1981.

7. Fox, B. H. and Newberry, B. H., Eds., *Impact of Psychoendocrine Systems in Cancer and Immunity,* C. J. Hogrefe, Toronto, 1983.

8. Levy, S. M., Ed., *Biological Mediators of Behavior and Disease: Neoplasia,* Elsevier, Amsterdam, 1982.

9. Riley, V., Psychoneuroendocrine influences on immunocompetence and neoplasia, *Science,* 212, 1100, 1981.

10. Stoll, B. A., Ed., *Mind and Cancer Prognosis,* John Wiley & Sons, New York, 1979.

11. de Wied, D., Bohus, B., Gispen, W. H., Urban, I., and van Wimersma Greidanus, T. B., Hormonal influences on motivational, learning, and memory processes, in *Hormones, Behavior, and Psychopathology,* Sachar, E. J., Ed., Raven Press, New York, 1976, 1.

12. Snyder, S. H., Brain peptides as neurotransmitters, *Science,* 209, 976, 1980.

13. Besedovsky, H. D., Del Ray, A., Sorkin, E., Da Prada, M., and Keller, H. H., Immunoregulation mediated by the sympathetic nervous system, *Cell. Immunol.,* 48, 346, 1979.

14. Bulloch, K., and Moore, R. Y., Innervation of the thymus gland by brain stem and spinal cord in mouse and rat, *Am. J. Anat.,* 162, 157, 1981.

15. Calvo, W., The innervation of the bone marrow in laboratory animals, *Am. J. Anat.,* 123, 315, 1968.

16. Fujiwara, M., Muryobayshi, T., and Shimamoto, K., Histochemical demonstration of monoamines in the thymus of rats, *Jpn. J. Pharmacol.,* 16, 493, 1966.

17. Singh, U., Millson, D. S., Smith, P. A., and Owen, J. J. T., Identification of β-adrenoreceptors during thymocyte ontogeny in mice, *Eur. J. Immunol.,* 9, 31, 1979.

18. Strom, T. B., Lundin, A. P., and Carpenter, C. B., The role of cyclic nucleotides in lymphocyte activation and function, *Prog. Clin. Immunol.,* 3, 115, 1977.

19. Prasad, K., Involvement of cyclic nucleotides in transformation, in *The Transformed Cell,* Cameron, I. L. and Pool, T. B., Eds., Academic Press, New York, 1981, 236.

20. Keller, R. and Keist, R., Suppression of growth of P-815 mastocytoma cells *in vitro* by drugs increasing cellular cyclic 3′,5′-adenosine monophosphate, *Life Sci.,* 12(Part II), 97, 1973.

21. Auerbach, R. and Auerbach, W., Regional differences in the growth of normal and neoplastic cells, *Science,* 215, 127, 1982.

22. Donati, M. B., Poggi, A., Mussoni, L., de Gaetano, G., and Garattini, S., Hemostasis and experimental cancer dissemination, in *Cancer Invasion and Metastasis: Biologic Mechanisms and Therapy,* Day, S. B., Myers, W. P. L., Stansly, P., Garattini, S., and Lewis, M. G., Eds., Raven Press, New York, 1977.

23. Bull, J. M. C., Whole body hyperthermia as an anticancer agent, *CA,* 32, 123, 1982.

24. Cannon, J. G. and Kluger, M. J., Endogenous pyrogen activity in human plasma after exercise, *Science,* 220, 617, 1983.

25. Farber, E., Chemical carcinogenesis, *N. Engl. J. Med.,* 305, 1379, 1981.

26. Cimetidine for malignant melanoma, *Med. Sci. Bull.,* 5(9), 1, 1983.

27. Nomura, T., Comparative inhibiting effects of methylxanthines on urethan-induced tumors, malformations, and presumed somatic mutations in mice, *Cancer Res.,* 43, 1342, 1983.

28. Committee on Diet, Nutrition, and Cancer, *Diet, Nutrition, and Cancer,* National Academy Press, Washington, D.C., 1982.

29. Shapot, V. S., On the multiform relationships between the tumor and the host, in *Advances in Cancer Research,* Vol. 30, Klein, G. and Weinhouse, S., Eds., Academic Press, New York, 1979, 89.

30. Furth, J., Hormones as etiological agents in neoplasia, in *Cancer: A Comprehensive Treatise,* Vol. 1, Becker, F. F., Ed., Plenum Press, New York, 1975, 75.

31. Lippman, M., Interactions of psychic and endocrine factors with progression of neoplastic disease, in *Biological Mediators of Behavior and Disease: Neoplasia,* Levy, S. M., Ed., Elsevier, Amsterdam, 1982, 55.

32. Wissler, R. W., Dao, T. L., and Wood, S., Jr., Eds., *Endogenous Factors Influencing Host-Tumor Balance,* University of Chicago Press, Chicago, Ill., 1967.

33. Stone, J. R., Holtzman, S., and Shellabarger, C. J., Neoplastic response and correlated prolactin levels in diethylstilbestrol-treated ACI and Sprague-Dawley rats, *Cancer Res.,* 39, 773, 1979.

34. Bengtsson, M. and Rydström, J., Regulation of carcinogen metabolism in the rat ovary by the estrus cycle and gonadotropin, *Science,* 219, 1437, 1983.

35. Ciocca, D. R., Parente, A., and Russo, J., Endocrinologic milieu and susceptibility of the rat mammary gland to carcinogenesis, *Am. J. Pathol.,* 109, 47, 1982.

36. Gupta, P. and Rapp, F., Effect of hormones on herpes simplex virus type-2-induced transformation, *Nature (London),* 267, 254, 1977.

37. Liebelt, A. G. and Liebelt, R. A., Chemical factors in mammary tumorigenesis, in *Carcinogenesis: A Broad Critique,* M. D. Anderson Hospital and Tumor Institute, Williams & Wilkins, Baltimore, 1967, 315.

38. Parks, W. P., Scolnick, E. M., and Kozikowski, E. H., Dexamethasone stimulation of murine mammary tumor virus replication: a tissue culture source of virus, *Science,* 184, 158, 1974.

39. Claman, H. N., Corticosteroids and lymphoid cells, *N. Engl. J. Med.,* 287, 388, 1972.

40. Monaco, M. E., Kidwell, W. R., Kohn, P. H., Strobl, J. S., and Lippman, M. E., Neurohypophyseal hormones and cancer, in *Hormones and Cancer,* Iacobelli, S., King, R. J. B., Lindner, H. R., and Lippman, M. E., Eds., Raven Press, New York, 1980, 165.

41. Sato, G. H., Towards an endocrine physiology of human cancer, in *Hormones and Cancer,* Iacobelli, S., King, R. J. B., Lindner, H. R., and Lippman, M. E., Eds., Raven Press, New York, 1980, 283.

42. Yates, J., Couchman, J. R., and King, R. J. B., Androgen effects on growth, morphology, and sensitivity of S115 mouse mammary tumor cells in culture, in *Hormones and Cancer,* Iacobelli, S., King, R. J. B., Lindner, H. R., and Lippman, M. E., Eds., Raven Press, New York, 1980, 31.

43. Kirschbaum, A., Liebelt, A. G., and Falls, N. G., Influence of gonadectomy and androgenic hormone on the induction of leukemia by methylcholanthrene in DBA/2 mice, *Cancer Res.,* 15, 685, 1955.

44. Newberry, B. H., Liebelt, A. G., and Boyle, D. A., Variables in behavioral oncology: overview and assessment of current issues, in *Impact of Psychoendocrine Systems in Cancer and Immunity,* Fox, B. H. and Newberry, B. H., Eds., C. J. Hogrefe, Toronto, 1983, 86.

45. Baldwin, R. W. and Price, M. R., Neoantigen expression in chemical carcinogenesis, in *Cancer: A Comprehensive Treatise,* Vol. 3, Becker, F. F., Ed., Plenum Press, New York, 1975, 353.

46. Levine, A. J., Transformation-associated tumor antigens, in *Advances in Cancer Research,* Vol. 37, Klein, G. and Weinhouse, S., Eds., Academic Press, New York, 1982, 75.

47. Fidler, I. J. and Kripke, M. L., Tumor cell antigenicity, host immunity, and cancer metastasis, *Cancer Immunol. Immunother.,* 7, 201, 1980.

48. Old, L. J., Cancer immunology: the search for specificity, in *Research Frontiers in Aging and Cancer,* NIH Publ. No. 82-2436, U.S. Government Printing Office, Washington, D.C., 1982, 193.

49. Prehn, R. T., Tumor progression and homeostasis, in *Advances in Cancer Research,* Vol. 23, Klein, G. and Weinhouse, S., Eds., Academic Press, New York, 1976, 203.

50. Melief, C. J. M. and Schwartz, R. S., Immunocompetence and malignancy, in *Cancer: A Comprehensive Treatise,* Becker, F. F., Ed., New York, Plenum Press, 1975, 121.

51. Black, P. H., Shedding from the cell surface of normal and cancer cells, in *Advances in Cancer Research,* Vol. 32, Klein, G. and Weinhouse, S., Eds., Academic Press, New York, 1980, 75.

52. Lewis, M. G., Phillips, T. M., Rowden, G., and Jerry, L. M., Humoral immune factors in metastasis in human cancer, in *Cancer Invasion and Metastasis: Biologic Mechanisms and Therapy,* Day, S. B., Myers, W. P. L., Stansly, P., Garattini, S., and Lewis, M. G., Eds., Raven Press, New York, 1977, 245.

53. Keast, D., Immune surveillance and cancer, in *Stress and Cancer,* Bammer, K. and Newberry, B. H., Eds., C. J., Hogrefe, Toronto, 1981, 71.

54. Pavelić, K. and Vuk-Pavlović, S., Retarded growth of murine tumors in vivo by insulin- and glucagon-stimulated immunity and phagocytosis, *J. Natl. Cancer Inst.,* 66, 889, 1981.

55. Barseghian, G., Levine, R., and Epps, P., Direct effect of cortisol and cortisone on insulin and glucagon secretion, *Endocrinology,* 111, 1648, 1982.

56. Dolva, L. Ø., Hanssen, K. F., Flaten, O., Hanssen, L. E., and von Schenck, H., The effect of thyrotrophin-releasing hormone (TRH) on pancreatic hormone secretion in normal subjects, *Acta Endocrinol.,* 102, 224, 1983.

57. Marco, J., Calle, C., Román, D., Diaz-Ferros, M., Villanueva, M. L., and Valverde, I., Hyperglucagonism induced by glucocorticoid treatment in man, *N. Engl. J. Med.,* 288, 128, 1973.

58. Wise, J. K., Hendler, R., and Felig, P., Influence of glucocorticoids on glucagon secretion and plasma amino acid concentrations in man, *J. Clin. Invest.,* 52, 2774, 1973.

59. Herman, P. G., de Sousa, M., Schroeder, S., Godleski, J., Lapray, J.-F., Drummey, J., and Lazarus, H., Sex-related differences in tumor progression associated with altered lymphocyte circulation, *Cancer Res.,* 41, 2255, 1981.

60. Riley, V., Fitzmaurice, M. A., and Spackman, D. H., Psychoneuroimmunologic factors in neoplasia: studies in animals, in *Psychoneuroimmunology,* Ader, R., Ed., Academic Press, New York, 1981, 31.

61. Spreafico, F., Filippeschi, S., Malfiore, C., Noseda, S., Falautano, P., and Serraglia, N., Effect of medroxyprogesterone acetate on DMBA-induced rat mammary carcinoma and on immunological reactivity, *Eur. J. Cancer Clin. Oncol.,* 18, 45, 1982.

62. Evans, R. and Eiden, D. M., Concomitant inhibition of tumor-associated inflammatory responses and rapid enhancement of cyclophosphamide-induced tumor regression by hydrocortisone, *Cancer Res.,* 42, 4437, 1982.

63. Kalland, T. and Forsberg, J.-G., Natural killer cell activity and tumor susceptibility in female mice treated neonatally with diethylstilbestrol, *Cancer Res.,* 41, 5134, 1981.

64. Mathews, P. M., Froelich, C. J., Sibbit, W. L., Jr., and Bankhurst, A. D., Enhancement of natural cytotoxicity by β-endorphin, *J. Immunol.,* 130, 1658, 1983.

65. Oehler, J. R. and Herberman, R. B., Natural cell-mediated cytotoxicity in rats. III. Effects of immunopharmacologic treatments on natural reactivity and on reactivity augmented by polyinosinic-polycytidylic acid, *Int. J. Cancer,* 21, 221, 1978.

66. Parillo, J. E. and Fauci, A. S., Comparison of the effector cells in human spontaneous cellular cytotoxicity and antibody-dependent cellular cytotoxicity: differential sensitivity of effector cells to in vivo and in vitro corticosteroids, *Scand. J. Immunol.,* 8, 99, 1978.

67. Greenberg, A. H., Dyck, D. G., and Sandler, L. S., Opponent processes, neurohormones and natural resistance, in *Impact of Psychoendocrine Systems in Cancer and Immunity,* Fox, B. H. and Newberry, B. H., Eds., C. J. Hogrefe, Toronto, 1983, 225.

68. Pavlidis, N. and Chirigos, M., Stress-induced impairment of macrophage tumoricidal function, *Psychosom. Med.,* 42, 47, 1980.

69. Bammer, K. and Newberry, B. H., Eds., *Stress and Cancer,* C. J. Hogrefe, Toronto, 1981.

70. Bieliauskas, L. A. and Garron, D. C., Psychological depression and cancer, *Gen. Hosp. Psychiatr.,* 4, 187, 1982.

71. Fox, B. H., Premorbid psychological factors as related to cancer incidence, *J. Behav. Med.,* 1, 45, 1978.

72. Sklar, L. S. and Anisman, H., Stress and cancer, *Psychol. Bull.,* 89, 369, 1981.

73. Achterberg, J., Matthews-Simonton, S., and Simonton, O. C., Psychology of the exceptional cancer patient: a description of patients who outlive predicted life expectancies, *Psychother. Res. Pract.,* 14, 416, 1977.

74. Cunningham, A. J., Should we investigate psychotherapy for physical disease, especially cancer?, in *Biological Mediators of Behavior and Disease: Neoplasia,* Elsevier, Amsterdam, 1982, 83.

75. Simonton, O. C. and Simonton, S. S., Belief systems and management of the emotional aspects of malignancy, *J. Transpers. Psychol.,* 7, 29, 1975.

76. Borysenko, J. Z., Behavioral-physiological factors in the development and management of cancer, *Gen. Hosp. Psychiatr.,* 4, 69, 1982.

77. Laudenslager, M. L., Ryan, S. M., Drugan, R. C., Hyson, R. L., and Maier, S. F., Coping and immunosuppression: inescapable but not escapable shock suppresses lymphocyte proliferation, *Science,* 221, 568, 1983.

78. Lewis, M. G. and Phillips, T. M., The possible effects of emotional stress on cancer mediated through the immune system, in *Cancer, Stress, and Death,* Tache, J., Selye, H., and Day, S. B., Eds., Plenum Press, New York, 1979, 21.

79. Locke, S. E., Stress, adaptation, and immunity: studies in humans, *Gen. Hosp. Psychiatr.,* 4, 49, 1982.

80. Rosch, P. J., Stress and cancer: a disease of adaptation?, in *Cancer, Stress, and Death,* Plenum Press, New York, 1979, 187.

81. Visintainer, M. S., Volpicelli, J. R., and Seligman, M. E. P., Tumor rejection in rats after inescapable or escapable shock, *Science,* 216, 437, 1982.

82. Morrison, F. R. and Paffenbarger, R. A., Jr., Epidemiological aspects of biobehavior in the etiology of cancer: a critical review, in *Perspectives on Behavioral Medicine,* Weiss, S. M., Herd, J. A., and Fox, B. H., Eds., Academic Press, New York, 1981, 135.

83. Peters, L. J. and Mason, K. A., Influence of stress on experimental cancer, in *Mind and Cancer Prognosis,* Stoll, B. A., Ed., John Wiley & Sons, New York, 1979, 103.

84. Sklar, L. S. and Anisman, H., Stress and coping factors influence tumor growth, *Science,* 205, 513, 1979.

85. Curtis, G. C., Psychoendocrine stress response: steroid and peptide hormones, in *Mind and Cancer Prognosis,* Stoll, B. A., Ed., John Wiley & Sons, New York, 1979, 61.

86. Ahlqvist, J., Hormonal influences on immunologic and related phenomena, in *Psychoneuroimmunology,* Ader, R., Ed., Academic Press, New York, 1981, 355.

87. Berczi, I., Nagy, E., Kovacs, K., and Horvath, E., Regulation of humoral immunity in rats by pituitary hormones, *Acta Endocrinol.,* 98, 506, 1981.

88. Monjan, A. A., Stress and immunologic competence: studies in animals, in *Psychoneuroimmunology,* Ader, R., Ed., Academic Press, New York, 1981, 185.

INDEX

A

A, see Adrenaline
ABO blood group, 188
Accessory cells, 70, 79, 92, 230
Acetylcholine, 95, 101, 107, 110, 231—232
Acid phosphatase, 80
Acne, 31
Acquired hemolytic anemia, 52
Acral enlargement of head, 30
Acromegaly, 29—30, 45, 134, 143, 169
    insulin receptors, 146
ACTH, 29—31, 35, 111
    antitumor NK activity and, 307
    asthma, 69
    blood levels following GIF, increased, 244
    catecholamine synthesis, 100
    contact sensitivity reactions, 138, 167—168
    effects on man, 45
    glucocorticoid secretion, 228
    growth hormone inhibition by, 140
    human chorionic gonadotropin, 186
    humoral immune response, 136
    immune blockage, prevention of, 187
    immune system and, 274
    immunofluorescence with antibody to, 112
    immunosuppressive effect, 234
    release of, 236, 274
    reserve, 112
    rheumatoid arthritis, 52
    role, 228
    stress, 234
    thymosin fraction 5, 112
    treatment with, 50—53
    tuberculin hypersensitivity, 93
ACTH-adrenal axis, 110—111, 228—232, 234—235
ACTH-adrenocortical axis, 104—105, 110—113
ACTH-corticosteroid axis, 231
ACTH-secreting cells, 112
Activated macrophages, 306
Activating factors, 16
Active hepatitis, 277
Acute allergic alveolitis, 93
Acute infectious mononucleosis, 70
Acute inflammation, 9
Acute onset insulin dependent diabetes mellitus, 149
Acute phase proteins, 22
ADCC, see Antibody dependent cellular cytotoxicity
Addison's disease, 31, 58
Adenocarcinoma allografts, 95
Adenohypophyseal cells, 30, 167
Adenohypophysis, 28
Adenohypophysis hormones, 30
Adenoids, 12
Adenosine cyclase, 102
Adenosine diphosphate (ADP), 9, 88
Adenosine triphosphate (ATP), 9

Adenylate cyclase, 87, 100, 102, 104, 105, 144, 224
Adenyl cyclase, 36
ADH, see Antidiuretic hormone
Adherent cells, 76, 107, 230
Adipose tissue, 284
Adjuvant, 96
Adjuvant arthritis, 44, 111, 140—141, 167, 175—178, 216
    contact sensitivity to DNCB, 52
    follicle stimulating hormone, 187
    human chorionic gonadotropin, 186
    luteinizing hormone, 187
ADP, see Adenosine diphosphate
Adrenal adenoma, 58
Adrenal cortex, 162
Adrenal cortical hormones, 243
Adrenal corticosteroids, 45, 55, 307
Adrenalectomy, 110, 243
    acid protease, 62
    ACTH, 51
    circadian rhythm, 63
    corticosterone, 110
    eosinophilia, 104, 108
    glucocorticoid receptors, 56
    Hypox animals, 194
    immunocytes and immune responses and, 54—55
    mice, 232
    plasma corticosterone levels, 79
    rabbits, 112
    thymic lymphocytes, 193
    thymocytes, 61
    thymus regeneration, 228
Adrenalectomy and gonadectomy combined, 190—191
Adrenal glands, 59, 110, 194, 246, 284
Adrenal hormones, see also specific topics, 54—95
    adrenalectomy, 54—55
    glucocorticoids, 55—95
Adrenal hypertrophy, 110
Adrenalin, 100, 108—109, 234
Adrenal insufficiency, 66
Adrenal medulla, catecholamine synthesis, 100
Adrenal weight, 193
Adrenal zona fasciculata atrophy, 31
β-Adrenergic agents, 103
Adrenergic agonists, 101
α-Adrenergic agonists, 106
β-Adrenergic agonists, 106
α-Adrenergic antagonists, 106
β-Adrenergic antagonists, 102
α-Adrenergic blocking agents, 103
β-Adrenergic blocking agents, 103—104
β-Adrenergic drugs, 103
Adrenergic receptor, 214
α-Adrenergic receptor, 100, 102, 215
β-Adrenergic receptor, 87, 90, 100—101, 105, 215, 231

C

E receptor, 5, 53
E rosette, 4, 53, 57, 63, 65—66, 105, 107, 149,
    196
Erythrocyte-antibody-complement-rosette forming B
    cells, 149
Erythrocyte precursors, Ia antigens, 18
Erythrocytes, see Red blood cells
Erythroid cell, 222
Erythropoiesis, 135, 197, 199
Erythropoietin, 3, 60
Erythropoietin stimulating factor (ESF), 135
Escherichia coli, 113, 150, 163, 278—279
ESF, see Erythropoietin stimulating factor
ESP, see Eosinophil stimulation promoter
Essential amino acids, 21
Estradiol, 164, 187—188, 200, 278—279, 284—
    285, 288
    antibody response, 196
    binding reaction, 86
    DNA synthesis, 137, 192
    fetal thymus, 195—196
    glucocorticoid binding, 59
    IgA in uterus, 200
    IgG in uterus, 200
    immune reactions enhanced by, 233
    mitogenic response, 196
    mixed lymphocyte reactions, 192
    oral contraceptives, 202
    ovariectomy, 192, 194
    peripheral blood lymphocytes, 196
    PHA response, 196
    receptors, 187
    secretory component, 199
    suppressor cells, 200
    thymectomy, 193
    thymic sensitivity, 191
    thymocytes, effect on, 289
    uterine secretion of Ig, 193
β-Estradiol, 291
17-β-Estradiol, 289
Estradiol benzoate, 202
β-Estradiol-3-benzoate, 279
Estriol, 86, 194, 196, 284—285
Estriol-receptor complexes, 286
Estrogenic phase, 201
Estrogen/progestogen contraceptives, 201
Estrogens, 76, 164, 263, 265, 279, 284, 286
    antibody response, 94, 287
    antitumor NK activity, 306
    castration, 189
    diestrus, 191
    estrous, 191
    immune reactions enhanced by, 233
    immune system, effect on, 191—197, 296
    implants in castration, 292—293
    influence on immunity to infectious agents, 278—
        279
    inhibitors, 291
    Kurloff cells, 196
    mast cell degranulation, 197
    metabolism, 189, 285

    metestrus, 191
    postmenopausal women, 197
    proestrus, 191
    prolactin receptors, 194
    receptors, 187, 191, 195, 233, 285
    sex differences, 188—189
    sex hormone secretion, 203
    skin graft survival, 192
    synthetic, 201
    thymic atrophy, 186
    thymus size, 289
    thyroiditis, 194
    tumor immunity and, 306
Estrone, 191, 279, 284—286
Estrous, 191, 196
Estrous cycle, 191, 278, 286
Estrus, 193, 278
Ethynyl estradiol, 279
Ethynyltestosterone, 295
Eticholanolone, 286
Euthyroidism, 217
Exocytosis, 107
Exogenous agents, 304
Experimental allergic encephalitis, 52
Experimental allergic encephalomyelitis, 55, 110,
    190
Experimental allergic thyroiditis, 223
Extinction, 254
Eye complaints, 31

F

Fab fragment, 11
F(ab')₂ fragments, 11
Factor VIII related antigen, 88
Fat cell, 217
Fatigue, 31
Fc fragment, 11
Fc portions, 12
Fc receptor, 2, 4—10, 12, 19, 69, 112, 147, 163,
    217, 231, 266—267
Fc receptor augmenting factor (FRAF), 72, 74
FcR-IgG interactions, 90
Fd fragment, 11
Feedback control mechanisms, 288
Feedback mechanisms, 252
Feedback regulatory signals, 110
Feedback signals, 42, 236
Feedforward regulation, 251—259
Female, 188—189
    genital tract, 236
    sex hormones, 146
Fenoterol, 105, 109
Fertility, 267
α-Fetoprotein, 21
Fever, 51, 222, 274, 276
Fibrinolysis, 146
Fibroblast growth factor, 9
Fibroblasts, 9, 92
Fibrosarcoma, 305

H

H, see Heavy chain
H_1-histamine receptors, 111
H-2 antagonists, 102
H-2 gene complex, 58
H-2^d antigens, 101
H-2^k antigens, 101
Haemonchus contortus, 276
Haloperidol, 104, 187
Hamsters, 55, 223, 279
Haptens, 16
Hashimoto's disease, 217
Hashimoto's thyroiditis, 150
HCG, see Human chorionic gonadotropin
Headache, 32
Heat intolerance, 31
Heavy (H) chain, 11—14
Helper cells, 19, 62
Helper/inducer cells, 70
Helper/inducer subpopulation, 109
Helper/suppressor cell ratio, 149
Helper T cells, 2, 4, 19, 21, 61, 74, 91—92, 145,
    148, 150, 230
  cortisol, 68
  FC receptor, 5
  glucocorticoids, effect of, 70
  interleukin 2, 71
  Lyt 1$^+$2$^-$, 287
  target of GRMF, 79
  thyroid hormones, 215
Helper T lymphocytes, see Helper T cells
Hematological disease, 88
Hematopoietic cell, 22
Hemobartonella muris, 166
Hemoglobin iron, 79
Hemolysin formation, 200
Hemolytic anemia, 290
Hemophilia, 295
Hemopoiesis, 59—60
Hemopoietic system, 59
Heparin, 8, 61—62, 91, 230
Hepatic gluconeogenic enzyme, 79
Hepatic phagocytosis, 192
Hepatitis, 149, 275
Hepatitis-B virus, 277—278
Hepatoma, 306
Hereditary angioedema, 295
Hexoestrol, 279
Hexose monophosphate, 107
HGH, see Human growth hormone
Hibernating gland, 223
Hibernating ground squirrel, 223
High endothelial venules, 10, 65
Hirsutism, 31
Histamine, 8, 70, 93, 95, 109, 144
  biological effect, 236
  release, 84, 86, 89, 101, 106, 110, 111, 224
  thymocyte maturation, 175
  thymus cells, 102

Histamine H_1-receptor agonist, 111
Histamine H_2-receptor agonist, 111
Histiocyte formation, 6
Histocompatibility, 18, 306
Histocompatibility antigens, 17—19, 188
Histoplasmin, 94
HLA-B7, 70
HLA-B12, 70
Hoarse voice, 31
Homeostasis, 28
Homeostatic mechanisms, 242, 247
Homocytotropic antibody, 14
Hooved animals, 163
Hormonal immunoregulation, see Immunoregulation
Hormonal manipulations, 308
Hormone receptors, 34—35
Hormones, see also specific types, 34—37
Host defense, 22
Host resistance, 8, 275—280
HPL, see Human placental lactogen
Human, see also Man
  autoimmune diseases, susceptibility to, 284
  B cells, 101, 145
  females, susceptibility to autoimmune diseases,
      284
  lung, 110
  lupus, 295—296
  monocytes, 59
  mononuclear phagocytes, 222
  peripheral blood lymphocytes, 101, 216, 224,
      244
  placenta, 263
  platelets, 102
  T cells, 101
Human calcitonin, 222
Human chorionic gonadotropin (HCG), 186, 263
Human eosinophils, 231
Human growth hormone (HGH), 143
Human histocompatibility antigen, see HLA
Human leukemia IM-9 cell line, 144
Human leukocytes, 57
Human lymphoblastic cell lines, 222
Human lymphocytes, 134, 150, 228
Human placental lactogen (HPL), 167, 176, 179
Humoral immune response, 199, 230
  alloxan, 147
  corticosterone, 111
  spleen, 42
  testosterone, 199
  thymus, 42
Humoral immunity, see also Immunoglobulins, 2,
      11—16, 99, 137, 144, 192, 228, 276
Humoral immunodeficiency, 149
Hydatidiform mole, 32
20β-Hydrocortisol, 88
Hydrocortisone, 51, 58, 275
  B lymphocytes, 77
  chemotaxis, 87
  concanavalin A, 62
  cytolytic effect in vitro, 63
  cytotoxic T lymphocyte precursors, 61

331

properties, 4
recirculation, 63—67, 231
Leukocytic pyrogen, 222
Levan, 6
Levodopa, 143
Lewis blood group, 188
Leydig cells, 202—203
LH, see Luteinizing hormone
LH-RH, see Luteinizing hormone releasing hormone
Libido, 32
LiCl, taste aversion, 253
Light (L) chain, 11—14
Lipolysis, 30
Lipopolysaccharide (LPS), see also Bacterial lipopo-
    lysaccharide; Mitogens, 6, 15, 17, 78, 90,
    146, 224, 274—275
  blastogenic responsiveness to, 191
  chemotaxis, 88
  cortisol acetate, 68, 75
  dexamethasone, 88, 91
  diethylstilbestrol, 193
  DNA synthesis, 62
  elastase, 87
  interleukin 1 stimulation, 71
  lactogenic receptors, 162
  lymphocytes, 103
  ovariectomy, 192
  splenocyte response to, 306
  steroidogenesis, 113
Lipoprotein lipase, 36
Lipoproteins, 17, 21, 79
β-Lipotrophin, 29—31, 53
Liver, 76
  cytoplasmic receptor, 58
  erythropoietic cells, 59
  granulomas, 224
  immune complexes, 166
  prolactin receptors, 162
Lizards, 162, 274
Local immune suppression, gestational hormones,
    264—265
Lorain-Levi's syndrome, 30
β-LPH, see β-Lipotrophin
LPS, see Bacterial lipopolysaccharide;
    Lipopolysaccharide
Lung lesions, 9, 76
Lupus erythematosus, 84
Luteinizing hormones (LH), 29—32, 35, 187, 263,
    284
  catecholamines, 100
  Hypox animals, 194
  ovine, 187
  release of, 236
  sex hormone secretion, 202
Luteinizing hormone releasing factor (LHRH), 33—
    35, 236, 284
Luteotropic factors, 203
Luteotropic hormone, 43
Luteotropin (LH), see Luteinizing hormone
Ly-1 antigens, 101

Ly-2 antigens, 101
Ly-3 antigens, 101
Ly-4 antigens, 101
Ly-5 antigens, 101
Ly-7 antigen, 101
Lymphadenopathy, 290
Lymphatic hyperplasia, 45, 134
Lymphatic tissue involution, 55
Lymph node cells, 166
Lymph nodes, 3, 10, 223
  adrenalectomy, 54
  anaphylactoid inflammation promoting factor, 146
  B lymphocytes, 6, 229
  cortisol, 86
  dendritic cells, 6—7
  dexamethasone, 75
  enlargement, 290
  estrous cycle, 191
  glucocorticoid receptors, 56
  glucocorticoids, 67
  growth hormone, 134—136
  growth hormone receptors, 135
  hydrocortisone acetate, 59—60
  immunosuppressive effect of ACTH, 234
  insulin dependent diabetes, 148
  lactogenic receptors, 162
  mast cells, 8
  mesenteric, 174
  orchidectomy, 190
  oxazolone, 92
  pituitary dwarfism, 42
  plaque forming cells, 88
  popliteal, 255—256
  prednisolone, 65
  pregnancy, 165
  T lymphocytes, 4
Lymphocyte β-adrenergic receptor defect, 106
Lymphocytes, see also B lymphocytes; T lympho-
    cytes, 3—6, 10, 15, 265—266
  adenylate cyclase, 224
  anaphylactoid inflammation promoting factor, 146
  androstenedione, 200
  antigen specific activation of, 234
  blood, 64, 69
  bone marrow, 165
  catecholamine receptors, 103, 231
  circulating, 64, 192
  cytotoxic, see Killer cells
  cytotoxicity against fibrosarcoma, 305
  DNA synthesis, 222
  effector, 4
  epinephrine, 104
  Fc receptor bearing, 66
  fetal, 144
  genetically diabetic animals, 148
  human, 224, 244
  human blood, 216
  human infant, 150
  human neonatal, 203
  ^{125}I-HYP, 101
  Ia antigens, 18

IgG Fc receptor bearing, 81, 84
IgE Fc receptors, 14
insulin dependent diabetes, 148
insulin receptors, 232
isoproterenol, 104
kinetics, cortisol, 65
mesenteric, 164
metaproterenol, 106
mitogenic response, 196
mouse, 189
murine, 107
nonadherent, 222
norepinephrine, 104
opiate receptors, 53
peripheral blood, 57, 67, 101, 105, 148, 196, 216
prolactin receptors, 233
proliferation, 263
recirculation, 51—52
secondary response, 189
somatostatin, 144
spontaneous diabetes, 151
subpopulations, sex hormones, 287—288
theophylline, 106
thoracic duct, 51, 64
toxicity to, 92
transfer, 166
transformation in vitro, 149
trapping, 65
Lymphocytic hypophysitis, 167
Lymphocytic infiltration, 167
Lymphocytopenia, 60, 65, 70, 93
Lymphocytosis, 66, 104
Lymphoid cells, 3, 222
  catecholamine receptors, 100—103
  prolactin receptors on, 162—163
Lymphoid organs, see also Primary lymphoid organs; Secondary lymphoid organs
  ACTH treatment, 228
  dexamethasone, 59
Lymphoid tissue
  glucocorticoid receptors in, 56—59
  sex hormone receptors, 187—188
Lymphokines, 3—5, 9, 16—17, 22, 229, 234, 242, 245
  adrenal gland, 112
  B cell secretion, 6
  biological effect, 236
  corticosterone, 111
  insulin dependent diabetes, 148
  platelet aggregation and release, 10
  production, 274
  receptors, 7
  thymic hormones, 112
Lymphoma, 81, 145, 162, 193, 306
Lymphopenia, 52, 54, 66, 93, 97, 104, 200
  ACTH, 50
Lymphopoiesis, 59—60
Lymphopoietic system, 59
Lymphosarcoma, 63, 306
Lymphotoxin, 16

Lymphotropic effect, 174
Lynestrenol, 202
Lysolecithin, 150
Lysosomal acid lipase, 216
Lysosomal enzyme discharge, 87, 90
Lysosomal enzymes, 9
Lysosomes, 6, 80, 93, 146
Lyt-1$^+$ cells, 192
Lyt-1.2 antigen, 190
Lyt-2 antigen, 74
Lyt surface antigens, 287

M

Macaca mulatta, 280
Macaca speciosa, 197, 280
Macrophage activating factor, 113
Macrophage aggregating factor (MAF), 80, 83, 93, 99
Macrophage chemotactic factor (MCF), 72—74
Macrophage migration inhibitory factor (MIF), 72, 74, 97
Macrophage mitogenic factor (MMF), 72, 80, 83, 232
Macrophages, 2—4, 6—7, 9, 22, 74, 109, 151, 298
  alveolar, 57, 59, 65, 80, 107
  antitumor activity of, and adrenal corticosteroids, 307
  arming, 79
  cortisol, 64, 80
  cytotoxic, 232
  dexamethasone, 63, 68
  effector, 72
  endocytic function, 147
  endogenous pyrogen, 112
  Fc receptors, 147
  fenoterol, 105
  fetal, human, 80
  functions, 91
  glucocorticoid receptors, 56
  glucocorticoids, effect of, 76, 79—83
  guinea pig, 224
  IgE Fc receptors, 14
  immune complex clearance, 292
  lymphocytic hypophysitis, 167
  migration, 196, 224
  mouse granulosa cells, 203
  peritoneal, 59, 79, 113, 192
  properties, 4
  pulmonary, 64
  sex hormones, effect of, 297
  somatostatin stimulated, 144
  suppression, 94
  testes, 187
  tumoricidal, 193
MAF, see Macrophage aggregating factor
Magnesium ions, 61
Major histocompatibility (MHC) antigens, 17—19, 262

Met-enkephalin, see also Endogenous opioids, 53,
        306
Metestrus, 191
L-Methionine, 101
^{35}S-Methionine, 61, 63
Methylated bovine serum albumin (MBSA), 292
Methyldopa, 45
3-O-Methylglucose, 215
2-Methylhistamine, 111
Methylprednisolone (MP), 275
    antigen presentation, 81
    asthma, 69
    granulocytes, 87, 90
    immune reactions, effect on, 97—99
    kidney graft rejection, 92
    killer cells, 95
    macrophages, effect on, 82—83
    mast cells, effect on, 90
    mixed lymphocyte cultures, 72
    monocytes, effect on, 82—83
    mononuclear cells, 70
    neutrophils, 87, 93
    potency, 88
    rheumatoid arthritis, 94
    spleen weights, 93
Methylprednisolone acetate, 93, 98
Methylprednisolone sodium succinate, 73, 87, 98
Methylprednisolone succinate, 80
Methysergide, 101
Metritis, 279
Metyrapone, 54
MHC, see Major histocompatibility complex
Mice, see Mouse
Microadenomas, 32
Microelements, 21
Microfilaments, 4
β_2-Microglobulin, 18
Microsomal antibodies, 168
Microsomal autoantibodies, 149
Microtubules, 4
MIF, see Macrophage migration inhibitory factor;
        Migration inhibitory factor
Migration inhibition, 277
Migration inhibitory factor (MIF), 72, 83, 99,
        148—149, 196
Milk, 163, 166, 186
Mineralocorticoids, 31, 87
Mitochondria, 61
Mitochondrial activation, 214
Mitochondrial T$_3$ receptors, 214
Mitogenesis, 193, 274
Mitogenic signals, 21
Mitogen responses, 150, 192, 196, 200—201, 215,
        231, 286
Mitogens, 4, 42—43, 99, 166
    ACTH, 52
    adrenalectomy, 54
    B lymphocyte, 5—6
    cortisol, 70
    glucocorticoid receptors, 58
    growth hormone effect on immunity, 135

insulin dependent diabetes, 148
insulin receptors, 145
interleukin 1, 62
prolactin, 169
spleen cells, 191
T lymphocyte stimulation, 5
Mitogen stimulation, insulin dependent diabetes,
        149
Mitomycin C, 145
Mixed lymphocyte culture (MLC), 74, 136
    arming factor, 79
    cortisone, 92
    insulin dependent diabetes, 148
    methylprednisolone, 72
    mitogenic response, 196
    progesterone, 200
Mixed lymphocyte reaction (MLR), 45, 99, 143,
        146, 166
    estradiol, 192
    estrogens, 197
    human chorionic gonadotropin, 186
    prednisone, 94
    prolactin, 169
    sex differences, 189
MLC, see Mixed lymphocyte culture
MLR, see Mixed lymphocyte reaction
MMF, see Macrophage mitogenic factor
Monkeys
    cynomolgus, 112
    immune-derived factors, 236
    macaques, 112
    New World, 59
    Old World, 59
    progesterone, 201, 280
    progestoids, 201
    prolactin receptors, 162
    prosimians, 59
    steroid resistant, 55
    stump-tail, 197
Monoamines, 36
Monoclonal antibodies, 215
Monocyte-macrophages, 15, 19, 22, 81, 229, 274
    Ia antigens, 18
    suppressor cells, 192
Monocytes, 2, 6—7, 57, 196, 216, 222, 229—230,
        275
    adherent, 222
    aminoglutethimide phosphate, 79
    blood, 64
    chemiluminescence, 222
    circulating, 63—64, 200
    complement receptors, 197, 200
    cortisol, effect of, 80
    diethylstilbestrol, 192
    epinephrine, 104
    fibrinolysis, 146
    glucocorticoids, effect of, 76, 79—83
    human, 59
    IgG Fc receptor, 80, 197
    IgG receptor, 200
    IgM Fc receptors, 200

N